Atlas of
Thoracic Surgical Techniques

Other Volumes in the Surgical Techniques Atlas Series

Atlas of
Thoracic Surgical Techniques
A Volume in the Surgical Techniques Atlas Series

Editor
Joseph B. Zwischenberger, MD
Johnston-Wright Professor and Chair
Department of Surgery
The University of Kentucky College of Medicine
Lexington, Kentucky

Series Editors
Courtney M. Townsend, Jr., MD
Professor and John Woods Harris Distinguished Chairman
Department of Surgery
The University of Texas Medical Branch
Galveston, Texas

B. Mark Evers, MD
Professor of Surgery
Director
Lucille P. Markey Cancer Center
Markey Cancer Foundation Endowed Chair
The University of Kentucky College of Medicine
Lexington; Kentucky

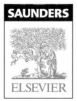

SAUNDERS

ELSEVIER

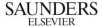

1600 John F. Kennedy Boulevard
Suite 1800
Philadelphia, PA 19103-2899

ATLAS OF THORACIC SURGICAL TECHNIQUES   ISBN: 978-1-4160-4017-0

Library of Congress Cataloging-in-Publication Data
Atlas of thoracic surgical techniques / editor, Joseph B. Zwischenberger. — 1st ed.
    p. ; cm. — (Surgical techniques atlas series)
  Includes bibliographical references.
  ISBN 978-1-4160-4017-0
  1. Chest—Surgery—Atlases.   I. Zwischenberger, Joseph B.   II. Series: Surgical techniques atlas series.
  [DNLM: 1. Thoracic Diseases—surgery—Atlases.   2. Thoracic Surgical Procedures—Atlases.
WF 17 A8814 2010]
  RD536.A782 2010
  617.5′4059—dc22
                                                                    2010012918

Publishing Director: Judith Fletcher
Developmental Editor: Rachel Miller
Publishing Services Manager: Tina Rebane
Senior Project Manager: Amy L. Cannon
Design Director: Steven Stave

Printed in China

Last digit is the print number: 9 8 7 6 5 4 3 2 1

To my wife, Sheila, who has supported me and been by my side for 33 years, putting up with all my antics; to my children, Brittany, Andrea, Christina, and Charlie, of whom I am very proud; to my team at work, whose advice and support have been instrumental to my successes and achievements; to my mentors and advisors who have guided me along the way, demonstrating the hard work, long hours, and dedication required to be an academic surgeon; and to all the medical students, residents, and interns who are embarking on the same journey that the surgeon–authors of this book have traveled—good luck and enjoy the ride.

CONTRIBUTORS

Mark S. Allen, MD
Chair, Division of General Thoracic Surgery,
  Department of Surgery, Mayo Clinic, Rochester,
  Minnesota
*Surgical Management of Bronchopleural Fistula; Chest Wall
Resection*

Omar Awais, DO
Thoracic Surgeon, The Heart, Lung and Esophageal
  Surgery Institute, University of Pittsburgh Medical
  Center, Presbyterian University Hospital, Pittsburgh,
  Pennsylvania
Minimally Invasive Esophagectomy

S. Scott Balderson, PA-C
Physician Assistant, Division of Thoracic Surgery,
  Department of Surgery, Duke University Medical
  Center, Durham, North Carolina
*Video-Assisted Thoracoscopic Surgery for Mediastinal Lymph
Node Dissection*

Daniel J. Boffa, MD
Assistant Professor, Thoracic Surgery, Yale University
  School of Medicine, New Haven, Connecticut
Transthoracic Esophagectomy

Mark R. Bonnell, MD
Assistant Professor, Division of Cardiothoracic
  Surgery, Department of Surgery; Director,
  Mechanical Circulatory Support, University of
  Kentucky College of Medicine, Lexington,
  Kentucky
Lung Transplantation

Ayesha S. Bryant, MSPH, MD
Assistant Professor, Division of Cardiothoracic
  Surgery, Department of Surgery, University of
  Alabama at Birmingham, Birmingham, Alabama
Techniques for Partial and Sleeve Pulmonary Artery Resection

Robert J. Cerfolio, MD
Professor, Department of Surgery, Division of
  Cardiothoracic Surgery, University of Alabama at
  Birmingham, Birmingham, Alabama
Techniques for Partial and Sleeve Pulmonary Artery Resection

Thomas A. D'Amico, MD
Professor of Surgery and Section Chief, Thoracic
  Surgery, Duke University Medical Center, Durham,
  North Carolina
*Video-Assisted Thoracoscopic Surgery for Mediastinal Lymph Node
Dissection*

Philippe G. Dartevelle, MD, PhD
Full Professor, Thoracic and Cardio-Vascular Surgery,
  Paris Sud University, Paris; Head of Department,
  Department of Thoracic and Vascular Surgery and
  Heart-Lung Transplantation, Marie-Lannelongue
  Hospital, Le Plessis Robinson, France
Bronchial and Pulmonary Arterial Sleeve Resection

Malcolm M. DeCamp, MD
Visiting Associate Professor Surgery, Department of
  Surgery, Harvard Medical School; Chief, Division of
  Cardiothoracic Surgery, Department of Surgery,
  Beth Israel Deaconess Medical Center, Boston,
  Massachusetts
Radiofrequency Ablation

Jean Deslauriers, MD, FRCSC
Professor of Surgery, Department of Thoracic Surgery,
  Laval University, Quebec City, Quebec, Canada
Diaphragmatic Eventration and Paralysis

Frank C. Detterbeck, MD
Professor and Chief, Thoracic Surgery, Yale University
  School of Medicine; Professor and Chief, Thoracic
  Surgery, Yale New Haven Hospital; Associate
  Director, Yale Cancer Center; Surgical Director, Yale
  Cancer Center Thoracic Oncology Program, New
  Haven, Connecticut
Pancoast Tumors

Almudena Moreno Elola-Olaso, MD, PhD
Research Fellow, Department of Surgery, Center for
  Minimally Invasive Surgery, University of Kentucky,
  Lexington, Kentucky
Robotic Esophagectomy

Aaron D. Fain, BS
University of Kentucky Medical School, Lexington,
  Kentucky
Giant Bullous Emphysema

David J. Finley, MD
Assistant Attending Surgeon, Thoracic Service,
  Department of Surgery, Memorial Sloan-Kettering
  Cancer Center, New York, New York
Carinal Resections

Raymond J. Gagliardi, MD
Associate Professor, Department of Surgery,
  University of Kentucky College of Medicine,
  Lexington, Kentucky
Robotic Esophagectomy

Priya Gaiha, MD
General Surgery Resident, University of Kentucky,
  Lexington, Kentucky
Resection of Benign Esophageal Tumors

Jonathan G. Hobbs, BS
University of Kentucky College of Medicine,
  Lexington, Kentucky
Lung Volume Reduction Surgery: Thoracoscopic

James Hoskins, BS
Information Technology Manager, University of
  Kentucky College of Medicine, Lexington,
  Kentucky
Pectus Excavatum: Minimally Invasive Nuss Procedure

Aaron B. House, MD
General Surgery Resident, University of Kentucky
  College of Medicine, Lexington, Kentucky
*Techniques of Esophageal Preservation for High-Grade Barrett
Esophagus*

Michael Kuan Yew Hsin, MBBChir, FRCS
Assistant Professor, Department of Surgery, Chinese
  University of Hong Kong; Assistant Professor,
  Department of Surgery, Prince of Wales Hospital,
  Shatin, New Territories, Hong Kong
*Video-Assisted Thoracic Surgery for Major
Pulmonary Resection*

Li Guang Hu, MD
Staff Thoracic Surgeon, First Teaching Hospital of
  Jilin University, Changchun, China
Diaphragmatic Eventration and Paralysis

Brannon R. Hyde, MD
General Surgery Resident, Department of Surgery,
  University of Kentucky College of Medicine,
  Lexington, Kentucky
*Lung Volume Reduction Surgery: Open Technique; Lung Volume
Reduction Surgery: Thoracoscopic*

Joseph A. Iocono, MD
Associate Professor of Surgery and Pediatrics, Division
  of Pediatric Surgery; Director, Surgery Pre-Doctoral
  Education; Surgical Director, Pediatric Trauma
  Program; Surgical Director, Pediatric ECMO
  Program; Associate Director, Minimally Invasive
  Surgery Center, University of Kentucky College of
  Medicine, Lexington, Kentucky
Pectus Excavatum: Minimally Invasive Nuss Procedure

Kiasha James, MD
University of Kentucky College of Medicine,
  Lexington, Kentucky
Transhiatal Esophagectomy

Dawn E. Jaroszewski, MD, MBA
Senior Consultant and Assistant Professor of Surgery,
  Division of Cardiothoracic Surgery, Mayo Clinic
  College of Medicine, Phoenix, Arizona
*Sternal-Splitting Approaches to Thymectomy for Myasthenia
Gravis and Resection of Thymoma*

Scott B. Johnson, MD
Head, Section of General Thoracic Surgery, Division
  of Cardiothoracic Surgery, Department of Surgery,
  University of Texas Health Science Center at San
  Antonio, San Antonio, Texas
Esophageal Reconstruction

Alexandros N. Karavas, MD
Cardiothoracic Surgery Resident, Department of
  Thoracic Surgery, Vanderbilt University;
  Cardiothoracic Surgery Resident, Thoracic Surgery,
  Vanderbilt University Medical Center, Nashville,
  Tennessee
Esophageal Diverticulum Excision and Repair

Michael S. Kent, MD
Instructor, Harvard Medical School; Surgeon, Division
  of Cardiothoracic Surgery, Beth Israel Deaconess
  Medical Center, Boston, Massachusetts
Radiofrequency Ablation

Kemp H. Kernstine, MD, PhD
Professor and Chief, Division of Thoracic Surgery;
  Director, Lung Cancer and Thoracic Oncology
  Program, City of Hope National Medical Center and
  Beckman Research Institute, Duarte; Clinical
  Professor of Surgery, University of California, San
  Diego, California
Robotic Lobectomy

Joseph M. Kinner, MD
Trainee, Training Program for Clinical Scholars in
  Cardiovascular Science, University of Kentucky
  College of Medicine, Lexington, Kentucky
Lung Volume Reduction Surgery: Open Technique

Mark J. Krasna, MD
Program on Health Policy, University of Maryland
  School of Medicine, Baltimore; Medical Director,
  Cancer Institute, Saint Joseph Medical Center,
  Towson, Maryland
Thoracoscopic Sympathectomy

Rodney J. Landreneau, MD
Professor of Surgery, The Heart, Lung and
  Esophageal Surgery Institute, University of
  Pittsburgh Medical Center; Director, Comprehensive
  Lung Center, The Heart, Lung and Esophageal
  Surgery Institute, Shadyside Medical Center,
  Pittsburgh, Pennsylvania
Anatomic Segmentectomy

Moishe Liberman, MD, PhD
Marcel and Rolande Gosselin Chair in Thoracic
  Surgical Oncology, Division of Thoracic Surgery,
  Centre Hospitalier de l'Université de Montréal,
  Montreal, Quebec, Canada
Tracheal Resection and Reconstruction

Virginia R. Litle, MD
Associate Professor, Department of Surgery,
  University of Rochester and Strong Memorial
  Hospital, Rochester, New York
Laparoscopic Myotomy and Fundoplication for Achalasia

James D. Luketich, MD
Henry T. Bahnson Professor Cardiothoracic Surgery,
  University of Pittsburgh; Chair, The Heart, Lung
  and Esophageal Surgery Institute, University of
  Pittsburgh Medical Center Presbyterian; Chief,
  Division of Thoracic and Foregut Surgery,
  University of Pittsburgh Medical Center, Pittsburgh,
  Pennsylvania
Minimally Invasive Esophagectomy

James E. Lynch, MD
General Surgery Resident, Department of Surgery,
  University of Kentucky College of Medicine,
  Lexington, Kentucky
*Transhiatal Esophagectomy; Resection of Benign
Esophageal Tumors*

Mitchell J. Magee, MD
Director, Thoracic Surgical Oncology; Chief,
  Cardiothoracic Surgery; Director, Minimally
  Invasive Surgical Institute for Lung Esophagus,
  Medical City Dallas Hospital, Dallas, Texas
Surgical Management of Empyema

Douglas J. Mathisen, MD
Chief, General Thoracic Surgery and Program
  Director, Department of Thoracic Surgery,
  Massachusetts General Hospital, Harvard Medical
  School, Boston, Massachusetts
Tracheal Resection and Reconstruction

Robert J. McKenna Jr, MD
Chief, Thoracic Surgery, Cedars Sinai Medical Center,
  Los Angeles, California
Right Upper Lobectomy

Daniel L. Miller, MD
Kamal A. Mansour Professor of Thoracic Surgery,
  Division of Cardiothoracic Surgery, Department of
  Surgery, Emory University School of Medicine;
  Co-Chair, Respiratory Center, Emory University
  Healthcare, Atlanta, Georgia
Extrapleural Pneumonectomy

Christopher R. Morse, MD
Instructor in Surgery, Division of Thoracic Surgery,
  Massachusetts General Hospital, Boston,
  Massachusetts
*Resection of Solitary Pulmonary Nodule: Open and Video-Assisted
Thoracoscopic Surgery*

Jacob E. Perry, MD
General Surgery Resident, Department of Surgery,
  University of Kentucky College of Medicine,
  Lexington, Kentucky
Pectus Excavatum: Minimally Invasive Nuss Procedure

Jonathan P. Pearl, MD
Department of Surgery, National Naval Medical
  Center, Bethesda, Maryland
Endoscopic Treatment for Gastroesophageal Reflux

Brian L. Pettiford, MD
Clinical Assistant Professor, Heart, Lung and
  Esophageal Surgery Institute, University of
  Pittsburgh Medical Center, Shadyside Medical
  Center, Pittsburgh, Pennsylvania
Anatomic Segmentectomy

Jeffrey L. Ponsky, MD
Oliver H. Payne Professor and Chairman, Department
  of Surgery, Case Western Reserve University School
  of Medicine, Cleveland, Ohio
Endoscopic Treatment for Gastroesophageal Reflux

Joe B. Putnam, MD
Chairman, Ingram Professor of Cancer Research,
  Professor of Biomedical Informatics, Department of
  Thoracic Surgery, Vanderbilt University; Chairman,
  Department of Thoracic Surgery, Vanderbilt
  University Medical Center, Nashville, Tennessee
Esophageal Diverticulum Excision and Repair

John Scott Roth, MD
Associate Professor of Surgery, Division of General
    Surgery, University of Kentucky College of
    Medicine; Chief, Gastrointestinal Surgery and
    Director, Minimally Invasive Surgery, Department
    of Surgery, University of Kentucky Medical Center,
    Lexington, Kentucky
*Transthoracic Antireflux Surgery Procedures; Laparoscopic Collis
Gastroplasty and Fundoplication*

Valerie Rusch, MD
Chief, Thoracic Service, Department of Surgery,
    Miner Family Chair in Intrathoracic Cancers,
    Memorial Sloan-Kettering Cancer Center, New
    York, New York
Carinal Resections

Adham R. Saad, MD
Research Fellow, Division of Cardiothoracic Surgery,
    Department of Surgery, University of Texas Health
    Science Center at San Antonio, San Antonio, Texas
Esophageal Reconstruction

Joshua R. Sonett, MD
Chief, General Thoracic Surgery; Surgical Director,
    Lung Transplant Program, New York-Presbyterian
    Hospital/Columbia University Medical Center;
    Professor of Clinical Surgery, Columbia University
    College of Physicians and Surgeons, New York,
    New York
Surgical Management of Empyema

Victor F. Trastek, MD, MBA
Chief Executive Officer and Professor of Surgery,
    General Thoracic Surgery, Mayo Clinic College of
    Medicine, Phoenix, Arizona
*Sternal-Splitting Approaches to Thymectomy for Myasthenia
Gravis and Resection of Thymoma*

Thomas J. Watson, MD
Associate Professor of Surgery, Division of Thoracic
    and Foregut Surgery, University of Rochester School
    of Medicine and Dentistry; Chief of Thoracic
    Surgery, Strong Memorial Hospital, Rochester,
    New York
Laparoscopic Myotomy and Fundoplication for Achalasia

Liu Wei, MD
Associate Director, Department of Thoracic Surgery,
    First Teaching Hospital of Jilin University,
    Changchun, China
Diaphragmatic Eventration and Paralysis

Joseph J. Wizoreck, MD
The Heart, Lung and Esophageal Surgery Institute,
    University of Pittsburgh Medical Center,
    Presbyterian University Hospital, Pittsburgh,
    Pennsylvania
Minimally Invasive Esophagectomy

Cameron D. Wright, MD
Associate Professor of Surgery, Division of Thoracic
    Surgery, Massachusetts General Hospital, Boston,
    Massachusetts
*Resection of Solitary Pulmonary Nodule: Open and Video-Assisted
Thoracoscopic Surgery*

Bedrettin Yıldızeli, MD
Associate Professor, Department of Thoracic Surgery,
    Marmara University School of Medicine, Istanbul,
    Turkey
Bronchial and Pulmonary Arterial Sleeve Resection

Anthony P. C. Yim, MD
Honorary Clinical Professor, Department of Surgery,
    The Chinese University of Hong Kong, China
Video-Assisted Thoracic Surgery for Major Pulmonary Resection

Lei Yu, MD
Assistant Professor, Department of Thoracic Surgery,
    Beijing Tongren Hospital, Capital Medical
    University, Beijing City, China
Thoracoscopic Sympathectomy

Joseph B. Zwischenberger, MD
Johnston-Wright Professor and Chair, Department of
    Surgery; Professor of Pediatrics, Diagnostic
    Radiology, and Pediatrics; Directo University of
    Kentucky Transplant Center, University of
    Kentucky College of Medicine, Lexington, Kentucky
*Giant Bullous Emphysema; Lung Volume Reduction Surgery: Open
Technique; Lung Volume Reduction Surgery: Thoracoscopic;
Transhiatal Esophagectomy; Techniques of Esophageal
Preservation for High-Grade Barrett Esophagus; Transthoracic
Antireflux Surgery Procedures; Resection of Benign Esophageal
Tumors*

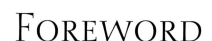

FOREWORD

"A picture is worth a thousand words."

Anonymous

This atlas is for practicing surgeons, surgical residents, and medical students for their review and preparation for surgical procedures. New procedures are developed and old ones are replaced as technologic and pharmacologic advances occur. The topics presented are contemporaneous surgical procedures with step-by-step illustrations, preoperative and postoperative considerations, and pearls and pitfalls, taken from the personal experience and surgical practices of the authors. Their results have been validated in their surgical practices involving many patients. Operative surgery remains a manual art in which the knowledge, judgment, and technical skill of the surgeon come together for the benefit of the patient. A technically perfect operation is the key to this success. Speed in operation comes from having a plan and devoting sufficient time to completion of each step, in order, one time. The surgeon must be dedicated to spending the time to do it right the first time; if not, there will never be enough time to do it right at any other time. Use this atlas; study it for your patients.

"An amateur practices until he gets it right; a professional practices until she can't get it wrong."

Anonymous

Courtney M. Townsend Jr, MD
B. Mark Evers, MD

PREFACE

"Medicine is the only profession that labours incessantly to destroy the reason for its own existence."

James Bryce, 1914

Surgery today is vastly different than it was even 20 years ago. New developments in technology and techniques allow major surgery to be performed using the smallest of incisions, causing less pain and shortening hospital stays. Even so, surgery is often accompanied by a sense of urgency. The surgeon holds in his hands the ability to change lives and give hope. Surgery is both a science and an art form, and mastery of both are required for the surgeon to be successful. The surgeon must wield skillfully a mega-array of delicate tools and instruments and be versed with the newest developments and technologies.

This textbook is a compilation of procedures and techniques as practiced by some of the best thoracic surgeons in America today. Although some surgical procedures outlined here may be done somewhat differently by another surgeon at a different institution, those described here have been tried and tested by the authors and found to be successful. I and the other authors offer you a snapshot of our experience. We hope one complete description and choreography of a successful approach will help as you develop your own successful techniques and nuances.

Joseph B. Zwischenberger, MD

Contents

Section III   Esophageal Cancer

Section IV   Esophageal Benign

Thoracic Cancer

CHAPTER 1

VIDEO-ASSISTED THORACOSCOPIC SURGERY FOR MEDIASTINAL LYMPH NODE DISSECTION

S. Scott Balderson and Thomas A. D'Amico

Mediastinal lymph node assessment is an integral component of a resection for all stages of non–small cell lung cancer (NSCLC).[1] Debate remains as to whether there is a therapeutic benefit to complete mediastinal lymph node dissection (MLND) compared with mediastinal lymph node sampling,[2] a question that may be answered by the American College of Surgeons Oncology Group Z0030 study.[3] Nevertheless, there is no debate that MLND improves the staging of patients with NSCLC at the time of resection by appropriately upstaging patients without clinically obvious lymph node involvement and enabling the use of adjuvant therapy, which may improve survival.[1]

Step 1. Surgical Anatomy

♦ Complete dissection of mediastinal lymph node stations is contingent on a thorough understanding of the anatomic considerations and meticulous surgical technique.
♦ Figure 1-1 demonstrates the most recent map of mediastinal lymph stations for lung cancer staging.[4,5]

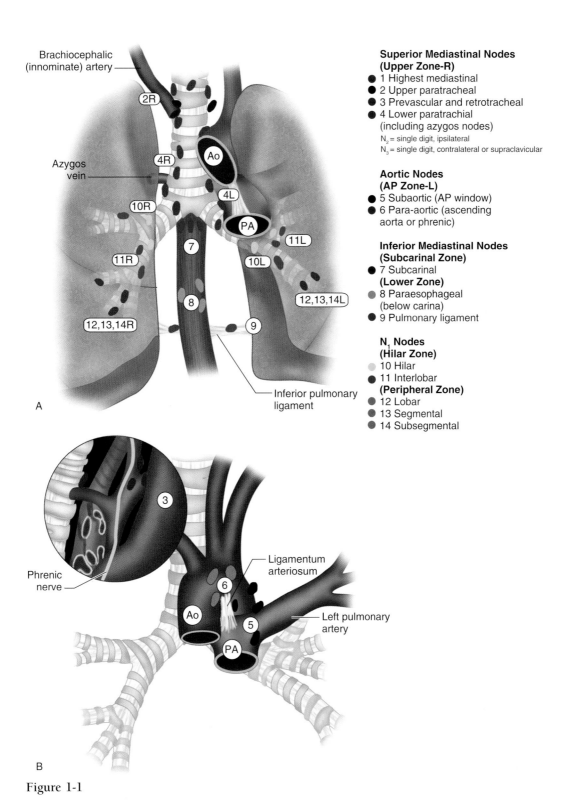

**Superior Mediastinal Nodes
(Upper Zone-R)**
● 1 Highest mediastinal
● 2 Upper paratracheal
● 3 Prevascular and retrotracheal
● 4 Lower paratrachial
   (including azygos nodes)
   N_2 = single digit, ipsilateral
   N_3 = single digit, contralateral or supraclavicular

**Aortic Nodes
(AP Zone-L)**
● 5 Subaortic (AP window)
● 6 Para-aortic (ascending
   aorta or phrenic)

**Inferior Mediastinal Nodes
(Subcarinal Zone)**
● 7 Subcarinal
   (Lower Zone)
● 8 Paraesophageal
   (below carina)
● 9 Pulmonary ligament

**N_1 Nodes
(Hilar Zone)**
○ 10 Hilar
● 11 Interlobar
   (Peripheral Zone)
● 12 Lobar
● 13 Segmental
● 14 Subsegmental

Figure 1-1

◆ The mediastinum may be subdivided into the following major regions: the right paratracheal stations (Fig. 1-2), the subcarinal station accessible from either the right or left (Fig. 1-3), and the left paraortic stations (Fig. 1-4). After incising the mediastinal pleura, the underlying lymph node stations can be visualized.

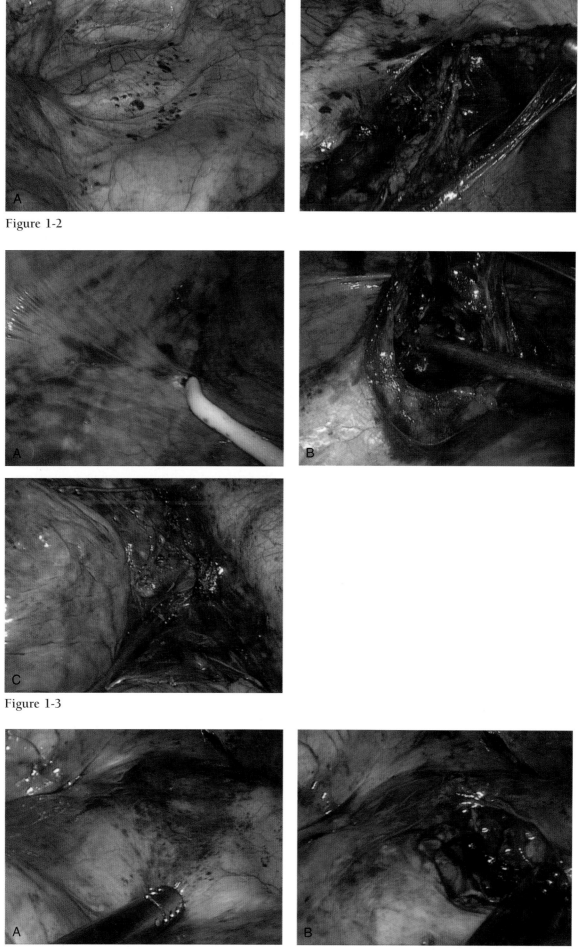

Figure 1-2

Figure 1-3

Figure 1-4

Step 2. Preoperative Considerations

◆ Most patients with clinical stage I NSCLC and selected patients with stage II NSCLC are candidates for thoracoscopic lobectomy, including thoracoscopic MLND, with outcomes equivalent to conventional thoracotomy.[6-9] Previous thoracic procedures are not contraindications to the thoracoscopic approach to lobectomy with MLND.

◆ Cervical mediastinoscopy with mediastinal lymph node biopsy should precede surgical resection and MLND in appropriate patients, including those with clinical stage IB, stage II, or stage III disease.[1]

Step 3. Operative Steps

◆ After establishing single-lung ventilation with the patient in the lateral decubitus position, thoracoscopic exploration can be performed using various thoracoscopic instruments.

◆ Mediastinal lymphadenectomy can be performed before or after the lobectomy is completed, according to the surgeon's preference. However, node dissection before hilar vessel dissection may facilitate the procedure.[10]

◆ Node dissection can be accomplished using a combination of blunt and sharp techniques, and hemostasis can be accomplished with clips or energy sources, such as electrocautery, bipolar thermal energy, or ultrasonic devices.

1. Right Paratracheal Dissection

◆ Dissection of the right paratracheal lymph nodes (stations 2R and 4R) usually includes dissection of the azygos lymph nodes (station 10) and is facilitated by ligation of the azygos vein using a stapling device.

◆ The margins of the resection include the superior vena cava (anterior), the trachea (posterior), and the pericardium (medial). Cephalad dissection to the level of the innominate artery is performed, taking care to avoid the right recurrent laryngeal nerve. Caudally, dissection includes all lymph nodes at the hilum (Fig. 1-5).

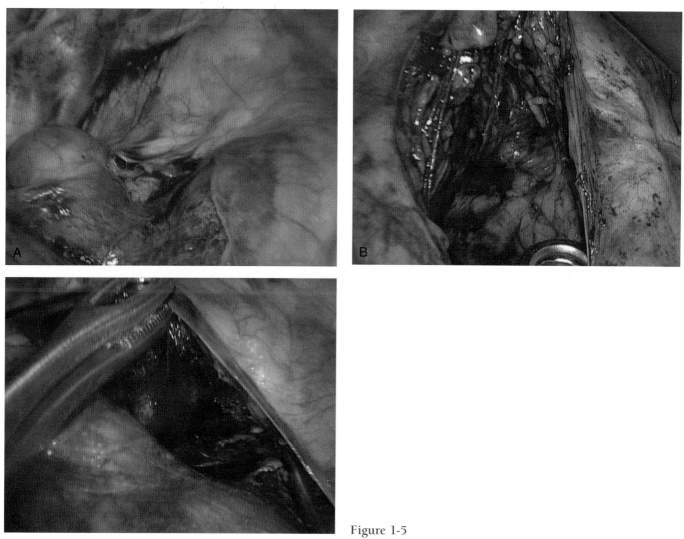

Figure 1-5

2. Right Subcarinal Dissection

- Dissection of the subcarinal space is facilitated if lower lobectomy has already been performed, including stapling of the inferior pulmonary vein; however, dissection with this vein intact is certainly feasible.
- The margins of resection include the esophagus (posterior), the right bronchus (anterior), and the pericardium and left bronchus (medial). Cephalad dissection to the level of the carina is performed while taking care to avoid injury to the membranous trachea (Fig. 1-6).

3. Paraortic Dissection

- Dissection of the para-aortic region includes the aortopulmonary window lymph nodes (level 5) and paraortic lymph nodes (level 6). The margins of resection include the descending aorta (posterior), the phrenic nerve (anterior), and the left pulmonary artery (medial).
- Cephalad dissection to the level of the aortic arch is performed with care to avoid injury to the left recurrent laryngeal nerve (Fig. 1-7). Visualization of the nerve is facilitated by the magnification afforded by the video camera and monitor.

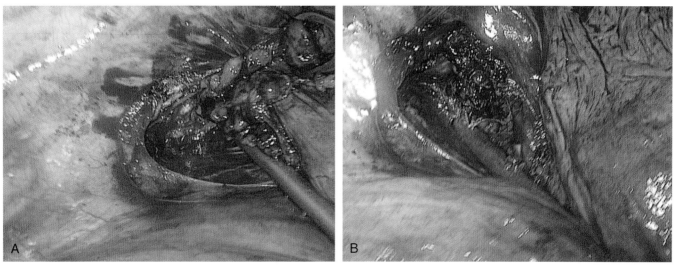

Figure 1-6

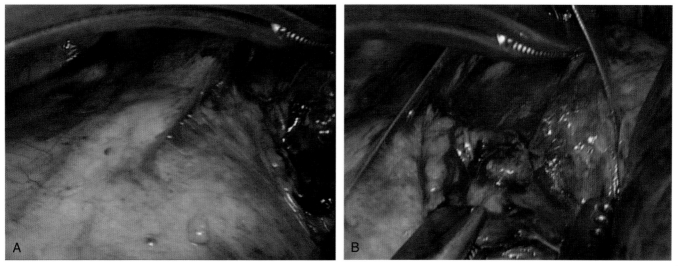

Figure 1-7

4. Left Subcarinal Dissection

- The left subcarinal dissection is the most difficult of the major regions. Dissection of the left subcarinal space is facilitated if lower lobectomy has already been performed, including stapling of the inferior pulmonary vein; however, dissection with this vein intact is certainly feasible. The margins of resection include the aorta (posterior), the left bronchus (anterior), and the pericardium and right bronchus (medial). Cephalad dissection to the level of the carina is performed with care to avoid injury to the membranous trachea (Fig. 1-8).
- After completion of nodal dissection, the fields are examined for hemostasis before placement of a chest tube and closure. In most cases, a single tube (24-28 French) will suffice.

Step 4. Postoperative Care

- Postoperatively, chest tube output is monitored and the chest tube is removed when there is no air leak and minimal drainage of serosanguineous fluid. Whereas a daily output of 150 mL or less has been historically used, removal with daily output less than 300 mL is usually successful.
- Postoperative chylothorax, defined as triglyceride level in the pleural fluid greater than 110 mg/dL or positive Sudan stain, rarely results. Nonoperative management is usually successful, and thoracic duct ligation is infrequently required.

Step 5. Pearls and Pitfalls

- The most important complications of lymphadenectomy, including phrenic or recurrent nerve injury, tracheobronchial or esophageal injury, and chylothorax are rare.[11] The use of video techniques improves the visualization of vital structures, which may lower the complication rate.
- The performance of thoracoscopic lobectomy is facilitated by lowering the tidal volume (250 mL), creating a larger thoracic space. During node dissection, increasing the tidal volume may make mediastinal lymph nodes more accessible, especially in the subcarinal regions.
- The use of long, curved thoracoscopic instruments allows several instruments to be used, without interference, through the anterior access incision.
- Energy sources may facilitate dissection, but the surgeon must be aware that the energy sources may create collateral damage.
- During the right paratracheal lymphadenectomy along the innominate artery, care must be taken because the right recurrent laryngeal nerve may be closer to the field than anticipated.
- During the subcarinal lymphadenectomy, circumferential mobilization is performed; at the apex of the lymph node, bronchial arterial branches enter the nodal tissue. At this stage of the dissection, the arterial branches should be ligated, using either a clip or an energy source.
- The subcarinal lymphadenectomy is facilitated by rotating the operative table anterior, creating anterior traction on the hilum.

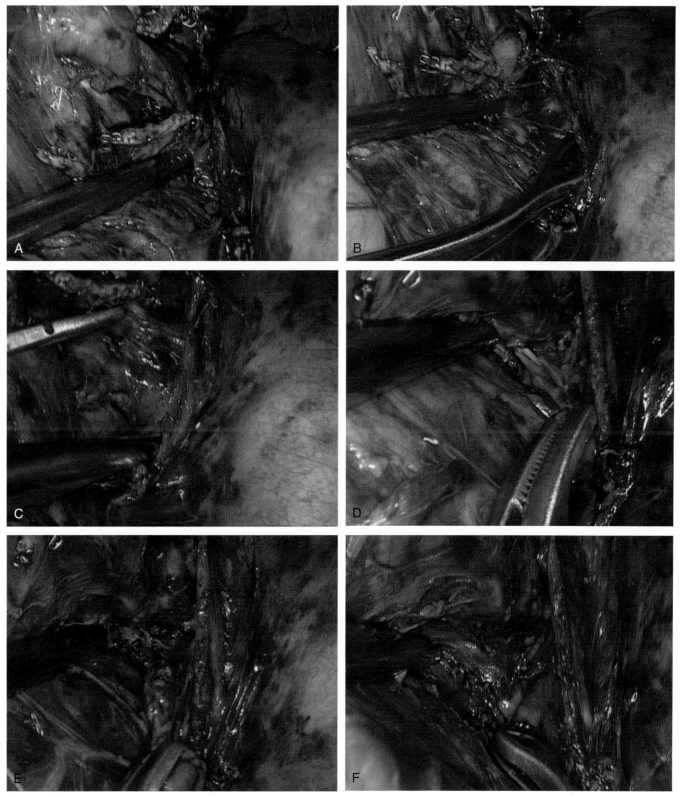

Figure 1-8

- ◆ The boundaries of the para-aortic dissection are the most indistinct because there is considerable adipose tissue in the anterior mediastinum. Nevertheless, close attention to the phrenic nerve (anterior margin) allows safe lymphadenectomy at levels 5 and 6.
- ◆ Another option for subcarinal lymphadenectomy, particularly for left upper lobectomy, is to perform the resection of the level 7 lymph nodes during mediastinoscopy, using the technique of transcervical extended mediastinal lymphadenctomy[12] or video-assisted mediastinoscopic lymphadenectomy.[13]
- ◆ Recently, it was demonstrated that thoracoscopic lobectomy and MLND are safe and effective after induction therapy.[14] In these patients, thoracoscopic restaging at the time of resection is an effective strategy of mediastinal lymph node assessment.[15]

References

1. Ettinger DS, Akerly W, Bepler G, et al. National Comprehensive Cancer Network (NCCN). Non–small cell lung cancer clinical practice guidelines in oncology. J Natl Compr Canc Netw 2008;6:228-269.
2. Whitson BA, Groth SS, Maddaus MA. Surgical assessment and intraoperative management of mediastinal lymph nodes in non–small cell lung cancer. Ann Thorac Surg 2007;84:1059-1065.
3. Allen MS, Darling GE, Pechet TT, et al. Morbidity and mortality of major pulmonary resections in patients with early-stage lung cancer: Initial results of the randomized, prospective ACOSOG Z0030 trial. Ann Thorac Surg 2006;81:1013-1019.
4. Mountain CF, Dresler CM. Regional lymph node classification for lung cancer staging. Chest 1997;111:1718-1723.
5. Rusch VW, Crowley J, Giroux DJ, et al. The IASLC lung cancer staging project: Proposals for the revision of the N descriptors in the forthcoming seventh edition of the TNM classification for lung cancer. J Thorac Oncol 2007;2:603-612.
6. Onaitis MW, Petersen PR, Balderson SS, et al. Thoracoscopic lobectomy is a safe and versatile procedure: Experience with 500 consecutive patients. Ann Surg 2006;244:420-425.
7. McKenna RJ, Houck W, Fuller CB. Video-assisted thoracic surgery lobectomy: Experience with 1,100 cases. Ann Thorac Surg 2006;81:421-426.
8. Sugi K, Kaneda Y, Esato K. Video-assisted thoracoscopic lobectomy achieves a satisfactory long-term prognosis in patients with clinical stage IA lung cancer. World J Surg 2000;24:27-31.
9. Watanabe A, Koyanagi T, Ohsawa H, et al. Systematic node dissection by VATS is not inferior to that through an open thoracotomy: A comparative clinicopathologic retrospective study. Surgery 2005;138:510-517.
10. Burfeind WR, D'Amico TA. Thoracoscopic lobectomy. Operative Techniques in Thoracic and Cardiovascular Surgery. 2004;9:98-114.
11. D'Amico TA. Complications of mediastinal surgery. In Little AG, ed. Complications in Cardiothoracic Surgery. Elmsford, NY: Blackwell; 2004.
12. Kuzdzal J, Zielinski M, Papla B, et al. The transcervical extended mediastinal lymphadenectomy versus cervical mediastinoscopy in non-small cell lung cancer staging. Eur J Cardiothorac Surg 2007;31:88-94.
13. Leschber G, Holinka G, Linder A. Video-assisted mediastinoscopic lymphadenectomy (VAMLA)—a method for systematic mediastinal lymph node dissection. Eur J Cardiothorac Surg 2003;24:192-195.
14. Petersen RP, Pham DK, Toloza EM, et al. Thoracoscopic lobectomy: A safe and effective strategy for patients receiving induction therapy for non-small cell lung cancer. Ann Thorac Surg 2006;82:214-219.
15. Jaklitsch MT, Gu L, Harpole DH, et al. Prospective phase II trial of pre-resection thoracoscopic (VATS) restaging following neoadjuvant therapy for IIIA(N2) non-small cell lung cancer (NSCLC): Results of CALGB 39803. Proc Am Soc Clin Oncol 2005;24 [abstract 7065].

CHAPTER 2

RESECTION OF SOLITARY PULMONARY NODULE: OPEN AND VIDEO-ASSISTED THORACOSCOPIC SURGERY

Christopher R. Morse and Cameron D. Wright

Definition and Etiology

- ◆ Solitary pulmonary nodule (SPN)
  - ▲ No standard definition is available for SPN. Size criteria vary, but they are usually considered smaller than 3 cm in diameter. Other definitions include characteristics of density on computed tomography (CT) imaging and the absence of cavitation and air bronchograms leading to lesion.
  - ▲ There must be an absence of additional radiographic findings on imaging (e.g., no lymphadenopathy, other nodules).
  - ▲ SPNs are within the lung parenchyma and either peripheral or central within the lung, often determining the operative approach.
- ◆ The causes of SPNs are many:
  - ▲ Malignant processes comprise 70% to 80% of SPNs.
    - ● Non–small cell lung cancer
    - ● Small cell lung cancer (rarely)
      - ■ Metastatic lesions to the lung (e.g., sarcoma, colon cancer, breast cancer, renal cell cancer) can present as SPN, although are often found as multiple nodules.
    - ● Pulmonary carcinoid tumors
  - ▲ Infectious
    - ● Infectious granulomas (e.g., histoplasmosis, coccidioidomycosis, blastomycosis, aspergillosis)
    - ● *Mycobacterium* spp.
    - ● Pneumocystis (immunocompromised patients)
  - ▲ Benign
    - ● Hamartoma
    - ● Lipoma, leiomyoma
    - ● Noncalcified lymph node

Step 1. Surgical Anatomy

◆ Location of the SPN within lung parenchyma is critical in planning the resection of the nodule.
  ▲ Peripheral nodules allow for wedge resection (Fig. 2-1). With peripheral pulmonary nodules, a margin must be maintained around the lesion and the lesion not compromised with the resection.
  ▲ More central nodules may require anatomic resection (Fig. 2-2) in the form of either a lobectomy or segmentectomy.

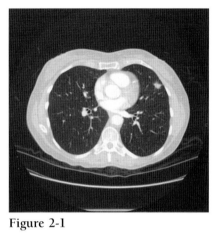

Figure 2-1

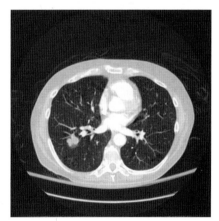

Figure 2-2

Step 2. Preoperative Considerations

- ◆ Several standardized management algorithms are available; included here is the Massachusetts General Hospital algorithm (Fig. 2-3).
  - ▲ If available, all current imaging must be compared with any previous imaging.
    - It allows for assessment of growth or change in the characteristics of the nodule. With an increase in size, one must consider intervention in the form of resection.
    - With no previous imaging available, the first choice is CT, and a thorough clinical evaluation always includes a history of malignancy and current and previous tobacco history.
    - Positron emission tomography may have a role in the evaluation of SPNs larger than 1 cm in diameter, with a reasonably high sensitivity for malignancy but a low specificity.
- ◆ Preoperative localization of lesion (video-assisted thoracoscopic surgery [VATS])
  - ▲ It may be difficult to visualize or palpate the nodule during the VATS procedure.
  - ▲ Preoperative guidance can come in several forms, often placed before the procedure:
    - CT-guided wire-hook placement
    - Placement of metallic microcoils
    - Navigational bronchoscopy
    - Percutaneous staining of lesion with methylene blue
    - Intraoperative ultrasound guidance
    - Transthoracic injection of radiolabeled tracer with intraoperative localization
    - Intraoperative real-time CT imaging

Step 3. Operative Steps

- ◆ VATS resection of SPN
  - ▲ For any VATS procedure, ipsilateral, single-lung ventilation with a double-lumen endotracheal tube is mandatory.
    - Occasionally, carbon dioxide (CO_2) insufflation can expedite collapse of the lung. Insufflating pressures should be kept below 6 mm Hg to minimize hemodynamic compromise.
  - ▲ The patient is placed in the full lateral decubitus position.
  - ▲ Dedicated VATS instrumentation is not necessary for most procedures, and standard open instruments can be used to manipulate the lung, including ring clamps and Duval clamps.
  - ▲ A 5-mm or 10-mm 30-degree thoracoscope is used for visualization. A 30-degree thoracoscope carries the advantage of increased visualization of the thorax, although it does take practice for the surgeon to become oriented to using the scope.

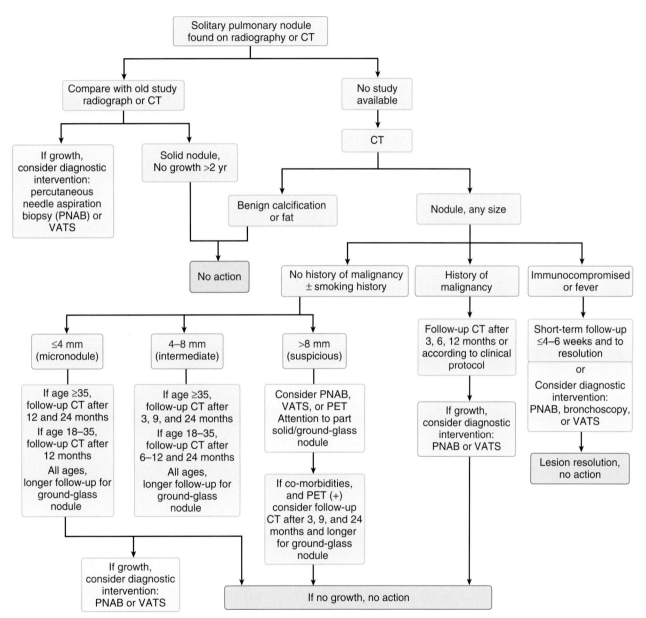

Figure 2-3

- Thoracoscopic port placement (Fig. 2-4) in the resection of peripheral SPNs is fairly standard, with the goal being to triangulate around the lesion.
  - ▲ Port placement may vary slightly based on location of the lesion, and the ports may be placed higher or lower in the chest.
  - ▲ The initial camera port (1- to 2-cm incision) is placed at the eighth or ninth intercostal space at the midaxillary line.
  - ▲ The use of a trocar, either hard or soft, at the camera site assists in keeping the camera clear and allows for easy entrance and exit from the chest.
  - ▲ If CO_2 insufflation is to be used, airtight trocars, such as those used in laparoscopy, should be used to maintain a seal.
    - ● Two additional ports are placed to triangulate around SPNs:
      - ■ The anterior port (1- to 2-cm incision) is placed in the fifth interspace at the midclavicular line. A trocar is often not used in this location, and the incision must be large enough to allow entrance of instruments and palpation of lung with a finger. Palpation of the lung is often essential in locating a subpleural SPN.
      - ■ The posterior port (1- to 2-cm) is placed at the fifth or sixth interspace, slightly posterior to the midaxillary line. This access port is most often placed in line with the incision for a standard posterolateral thoracotomy, below the scapula.
- A more anterior incision is slightly preferable because interspaces are narrower posteriorly.
  - ▲ Locating the SPN is critical and can be difficult from a VATS approach. Options for locating the nodule include the following:
    - ● Visualizing the subpleural nodule with the thoracoscope. Often, "tenting" of the pleura is present at the SPN.
    - ● Correlation of the location and anatomy with CT imaging
    - ● Palpation of the lesion with a finger is critical. A finger can be placed through one of the access ports and a clamp placed through the other to manipulate the lung for palpation (Fig. 2-5).
    - ● Preoperative localization of the lesion (as listed earlier)
  - ▲ After the SPN is identified and localized, it is wedged out using an endoscopic stapler. Either a 4.8-mm stapler (thick tissue) or a 3.6-mm stapler is used for the resection.
    - ● A ring forceps is brought through an access port and used to elevate the mass (Fig. 2-6). Caution must be exercised not to crush or manipulate the SPN so as to not affect the pathologic interpretation.
    - ● The stapler is often maneuvered between several of the access ports to complete the wedge resection.
  - ▲ A resection can also be performed using electrocautery, the cautery being used to excise the mass. Following the resection, the lung parenchyma is closed with intracorporeal suture techniques.

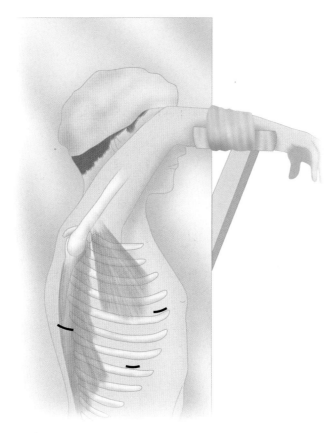

Figure 2-4

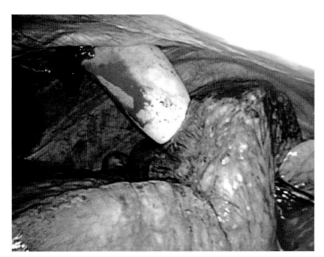

Figure 2-5

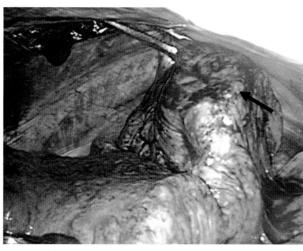

Figure 2-6

▲ Extraction of resected lesions from the thoracic cavity is best accomplished with the assistance of a retrieval bag device so as not to potentially contaminate the access port.

▲ A single chest tube is placed at the conclusion of procedure.

◆ Open-resection of SPN can be achieved using several different approaches, including a standard posterolateral thoracotomy or several hybrid techniques.

▲ Single-lung ventilation with double-lumen endotracheal tube is most often used, although it is not mandatory in open resections.

▲ The patient is positioned in the full lateral decubitus position, similar to the VATS procedure.

▲ A standard posterolateral thoracotomy (muscle-sparing) can be used (Fig. 2-7).

● This is often a hybrid procedure with a VATS camera port at the eighth interspace midaxillary line to improve visualization and light within the chest to allow for a slightly smaller incision.

● A thoracotomy allows for direct palpation of lung. This is particularly useful for nodules that are difficult to identify and palpate when using the VATS approach.

▲ An anterior thoracotomy may be appropriate for certain SPNs (Fig. 2-8).

● An incision is made anterior to the axilla in the line of the desired interspace.

● The latissimus dorsi muscle is retracted posteriorly without being divided.

● The serratus muscle is spread in the direction of its fibers.

■ Care must be taken not to injure the long thoracic nerve.

■ The intercostal muscles are divided from the superior aspect of the rib.

◆ A small chest spreader may be used to increase exposure. Alternatively, several Weitlaner retractors can be used to retract the soft tissues without spreading the ribs.

▲ The wedge resection is performed using an endoscopic articulating stapler.

● The stapler can be introduced via the camera port for difficult staple angles and may allow for a smaller incision.

▲ A resection can also be performed with the cautery and suture closure of lung parenchyma performed after the resection.

▲ A single chest tube is placed at the conclusion of procedure.

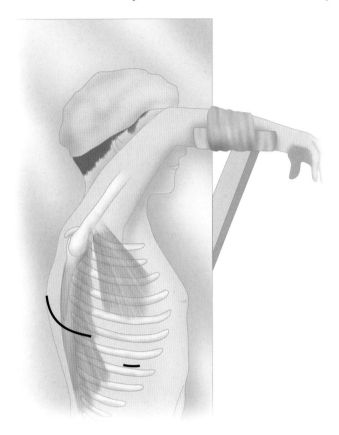

Figure 2-7

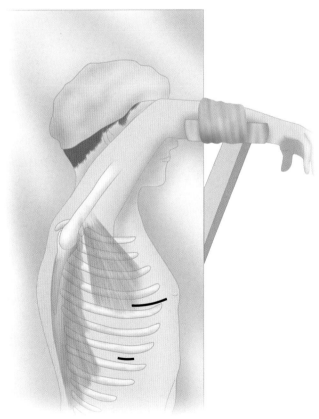

Figure 2-8

Step 4. Pearls and Pitfalls

- ◆ Deep parenchymal nodules may be difficult to localize with VATS. Preoperative localization techniques are available.
- ◆ Deep parenchymal nodules may require an anatomic resection.
    - ▲ Segmentectomy
    - ▲ Lobectomy
    - ▲ Both can be accomplished thoracoscopically

Suggested Readings

Gould MK, Maclean CC, Kuschner WG, et al. Accuracy of positron emission tomography for diagnosis of pulmonary nodules and mass lesions: A meta-analysis. JAMA 2001;285:914-924.

International Early Lung Cancer Action Program Investigators, Henschke CI, Yankelevitz DF, et al. Survival of patients with stage I lung cancer detected on CT screening. N Engl J Med 2006;355:1763-1771.

CHAPTER 3

RIGHT UPPER LOBECTOMY

Robert J. McKenna Jr

Step 1. Surgical Anatomy

- The anatomy for the right upper lobe (RUL) is consistent, thus the approach to a right upper lobectomy generally is consistent. The RUL vein is the most anterior structure. Posterior to the vein is the RUL bronchus. The arteries are superior and inferior to the bronchus, as seen in the accompanying figures.

Step 2. Preoperative Considerations

- The most common indication for a lobectomy is lung cancer, and the RUL is the most common lobe for lung cancer. Lung cancer affects 200,000 Americans each year, and it is the most common cancer killer in both men and women.
- For lung cancer, a wedge resection/segmentectomy has a 3- to 5-fold increase in local recurrence and a 20% lower cure rate than a lobectomy. The procedure should be a standard anatomic resection with individual ligation of the artery, vein, and bronchus and a lymph node dissection.
- Preoperative workup usually includes a chest computed tomography (CT) scan and a positron emission tomography (PET) scan. If the patient appears to have a higher stage of cancer or symptoms of metastatic disease, brain imaging is often performed. Pulmonary function tests are performed. Generally, expected postoperative forced expiratory volume in 1 second (FEV$_1$) should be greater than 800 mL or 40% predicted. If the patient is marginal, then a quantitative lung perfusion scan can be performed to determine the functionality of the area to be resected. If it is not functional, resection may still be undertaken.
- Mediastinoscopy with removal of lymph nodes in several stations is performed for patients other than stage 1A (T1N0) tumors, plus patients with synchronous primary lung cancers and patients with poor performance status. If the nodes are negative, pulmonary resection is undertaken.
- The video-assisted thoracoscopic surgery (VATS) procedure is performed using a double-lumen tube for single-lung ventilation. The patient is in the lateral decubitus position with a slight posterior tilt. The operating table is flexed so that the bend is at the level of the anterior superior iliac spine. This moves the hip out of the way and opens the intercostal space. In addition to general anesthesia, a long-acting local anesthetic is injected to block the intercostal nerves from T4-9.

Step 3. Operative Steps

1. The Overall Procedure

- The order of the steps of the operation are as follows: level 10 nodes, RUL vein, minor fissure, anterior trunk of the artery, posterior ascending artery, RUL bronchus, and the fissure. The incisions are the standard incisions with the utility incision placed directly up (lateral) from the superior pulmonary vein.

2. Incisions

- As seen in Figure 3-1, four incisions are used.
- The first incision is in the sixth intercostal space in the midclavicular line. The incision is tunneled posteriorly through the tissues so that the instruments through the incision point toward the major fissure, not straight down toward the pericardium.
- The 5-mm trocar and thoracoscope are placed through the eighth intercostal space in the posterior axillary line.
- The third incision is the utility incision. For an upper lobe, the incision begins at the edge of the latissimus muscle and extends anteriorly about 4 cm. The interspace is chosen by looking in the pleural space and retracting the lung posteriorly. This incision is made directly up from the superior pulmonary vein.
- The fourth incision is made 3 finger breadths below the tip of the scapula and halfway to the spine.

3. Level 10 Nodes

- Removal of the level 10 nodes defines the anatomy and facilitates the mobilization of the vessels for the lobectomy.
- The level 10 nodes are between the superior vena cava (SVC), azygos vein, and superior hilum of the lung (Fig. 3-2).
- Removing all the tissue in this triangle removes the level 10 nodes and exposes the right mainstem bronchus, anterior trunk, and SVC.

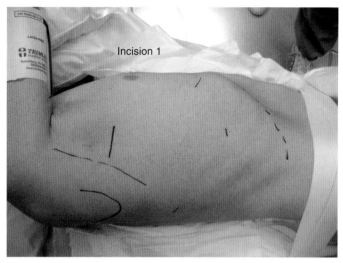

Figure 3-1

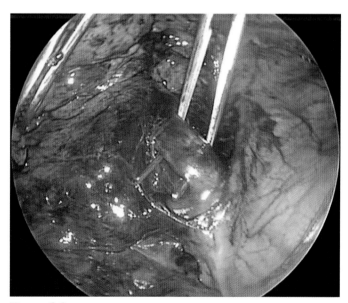

Figure 3-2

4. Right Upper Lobe Vein

- The RUL and right middle lobe (RML) veins are identified.
- Dissection is performed along the superior and inferior aspects of the RUL vein.
- The pulmonary artery is directly behind the vein.
- A right-angle clamp passes between the vein and the artery (Fig. 3-3).
- An endoscopic vascular stapler through incision 4 transects the RUL vein (Fig. 3-4).

5. Minor Fissure

- The minor fissure is now completed. To help define where the staples should be placed, there is usually at least a partially developed minor fissure on the lateral surface of the lung.
- For the first firing of the stapler, the anvil of the stapler should be pointed toward the venous confluence between the RUL and the RML veins (Fig. 3-5). The staple cartridge is placed in the minor fissure or pointed toward the minor fissure if it is incomplete. For the next firings, the anvil is placed on the surface of the artery.
- Ring forceps pull the lung parenchyma into the jaws of the endoscopic stapler with a 4.8-mm staple cartridge (Fig. 3-6).
- The jaws of the stapler are opened, and the lung parenchyma in the fissure is again pulled into the jaws with ring forceps.

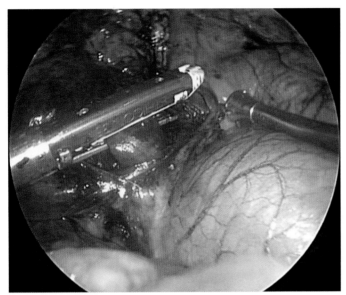

Figure 3-3

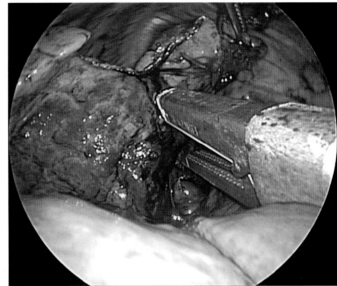

Figure 3-4

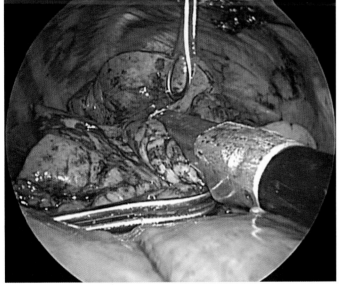

Figure 3-5

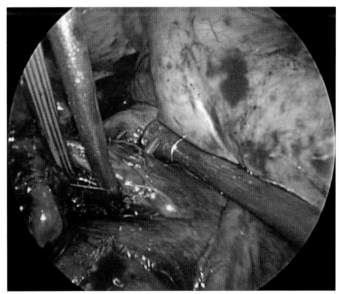

Figure 3-6

6. Anterior Trunk

- The anterior trunk is then prepared for stapling.
- The lymph nodes are removed from between the anterior trunk and the main right pulmonary artery.
- A right angle passes between the anterior trunk and the main pulmonary artery (Fig. 3-7).
- A stapler from incision 4 or incision 1 transects the artery (Fig. 3-8).

7. Posterior Ascending Artery

- Lobar nodes on the surface of the RUL bronchus are removed (Fig. 3-9).
- The posterior ascending artery can be seen inferior to the RUL bronchus.
- Metzenbaum scissors spread between the RUL bronchus and the posterior ascending artery (Fig. 3-10).
- The posterior ascending artery is clipped at its origin (Fig. 3-11). Do not place clips distally because they will be in the staple line.

8. Right Upper Lobe Bronchus

- Spreading the Metzenbaum scissors widely between the RUL bronchus and the posterior ascending artery creates a tunnel for the 4.8-mm stapler through incision 1 to staple the bronchus (Fig. 3-12).

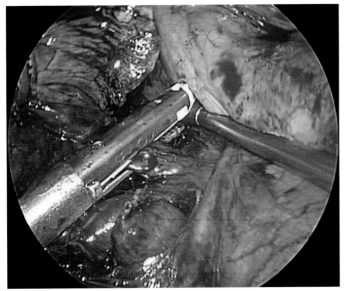

Figure 3-7

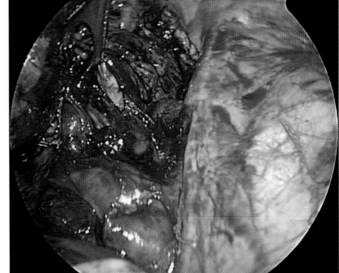

Figure 3-8

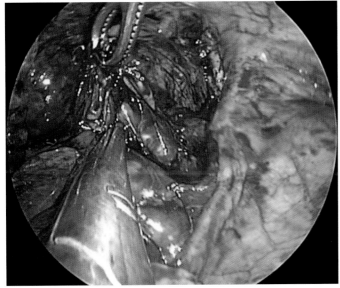

Figure 3-9

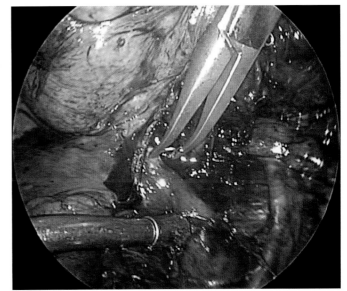

Figure 3-10

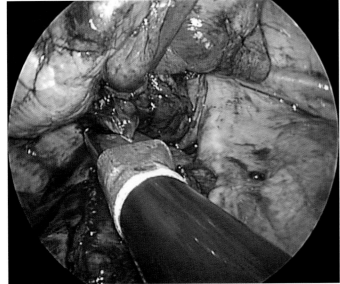

Figure 3-11

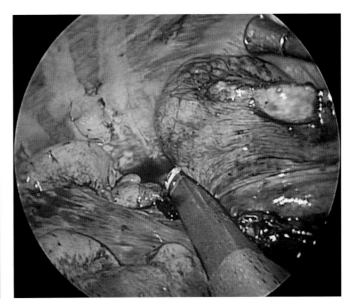

Figure 3-12

9. Completion of the Fissure

◆ Through incision 1, the endoscopic 4.8-mm stapler is fired several times to complete the fissure (Fig. 3-13).

10. Removal of the Lobe

◆ To minimize the chances of recurrent tumor in the incision, the RUL is placed into a bag for removal through the utility incision (Fig. 3-14).

Step 4. Postoperative Care

◆ Patients usually do not require care in the intensive care unit after undergoing a VATS lobectomy.
◆ Pain relief is usually by intraoperative intercostal nerve blocks, postoperative hydrocodone bitartate and acetaminophen (Vicodin), and subcutaneous hydromorphone HCl (Dilaudid). Occasionally, patient-controlled analgesia pumps are used.
◆ Chest drainage system is usually placed to water seal because suction prolongs air leaks.
◆ Early ambulation and pulmonary toilet are the keys to an uneventful postoperative course.
◆ In recent years, 46% of our patients have been discharged on the first or second postoperative day.

Step 5. Pearls and Pitfalls

◆ Work anteriorly to posteriorly with little manipulation of the lung.
◆ No posterior dissection is necessary.
◆ Complete resection of the tissue with the level 10 nodes exposes the right mainstem bronchus, SVC, and anterior trunk. During that dissection, the superior and posterior aspects of the anterior arterial trunk should be dissected well because it prepares the artery for transection later.

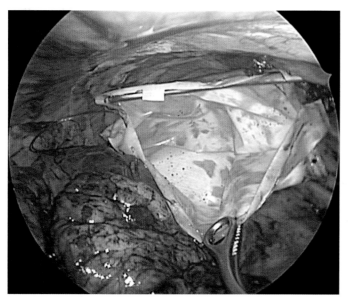

Figure 3-13

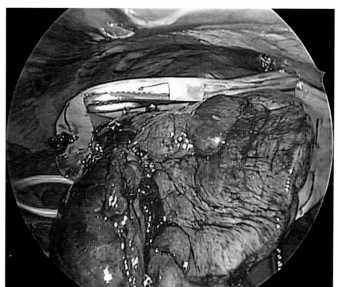

Figure 3-14

Suggested Readings

Alam N, Flores RM. Video-assisted thoracic surgery (VATS) lobectomy: The evidence base. ISLS 2007;1(3):368-374.

Gharagozloo F, Tempesta B, Margolis M, Alexander EP. Video-assisted thoracic surgery lobectomy for stage I lung cancer. Ann Thorac Surg 2003;76(4):1009-1014.

Flores RM, Alam N. Video-assisted thoracic surgery lobectomy (VATS), open thoracotomy, and the robot for lung cancer. Ann Thorac Surg 2008;85:S710-S715.

Houck WV, Fuller CB, McKenna RJ Jr. Video-assisted thoracic surgery upper lobe trisegmentectomy for early stage left apical lung cancer. Ann Thorac Surg 2004;78(5):1858-1860.

McKenna RJ Jr. Complications and learning curves for video-assisted thoracic surgery lobectomy. Thorac Surg Clin 2008;18(3):275-280.

McKenna RJ Jr, Houck W, Fuller CB. Video-assisted thoracic surgery lobectomy: Experience with 1,100 cases. Ann Thorac Surg 2006;91(2):421-425; discussion 425-426.

Ohtsuka T, Nomori H, Horio H, et al. Is major pulmonary resection by video-assisted thoracic surgery an adequate procedure in clinical stage I lung cancer? Chest 2004;125(5):1742-1746.

Walker WS, Codispoto M, Soon SY, et al. Long-term outcomes following VATS lobectomy for non–small cell bronchogenic carcinoma. Eur J Cardiothorac Surg 2003;23(3):397-402.

VIDEO-ASSISTED THORACIC SURGERY FOR MAJOR PULMONARY RESECTION

Michael Kuan Yew Hsin and Anthony P. C. Yim

Video-assisted thoracic surgery (VATS) in the management of lung cancer was first described in the early 1990s. Recent studies have shown that major lung resection by VATS has low perioperative morbidity and mortality rates and is associated with a good prognosis in patients with stage I non–small cell lung cancer (NSCLC).

Step 1. Surgical Anatomy

- Knowledge of thoracic anatomy is critical to VATS. Anatomic lung resection requires a dissection of the pulmonary hilum and ligation and division of the bronchus, pulmonary artery, and pulmonary vein to the involved pulmonary lobe. The rationale behind lung resection is a complete removal of tumor along with an en bloc resection of the lymph nodes from the mediastinum associated with the tumor.

Step 2. Preoperative Considerations

- All patients considered for VATS lung resection receive preoperative computed tomography (CT) scan of the thorax, bronchoscopy, and pulmonary function tests. Mediastinoscopy is performed if there is radiologic evidence of mediastinal lymphadenopathy (>1 cm) on preoperative CT scan of the thorax. Positron emission tomography is performed only when indicated. Patients with clinical stage I or II disease are considered for VATS lung resection. Patients with tumor size greater than 4 cm and bronchoscopic findings of endobronchial lesions are excluded.
- The standard setup for VATS consists of a videoscope, a light source, and a camera. A monitor is placed on each side of the operating table, near the head end of the patient. The cords and

cables of the videoscope are passed toward the head of the table in a standard fashion to minimize cluttering.

♦ The tower that contains the video components generally consists of, from top to bottom, a video monitor, which can be slaved to a second video monitor placed on the opposite side of the operating table; a camera processing unit; a light source; a Super VHS recorder; and a color printer.

♦ For major VATS lung resections, we use a 10-mm 30-degree videoscope. We endeavor to minimize the use of specially designed endoscopic instruments, with the exception of endoscopic stapling devices. The instruments in a standard thoracotomy set would suffice without modification. The advantages of conventional instruments are that they are light, easy to use, familiar to all surgeons, universally available, and inexpensive. Further, these instruments allow tactile feedback through instrument palpation.

♦ For VATS major lung resection, the patient will require general anesthesia and double-lumen intubation to achieve selective one-lung ventilation so as to collapse the side of the operation. A single-lumen endotracheal tube can be used with an endobronchial blocker as an alternative if double-lumen intubation is not feasible. It is good practice for the operating surgeon to perform on-table flexible bronchoscopy at this point to rule out endobronchial anomalies, if this has not been already performed.

Step 3. Operative Steps

1. Positioning of the Patient

♦ The positioning of the patient is in the lateral decubitus position, as per a posterolateral thoracotomy, because the surgeon should always be prepared to convert the procedure from a minimally invasive operation to an open conventional one. The patient is appropriately padded with one roll placed on either side of the chest and secured with straps. The operating table is flexed to allow the intercostal spaces of interest to be further opened to achieve better access as well as to bring the pelvis out of the way of the instruments.

♦ Typically the operating surgeon stands facing the front of the patient, as does the assistant holding the camera, with the scrub nurse standing facing the back of the patient.

2. VATS Port Strategy

- Our standard VATS port-site strategy uses a three-port technique, which consists of an inferior port for insertion of the videoscope, an anterior port, and a posterior port for placement of instruments. The anterior port is modified into an anteriorly placed utility mini-thoracotomy.
- In general, the sixth or seventh intercostal space in the midaxillary line is the position of choice for placement of the inferior port for videoscope access into the pleural cavity. This is the first port to be made, so it can be created only in a "blind" fashion; this care is taken to avoid injury to lung parenchyma, especially if the likelihood of pleural adhesions is high, and if necessary some blunt dissection may be needed. Digital palpation is recommended to confirm absence of adhesions.
- The videoscope is protected by a camera port, which prevents smudging of the camera lens. An assessment of the pleural cavity is made once the videoscope is positioned, and in cases of known or suspected malignant pathology, a special effort is made to look for pleural deposits, which may represent pleural metastases.
- The remaining anterior and posterior instrument ports are created under videoscopic vision. The precise location of the ports depends on the pathology and takes into account the location of the fissure as seen via the videoscope as well as the presence of any pleural adhesion.
- A typical port strategy is as follows: The second incision is placed after inspection of the intrathoracic anatomy, avoiding areas of adhesions. The anterior utility incision, 2 cm long, is placed in the fifth intercostal space starting at the anterior axillary line. The posterior incision is placed one or two intercostal spaces below and posterior to the tip of the scapula.
- As a general principle, an adequate distance should exist between the ports to avoid "fencing" of instruments. The instruments and the videoscope should all face the direction of the target pathology because "mirroring" may cause awkward handling of the instruments.
- We frequently perform a segmental rib resection for the anterior utility port for cases of VATS major lung resection. The segmental rib resection technique is especially advantageous in redo cases, when tumor size is larger than 3 cm, and in cases in which bidigital palpation is desirable.

- The skin incision is up to 5 cm long. The incision is carried down to the rib, which is then resected subperiosteally for the length of the incision (Fig. 4-1). With the use of a soft tissue retractor only (i.e., no rib spreading), a gap of up to 5 cm between ribs can be obtained underneath the wound to allow accurate bidigital palpation and retrieval of large specimens. At the time of wound closure, there is no need to reapproximate the ribs.
- The principles of VATS major lung resection will be illustrated with a right VATS pneumonectomy.

3. Right Pneumonectomy

Division of the Superior Pulmonary Vein

- The inferior pulmonary ligament is released to facilitate mobilization of the right lung. A sponge-holder clamp is passed via the posterior port to grasp the right lower lobe close to the inferior border to exert an upward traction. A rigid Yankauer sucker placed through the anterior port is used to depress the diaphragm, and a long-tipped diathermy is used to incise the inferior pulmonary ligament (Fig. 4-2), which is then further released with blunt dissection using a mounted peanut swab (Fig. 4-3).
- The right lung is then repositioned, with the posterior sponge-holder clamp grasping the right middle lobe close to its inferior border, giving it a posterior traction, which exposes the hilar structures.
- The superior pulmonary vein is exposed using a combination of sharp and blunt dissection. The upper and lower borders of the superior pulmonary vein are defined using a mounted peanut swab. The tip of a right angled clamp is passed round the back of the superior pulmonary vein, and a silk tie is slung around the superior pulmonary vein (Fig. 4-4). The space behind the superior pulmonary vein is further developed with a peanut swab mounted on a right-angled clamp.
- The videoscope is then repositioned through the anterior port, and an EndoGIA vascular stapler (Ethicon Endo Surgical Inc., Cincinnati, OH) is inserted through the inferior port. With slight tension on the silk tie, the flat blade of the vascular stapler is eased behind the superior pulmonary vein (Fig. 4-5). To help keep the tip of the stapler from emerging behind the superior pulmonary vein, it might be necessary to use a mounted peanut or a right-angled clamp to push out of the way any structure that could cause obstruction. The superior pulmonary vein is then divided.

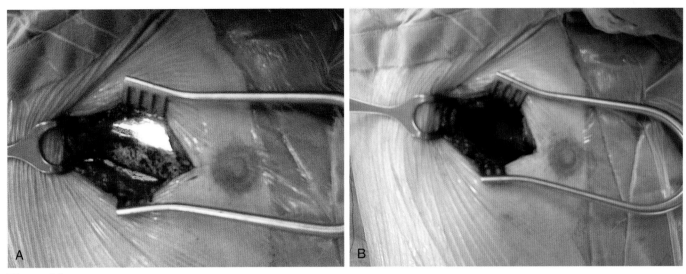

Figure 4-1

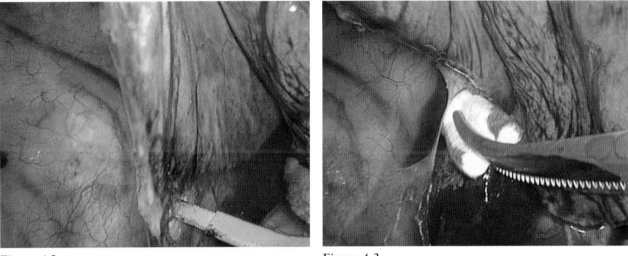

Figure 4-2

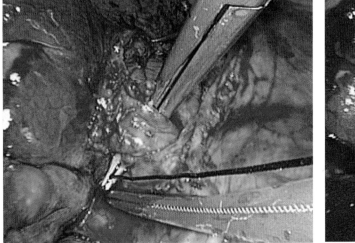

Figure 4-3

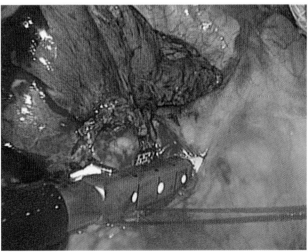

Figure 4-4

Figure 4-5

Division of the Right Pulmonary Artery

- The videoscope is returned to the inferior port position. Maintaining the same posterior traction using the posterior sponge-holder clamp, the right pulmonary artery is exposed with sharp and blunt dissection. Both upper and lower borders of the right pulmonary artery are defined using blunt dissection with a mounted peanut (Fig. 4-6).
- A right-angled clamp is passed behind the right pulmonary artery and a silk tie is slung around the vessel (Fig. 4-7). The space behind the right pulmonary artery is developed using a peanut mounted on a right-angled clamp.
- The videoscope is then repositioned through the anterior port, and an EndoGIA vascular stapler is inserted through the inferior port. With gentle traction on the silk tie, the flat blade of the vascular stapler is eased behind the right pulmonary artery, helped by a mounted peanut to displace any structure that might obstruct the tip of the stapler from emerging behind the right pulmonary artery (Fig. 4-8). The stapler is deployed when the trunk is secured between the jaws of the stapler and the right pulmonary artery is divided.
- Occasionally, there may be early branching of the truncus anterior, in which case this should be divided using the same principles.

Division of the Right Main Bronchus

- The videoscope is returned to the inferior port position. The fascia around the right pulmonary artery stump is cleared using sharp and blunt dissection. The right upper lobe bronchus is then exposed. By tracing this proximally, the right main bronchus is seen.
- The lower border of the right main bronchus is defined using blunt dissection with the tip of the rigid sucker and a mounted peanut. The plane below the right main bronchus is initially opened up with a right-angled clamp. A right-angled Rumel clamp is then passed behind the right main bronchus, and a silk tie is slung around the right main bronchus (Fig. 4-9). The space behind the right main bronchus is further developed with a peanut mounted on a right-angled clamp.
- An EZ-45 No-Knife endoscopic stapler (Ethicon Endo Surgical Inc., Cincinnati, OH) is then introduced via the anterior port, and the right main bronchus is engaged between the opened jaws of the stapler. This maneuver may require traction on the silk tie as well as counter-traction using a peanut mounted on a right-angled clamp to ensure the right main bronchus is securely grasped by the EZ-45 stapler (Fig. 4-10). The stapler is then deployed and the right main bronchus divided.

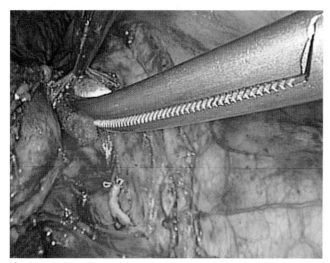

Figure 4-6

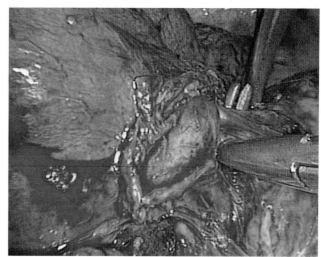

Figure 4-7

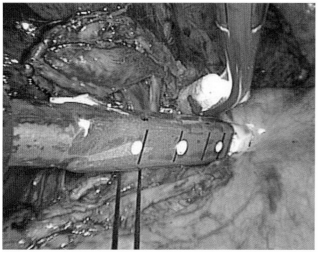

Figure 4-8

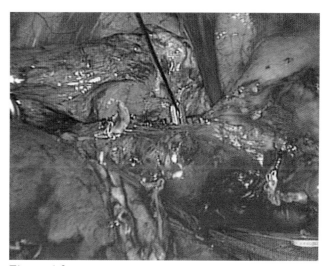

Figure 4-9

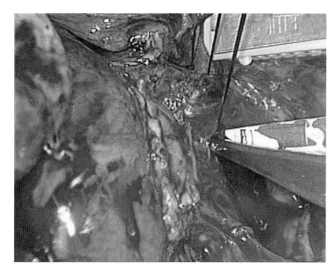

Figure 4-10

Division of the Inferior Pulmonary Vein

- The right lower lobe is elevated using the posterior ringed-clamp to grasp on the right lower lobe near the inferior margin. With upward traction on the right lower lobe, the inferior pulmonary vein is pulled taut. A right-angled clamp is used to pass behind the inferior pulmonary vein, and a silk tie is slung around the inferior pulmonary vein. The space behind the inferior pulmonary vein is further enlarged using a peanut mounted on a right-angled clamp (Fig. 4-11).
- An EndoGIA vascular stapler is introduced through the anterior port, and the flat blade of the vascular stapler is eased behind the inferior pulmonary vein, helped by gentle traction on the silk tie. Once it is confirmed that the inferior pulmonary vein is securely engaged by the vascular stapler, the inferior pulmonary vein is divided (Fig. 4-12).
- The right lung should now be free to mobilize. Any remaining attachment of the right lung to the hilum can be safely divided at this stage and the right lung specimen removed through the anterior port via a specimen bag. Medistinal lymph node sampling is performed as per routine.
- Hemostasis is performed, and intercostal infiltration of local anesthetic is given.
- The thoracic cavity is washed out with warm water, and following testing of the stump to sustained pressure (25 cm H_2O) under water for air leak, a 28 French chest drain is inserted under vision.
- The wounds are closed in layers using absorbable sutures.

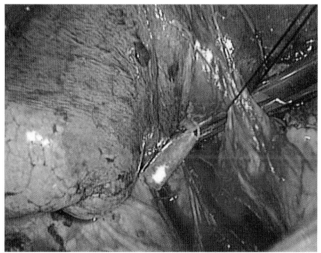

Figure 4-11

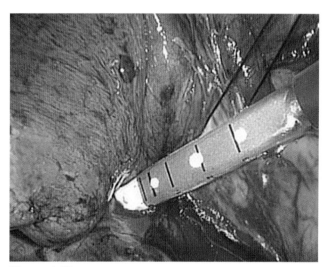

Figure 4-12

Step 4. Postoperative Care

- The patient is turned to the supine position and extubated in the operating room.
- The chest drain is left on free drainage into a chest drain bottle which is clearly marked "No Suction." A chest radiograph is taken in the recovery unit. The chest drain is removed on the first postoperative day.
- Adequate analgesia is given so that patients are encouraged to work with an incentive spirometer at hourly intervals. Chest physiotherapy and early mobilization are essential. Supplementary oxygen is given via nasal cannula as needed to keep O_2 saturation above 94%. Infrequently, patients require bedside flexible bronchoscopy for bronchial toileting.
- Daily chest radiograph is taken, and once the fluid level in the post-pneumonectomy space rises above the bronchial stump and the patient remains clinically well, the patient may be discharged to be seen in the outpatient clinic in 2 weeks.

Step 5. Pearls and Pitfalls

- ◆ Despite concerns regarding the safety and efficacy of VATS major lung resection, excellent outcomes have been demonstrated for patients with early-stage lung cancer.
- ◆ Even though the technique has yet to gain wide acceptance, there is accumulating evidence to show that the VATS approach may contribute to better preservation of human immune function.
- ◆ Surgical trauma induced by conventional (non-VATS) lung resection is believed to be associated with a certain degree of immunosuppression, which theoretically could lead to promotion of tumor growth and tumor recurrence.
- ◆ In treating an increasingly aging population who present with multiple co-morbidities, the minimally invasive approach of VATS may result in early mobilization and restoration of body function.

Suggested Readings

Roviaro G, Varoli F, Vergani C, et al. Minimal access cardiothoracic surgery. In Yim APC, Hazelrigg SR, Izzat MB, et al, eds. Anatomic Lung Resection. Philadelphia: WB Saunders; 2000:107-115.

Shigemura N, Hsin MK, Yim AP. Segmental rib resection for difficult cases of video-assisted thoracic surgery. J Thorac Cardiovasc Surg 2006;132:701-702.

Yim AP, Liu HP. Thoracoscopic major lung resection—indications, technique, and early results: Experience from two centers in Asia. Surg Laparosc Endosc 1997;7:241-244.

CHAPTER 5

ROBOTIC LOBECTOMY

Kemp H. Kernstine

Step 1. Surgical Anatomy

- A thorough understanding of the anatomy of the mediastinum, hilum, and lobes and their variations is necessary (Fig. 5-1)
- Figure 5-1 demonstrates the relationship between the mediastinal structures and the hila and lobes.

Step 2. Preoperative Considerations

- Lobectomy is most commonly performed for primary lung cancer. Of the available treatments, it provides the best rate of cure. The mean age of these patients is 70 years, and they often have numerous co-morbidities, potentially affecting the postoperative mortality, morbidity, hospital length of stay, and recovery.
- Performing a lobectomy for lung cancer reduces the local recurrence rate and appears to improve survival. Performing an anatomic lung resection, either lobectomy or bilobectomy along with resection of the ipsilateral hilum and at least two to four mediastinal lymph nodal groups counting at least 11 to 16 lymph nodes, including the contralateral mediastinum, appears to provide a survival advantage.[1-4]
- Lobectomy by thoracotomy is considered standard of care, and video-assisted thoracic surgical (VATS) resection may provide the same level of resection, less pain, reduced complications, shorter hospital stay, and earlier return to preoperative functional status than the open thoracotomy and additionally may provide a similar cure rate.[5-7] Computer-assisted technology or robotics may provide a superior resection compared to VATS to perform a wide lymph node resection, improved rate of complete resection with potentially less pain, and a reduced conversion rate.[8-10]
- Computed tomography of the chest with 2- to 5-mm cuts, including the lower liver to the angle of the jaw, provides sufficient information about the primary tumor, the health of the other lung, other lesions, hilar and mediastinal lymph node status, potential liver and adrenal metastases, and other staging information.
- Fluorodeoxyglucose (FDG)–positron emission tomography (PET) scan provides additional information about the primary tumor, status of the mediastinum, and potential of metastatic disease outside the chest.

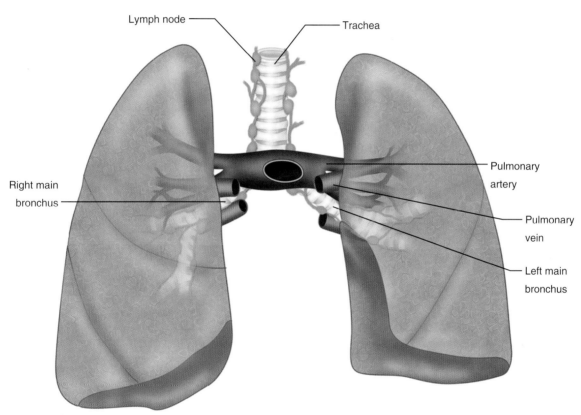

Figure 5-1

- Pulmonary function studies, including spirometry and diffusion capacity, provide information about the pulmonary reserve after lung resection.
- For patients with limited pulmonary reserve, forced expiratory volume in 1 second (FEV_1) or diffusing capacity of lung for carbon monoxide (DLCO) less than 40% of normal, a quantitative ventilation/perfusion scan and exercise pulmonary function study may assist in assessing the post–lung resection pulmonary reserve.
- A thorough evaluation of co-morbidities should be performed, especially cardiac, renal, and neurologic risks; if any are found, these should be appropriately addressed by obtaining specialty assistance as necessary.

Step 3. Operative Steps

1. Patient Position (Fig. 5-2)

- In the supine position, a double-lumen tube or bronchial blocker is placed for eventual single-lung ventilation.
- On a deflatable beanbag, the patient is then positioned in the lateral decubitus position and strapped to the operating table with the upper arm placed in an arm sling positioned close over the forehead, the lower arm axilla on a soft axillary roll, and the arm up and lateral.
- Once sufficiently arranged, the table is rotated 15 to 30 degrees posteriorly for upper and middle lobes and 15 to 30 degrees anteriorly for lower lobes. Patients with wide hips should have reverse mid-operating table flexion to provide sufficient chest exposure and range of motion of the robotic arms and videoport. Reverse Trendelenburg allows any of the minimal bleeding that occurs during the procedure to collect at the inferior aspect of the pleural space away from the operating location and allows for the subdiaphragmatic organs to fall away from the operative field, providing better access.

2. Thoracoport Placement (Fig. 5-3)

- Using an indelible marker, a 4- to 5-cm circle is drawn just anterior to the tip of the scapula, with the center 2 to 3 cm from the tip; this is the target of the dissection.
- Six puncture sites are then drawn onto the patient's chest, differing in location for the upper and lower lobes.
- For the upper and middle lobes, the videoport is placed in the seventh to eighth intercostal space, just lateral to the costal margin. From that port site a triangle is then drawn to the target serving as the base of the triangle. Then about 10 cm lateral to the right and left arm of the triangle, the two 8-mm robotic port sites are drawn to avoid later instrument collision. The two posterior sites are then drawn; the posterior-superior port site is at the level of the fourth intercostal space, just immediately adjacent to the longitudinal spinous muscle. The posterior inferior port site is located along the same parallel line, just immediately adjacent to the longitudinal spinous muscle at the lateral border of the 10th intercostal space. The final port site, the anterior superior site, is located at the fourth intercostal space in the midclavicular to lateral-third clavicular line.
- For the lower lobes, the video port site is marked to be about 6 to 8 cm lateral to the longitudinal spinous muscle in the ninth intercostal space. Again, a triangle is drawn between the video port site and the target. The left and right robotic arms are then placed outside the triangle, each approximately 10 cm away from the video port site. The leftward robotic arm

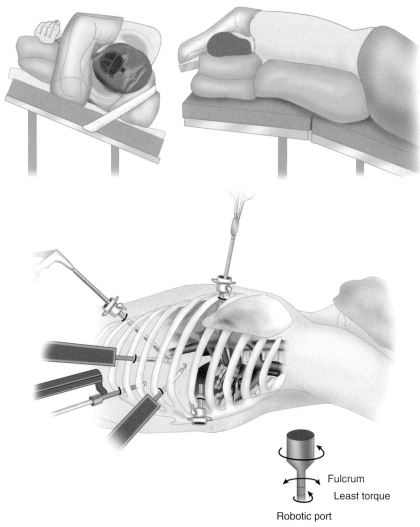

Fulcrum

Least torque

Robotic port

Figure 5-2

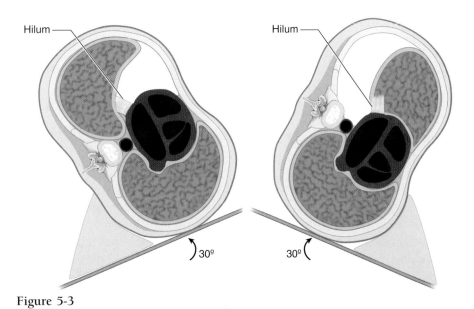

Hilum

Hilum

30º

30º

Figure 5-3

is just at or slightly medial to the lateral border of the longitudinal spinous muscle, and the rightward arm site is drawn at approximately the seventh to eighth intercostal space laterally. The posterior-superior port site and the anterior-superior port sites are in the same location as for the upper lobes. The anterior-inferior port site is placed at the sixth to seventh intercostal space 3 to 4 cm lateral to the costal margin.

- The chest is then sterilely prepared in the usual fashion, and surgical drapes are applied.
- The first incision made for either the upper or lower lobes is at the anterior-inferior port site. A small incision is made; then, using a tonsil clamp, the pleural space is entered after single-lung ventilation is initiated. A 10- to 12-mm thoracoport and the videoscope are then placed. The remaining ports will be placed under direct thoracoscopic vision to minimize injury to the intercostal bundle. First, the intrapleural location is verified and CO_2 is infused slowly, increasing to achieve sufficient access and visibility and avoid hemodynamic compromise.
- The two 8-mm robotic arms are placed, as well as the 10- to 12-mm thoracoports, aiming the direction of the thoracoports medially toward the hilum, where they will have the greatest function.
- The robotic chassis is then rolled into position. For the upper and middle lobes, the robot is brought posteriorly and obliquely over the neck and shoulder so that the base of the chassis is in line with the target and videoport site. For the lower lobes, the chassis is brought obliquely from the anterior aspect of the head, aiming it toward the target and the videoscope. The positioning of the robot chassis base in relation to the operating room table is important to optimize robotic arm and instrument function. The robot arms and instruments function optimally when they are aimed toward the base of the robot chassis. This is determined, and the first joint of the video port arm is within 10 to 12 cm from the base of the chassis after the arm has been attached to the video thoracoport.
- The videoscope arm is attached to the videoscope thoracoport, and the clutch button is used to guide the 0-degree scope into position to obtain visibility for the other arms to be placed.
- The right and left robotic arms are then attached. Using the "setup joint" buttons, the arms are positioned to raise the arm base up and lateral as much as possible to achieve maximal maneuverability of the arms for the dissection.
- In the left arm, a ProGrasp can be placed and in the right arm, a Harmonic scalpel. Using the clutch button, the arm instruments can be pushed into position so that the working parts can be visualized. Throughout the procedure, the instrument tips should be visible.

3. Dissection (Fig. 5-4)

- For the upper right lobe, a Landreneau ring clamp is passed through the posterior-superior thoracoport and grasps the lung parenchyma just lateral to the superior pulmonary vein, keeping it on stretch. The pleura is incised just lateral to the phrenic nerve, and all the hilar tissue around the base of the lobe, including beneath the azygos vein, is taken with the lobe.
- The superior pulmonary vein is identified and separated from the middle lobe vein, and all the adjacent hilar tissue around the vein is taken with the specimen. A 10- to 12-cm-long, heavy silk suture is passed around the vein and held by one of the robotic instruments. Then, from the posterior inferior thoracoport, a vascular endostapler is passed to divide the vein immediately adjacent to the middle lobe vein, but not obstruct it. Once the upper lobe venous drainage is divided, all the hilar tissue around the pulmonary artery trunk is dissected to expose the origin of the pulmonary arteries to the upper lobe. All the tissue can be resected en bloc or removed separately to achieve adequate exposure of the pulmonary arteries. A silk passed around each vessel may facilitate this process.

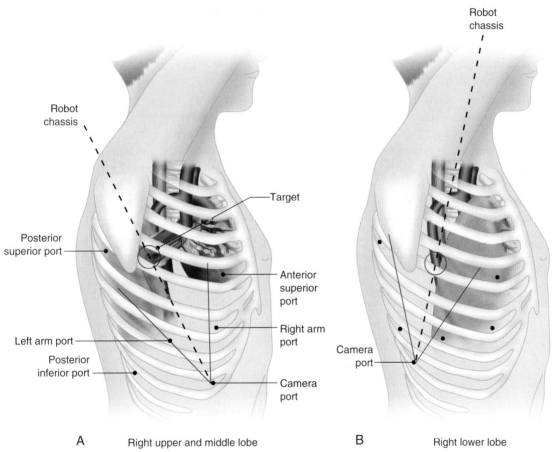

A   Right upper and middle lobe   B   Right lower lobe

Figure 5-4

- The vascular endostapler is brought through the same thoracoport, that is, the posterior-inferior thoracoport. The hilar tissue in front of the right mainstem and right upper lobe bronchi are dissected away with the specimen or separately removed. The right upper lobe bronchus is carefully dissected from adjacent structures, and the bronchus is encircled with a heavy silk. A 3.5- to 4.8-mm endostapler is used to divide the bronchus immediately adjacent to the mainstem airway. Before firing the stapler, to ensure that the correct bronchus is being taken, bronchoscopy can be performed and the remaining lobes inflated.

- In some cases, hilar scarring may be severe or severe inflammation or bulky adenopathy may be present at the base of the bronchus, making it difficult to be sure that the correct airway is being dissected. In these cases, a posterior view may be helpful and the lung retracted anteriorly to expose the posterior hilum. The pleura may then be resected over that area to expose the origin of the bronchus.

- Once the bronchus is divided, the remaining and immediately adjacent nodal tissue may be included in the specimen to expose the remaining minor fissure. Through the posterior-superior and anterior thoracoport sites, the fissure is completed. The hilar area is then submerged with saline and the ipsilateral airway ventilated. If air bubbles are seen, needle holders can be placed into the robotic arms to repair the defect, and adjacent vascular tissue can be brought into place to cover the defect as necessary. Further paratracheal mediastinal and subcarinal mediastinal tissue can be resected to complete the lymphadenectomy. The specimens are brought out through the anterior superior port site in an endobag. To prevent postoperative torsion of the right middle lobe, the middle lobe can be plicated to the lower lobe by stapling the very edges in one or two places as necessary.

- For the right middle lobectomy, the Landreneau ring clamp is placed just lateral to the middle lobe vein and the dissection is initiated as previously stated. First the vein is taken, and then the deep dissection of the hilum and adjacent lymphatic tissue is performed, exposing the right middle lobe pulmonary artery or arteries and the bronchus just at its origin from the bronchus intermedius. The major and minor fissures are then divided accordingly, and the remainder of the procedure is performed as with the upper lobe.

- For the left upper lobectomy, a similar sequence of events occurs. Typically, we take the aortopulmonary window lymph nodes, resecting all of the mediastinal tissue anterior and posterior to the phrenic nerve at that location.
  - ▲ After this is completed, the first one to two branches of the pulmonary artery to the left upper lobe are exposed and then divided. As for the right upper lobe, the vascular endostapler is brought in from the posterior inferior thoracoport site.
  - ▲ After division of the pulmonary artery branches, the superior pulmonary vein can be better dissected circumferentially. A heavy silk is passed around the superior pulmonary vein and divided in a similar fashion as were those in the right upper lobectomy. The adjacent hilar lymphatic tissue is then dissected to expose the left mainstem bronchus and the bifurcation between the upper and lower lobes. Dissection of the left upper lobe airway can be confirmed by identifying the pulmonary artery immediately behind it and continuing the dissection around the bifurcation.
  - ▲ The left upper lobe bronchus is then dissected away from the main pulmonary artery and a silk passed around the left upper lobe bronchus; it is divided with a 3.5- to 4.8-mm stapler brought in through the posterior inferior thoracoport. The Landreneau clamp is then repositioned to grasp the left upper lobe bronchus on the specimen side or the tissue adjacent to it, exposing the two to four pulmonary artery branches to the left upper lobe. Then, using an endostapler through the posterior inferior thoracoport, these are divided either as a group or individually. The fissure is divided with an endostapler. The remaining portion of the procedure is performed as with the right upper lobectomy.

- The right and left lower lobectomies are performed in similar fashion. The videoport site should be as low as possible to the lateral posterior reflection of the diaphragm from the chest wall and the two robotic arms placed fairly low and wide to achieve maximal function. The robotic chassis is brought in anteriorly and superiorly in an oblique fashion to the patient, as previously described.

▲ The Landreneau is placed through the anterior superior or posterior superior thoracoport and used to grasp the lung parenchyma low and close to the inferior pulmonary ligament origin at the lower lobe. The inferior hilum and inferior pulmonary ligament are widely resected with the specimen, including the pericardial and periesophageal lymph nodes. The dissection is continued posteriorly taking all the adjacent nodal tissue, exposing the posterior aspect of the inferior pulmonary vein and the adjacent bronchus.

▲ The inferior pulmonary vein is divided using an endostapler brought in through the anterior inferior thoracoport site. Then a plane is created between the bronchus and the pulmonary artery. For the left lower lobe, the bronchus can be fairly easily divided at the bifurcation between the upper and lower lobe once the bifurcation is identified by the pulmonary artery to the lower lobes sitting at the origin of the bifurcation.

▲ For the right lower lobe bronchial division, the right middle lobe can be obstructed if the angle of the superior segment from the basilar segments does not have sufficient distance from the staple line. In that case, where there is concern of obstructing a close right middle lobe, the superior segment can be divided separately from the basilar segment bronchus. Then the pulmonary artery to the lower lobe is divided using a vascular endostapler. The remainder of the procedure is performed as with the other lobectomies.

4. Closing

◆ With the lobe in an endobag pulled up snugly into the anterior port site, the robotic instruments are removed and the robot undocked and pushed away from the patient.

◆ As necessary, the anterior superior port site with the endobagged specimen in it is extended slightly and the endobag is pulled out of the site. Prior electrocautery incision of the intercostal parietal pleura, widely extending the intrathoracic portion of the anterior-superior thoracoport site, will allow much easier removal of the bagged specimen.

◆ Once the specimen is out of the chest, it is examined and nodal groups are resected from it, and the specimen is marked for the pathologists. It is then sent for frozen section to check the margins for microscopic disease.

◆ In the meantime, a long biopsy needle is used to inject the intercostal nerves from T2 to T10 with bupivacaine and epinephrine.

◆ Typically we use a single 19 French Blake drain through one of the port sites and guided to the apex. The lung is then reinflated under direct vision.

◆ The wounds are then closed with Vicryl sutures and Tegaderm dressings are applied.

Step 4. Postoperative Care

◆ Many of our patients are fully functional within a few hours of surgery and can ambulate.

◆ We reserve the diet until the next morning, as aspiration is common after intubation with a double-lumen endotracheal tube and after general anesthesia in older patients.

◆ We maintain a fluid restriction of less than 1500 mL daily until discharge.

◆ The patients are placed on telemetry until discharge.

◆ We minimize narcotics and encourage the use of acetaminophen and nonsteroidal anti-inflammatory drugs.

◆ The chest drain can be removed once the output is 400 mL or less and there is no air leak. If there is an air leak after the placement of a Blake drain, a connector to the drain can be attached to a chest drainage system.

Step 5. Pearls and Pitfalls

- ◆ The same and potentially greater rigor of dissection can be performed using the robotic approach.
- ◆ Careful placement of the thoracoports and preoperative planning can significantly reduce operative time.
- ◆ Lesions that are peripheral and smaller than 3 to 4 cm in diameter can be better approached using this technique. Larger and more central lesions can be resected with greater experience.
- ◆ The endobag should be very sturdy.

References

1. Ludwig MS, Goodman M, Miller DL, et al. Postoperative survival and the number of lymph nodes sampled during resection of node-negative non–small cell lung cancer. Chest 2005;128:1545-1550.
2. Robinson LA, Ruckdeschel JC, Wagner H Jr, et al. Treatment of non–small cell lung cancer—stage IIIA: ACCP evidence-based clinical practice guidelines (2nd edition). Chest 2007;132:243S-265S.
3. Ou SH, Zell JA. Prognostic significance of the number of lymph nodes removed at lobectomy in stage IA non–small cell lung cancer. J Thorac Oncol 2008;3:880-886.
4. Manser R, Wright G, Hart D, et al. Surgery for early stage non–small cell lung cancer. Cochrane Database Syst Rev 2005:CD004699.
5. Balderson SS, D'Amico T. Thoracoscopic lobectomy for the management of non–small cell lung cancer. Curr Oncol Rep 2008;10:283-286.
6. Swanson SJ, Herndon JE 2nd, D'Amico TA, et al. Video-assisted thoracic surgery lobectomy: Report of CALGB 39802—a prospective, multi-institution feasibility study. J Clin Oncol 2007;25:4993-4997.
7. Cheng D, Downey R, Kernstine K, et al. Video-assisted thoracic surgery in lung cancer resection, a meta-analysis and systematic review of controlled trials. Innovations 2007;2:261-292.
8. Park BJ, Flores RM, Rusch VW. Robotic assistance for video-assisted thoracic surgical lobectomy: Technique and initial results. J Thorac Cardiovasc Surg 2006;131:54-59.
9. Gharagozloo F, Margolis M, Tempesta B. Robot-assisted thoracoscopic lobectomy for early-stage lung cancer. Ann Thorac Surg 2008;85:1880-1885; discussion 1885-1886.
10. Anderson CA, Falabella A, Lau CS, et al. Robotic-assisted lung resection for malignant disease. Innovations 2007;2:254-258.

CHAPTER 6

ANATOMIC SEGMENTECTOMY

Brian L. Pettiford and Rodney J. Landreneau

The widespread use of high-resolution chest computed tomography (CT) has led to more frequent identification of small malignant pulmonary nodules. As the population ages, small peripheral lung cancers are frequently diagnosed in older patients with significant cardiopulmonary co-morbidities. Although sublobar resection has historically been reserved for patients with inflammatory or infectious disease states, such as bronchiectasis and tuberculosis, there has been a resurgent interest in its role for treating primary lung cancer patients with compromised cardiopulmonary function. Sublobar resection is also useful for the management of isolated pulmonary metastases such as occurs in sarcoma or colon cancer.

Anatomic segmentectomy is defined as the resection of a discrete portion of pulmonary parenchyma served by a specific segmental bronchovascular unit. Anatomic segmentectomy was proposed as a treatment of primary lung cancer in a review of 125 such procedures performed over a 12-year period. A 5-year actuarial survival rate of 56% was reported. These findings led to a debate regarding the utility of anatomic segmentectomy in treating lung cancer. The most widely accepted recommendations regarding the treatment of early-stage lung cancer came from the Lung Cancer Study Group, which reported higher local recurrence rates associated with sublobar resection. Landreneau and colleagues duplicated these results 2 years later. Despite a wide acceptance of lobectomy over sublobar resection, anatomic segmentectomy has become more common as a result of aggressive CT screening programs in Japan and the increased use of CT in the United States. Some series have reported 5-year survival and local recurrence rates similar to that of lobectomy.

Step 1. Surgical Anatomy

- Anatomic segmentectomy requires a thorough knowledge of the three-dimensional segmental bronchovascular relationships. During right upper lobe resections, the segmental vein is divided along the anterior hilum. The right upper lobe bronchus and its segmental branches are the most superior and posterior hilar structures. The segmental bronchus usually lies immediately posterior to the corresponding artery. The superior segmental artery lies opposite the middle lobe artery on the right and the lingular artery on the left. The inferior pulmonary vein subdivides into a basilar and superior segmental tributary. This arrangement should be considered when performing a lower lobe segmental resection because sacrifice of the entire inferior pulmonary vein will preclude anatomic segmentectomy.
- The left upper lobe vascular anatomy is the most variable of all lobes relative to size and number of segmental arteries. Although the left upper lobe segmental arterial branches are

the most superior hilar structures, their exposure is facilitated by upper lobe vein division. The lingular artery may arise as a single large vessel or, more commonly, as two medium-sized trunks. Nodal tissue is often interposed at bifurcation points at the segmental level. Careful nodal resection often reveals adjacent segmental arteries and bronchi.

Step 2. Preoperative Considerations

- The preoperative workup for patients undergoing anatomic segmentectomy mirrors that of patients undergoing lobectomy.
- High-resolution chest CT provides the target lesion size and location, which indicates resectability. CT and positron emission tomography scanning may be used to determine the need for mediastinoscopy to aid in pathologic staging.
- Patients with abnormal pulmonary function testing may require quantitative ventilation/perfusion scanning or exercise testing. Stress echocardiogram testing may identify patients with significant cardiac ischemia or ventricular dysfunction.

Step 3. Operative Steps

- Perioperative management includes flexible bronchoscopy to rule out endobronchial abnormalities and to confirm double-lumen tube or bronchial-blocker positioning. Patients are positioned in a semilateral decubitus position for vertical axillary thoracotomy and thoracoscopy.
- The target lesion location determines incision placement during thoracotomy. Upper and middle lesions require a muscle-sparing vertical axillary incision along the midaxilla beginning along the lower border of the hairline (Fig. 6-1, line A). The incision is placed along the midaxillary line beginning inferior to the hairline. The serratus anterior muscle fibers overlying the third rib are divided along the rib long axis. The pectoralis minor is mobilized along the lateral edge and reflected medially. The third rib is resected subperiosteally and the posterolateral aspect of the fourth rib is bivalved. The chest is entered through the third interspace.
- Lower lobe lesions are approached by placing the incision along the posterior axillary line beginning approximately 3 to 4 cm below the axilla, just anterior to the medial edge of the latissimus dorsi muscle (see Fig. 6-1, line B). The latissimus is reflected posteriorly, and the fatty avascular plane along the medial edge of the serratus anterior muscle is identified. The serratus is divided along the inferior margin of the wound in a radial fashion. The chest is entered through the fourth interspace. Transverse incision can also be used.
- Incision placement for thoracoscopic sublobar resection requires three port sites and one utility incision (Fig. 6-2). The camera port (B) is placed in the midclavicular line at the sixth or seventh interspace. A retraction port (D) is inserted along the posterior clavicular line, fourth interspace. Stapler passage through this port avoids excessive torque during vascular division. A vertical dissection port (C) is made in the midclavicular line, second interspace. The 3- to 4-cm utility incision (A) is made along the anterior axillary line fourth interspace. The vertical dissection port or utility incision may be extended to convert to a vertical axillary thoracotomy or lateral thoracotomy, respectively. Exposure can be improved by partial rib removal. Proper stapler application is facilitated by making a 1.5-cm "accessory" port-site incision through the sixth interspace along the posterior axillary line.

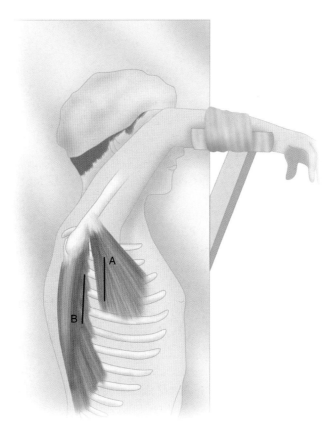

Figure 6-1

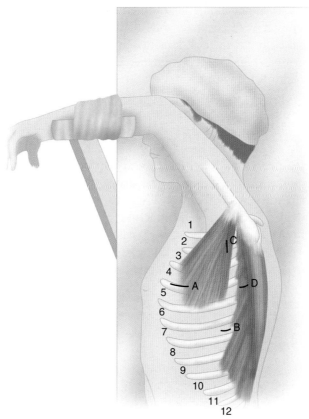

Figure 6-2

- With the exception of superior segmentectomy, the dissection commences along the anterior hilum. We favor stapling for fissure dissection over cautery or blunt dissection along a poorly developed fissure to minimize intraoperative hemorrhage and postoperative air leak. Bronchovascular dissection and division are facilitated by 0-silk placement around the structures and retraction to facilitate stapler application.
- The apical and posterior segments of the right upper lobe may be resected singly or together. The apical segmental vein is divided in the anterior hilum, exposing the upper lobe branch of the right pulmonary artery. The anterior segmental artery is spared along the truncus anterior as the apical segmental branch is divided. The apical segmental bronchus can be divided by a posterior hilar dissection (Fig. 6-3).
- The posterior segmental artery can be approached by exposing the interlobar pulmonary artery at the confluence of the horizontal and oblique fissures. An alternative method is to divide the posterior segmental bronchus from a posterior hilar approach. The segmental artery lies immediately anterior to the bronchus and may then be divided. Parenchymal division is then accomplished using a 45- or 60-mm endostapler with a 3.5-mm staple height. The specimen side of the divided bronchus is used as a reference point during parenchymal division (Fig. 6-4).
- Right upper lobe anterior segmentectomy is perhaps the most technically challenging of all forms of anatomic sublobar resection. The anterior segmental vein is divided along the anterior hilum. The anterior segmental artery is then isolated, taking care to avoid injury to the apical segmental branch or the truncus anterior (Fig. 6-5).
- The anterior segmental bronchus lies immediately posterior to the segmental artery and can be isolated and divided (Fig. 6-6). Parenchymal division requires division of the horizontal fissure, which is incomplete in approximately 90% of individuals. The right lower lobe superior segment can be approached by identifying the interlobar pulmonary artery and completing the oblique fissure posteriorly. The superior segmental arterial branch is seen opposite the posterior segmental branch to the upper lobe (see Fig. 6-6). The artery is divided between ties or with an endostapler. The superior segmental bronchus lies posterior to the artery. Following bronchial division, the parenchyma is divided using an endostapler, which decreases air-leak volume and duration. An increased incidence of airspace problems secondary to lung deformation has not been observed using this approach. Prior reports on segmentectomy advocate so-called finger fracture along the intersegmental plane during segmental parenchymal division; however, we make no attempt to identify the intersegmental vein during this phase. Alternatively, the bronchus can be divided along the posterior hilum, which exposes the corresponding artery located immediately anterior. Imprecise dissection around the bronchus from the posterior approach may result in arterial injury.

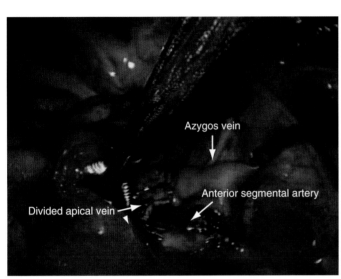

Figure 6-3
(From Pettiford BL, Schuchert MJ, Santos R, Landreneau RJ.
Role of sublobar resection [segmentectomy and wedge resection]
in the surgical management of non–small cell lung cancer.
Thorac Surg Clin 2007;17:175-190, with permission.)

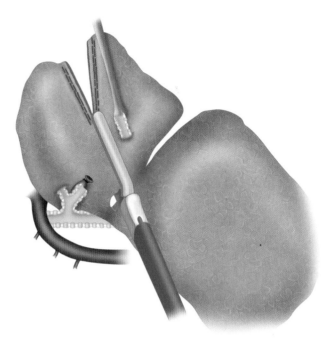

Figure 6-4

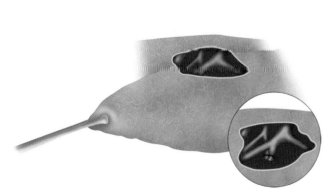

Figure 6-5

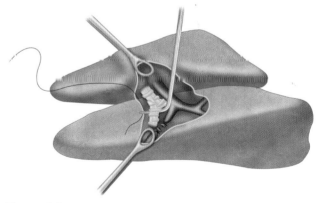

Figure 6-6

◆ Left upper division resection begins along the anterior hilum with division of the superior pulmonary venous drainage of the upper division (Fig. 6-7). The lingular branch is spared. Vein division exposes the underlying pulmonary artery. The anterior segmental branch is initially encountered and divided (Fig. 6-8). Exposure and ligation of the apical and posterior segmental branches are facilitated by division of the suprahilar tissues (Fig. 6-9). Complete upper division arterial ligation exposes the left upper lobe bronchus, which lies posterior to the interlobar artery. The upper division and lingular division bronchial branches are identified (Fig. 6-10). The upper division bronchus is divided using an endostapler with a 45-mm length and a 3.5-mm staple height (Fig. 6-11).

◆ Lingular arterial dissection may begin along the interlobar artery in patients with a well-developed fissure. Completion of the inferior aspect of the fissure identifies the "crotch" between the lingular and basilar segmental arteries (Fig. 6-12). Anterior retraction of the left upper lobe facilitates mobilization and division of the lingular segmental artery. The lingular bronchus is exposed within the fissure by gently retracting the interlobar pulmonary artery posteriorly. Removal of nodal tissue interposed between the lingular and upper division bronchi aid in exposing the lingular bronchus.

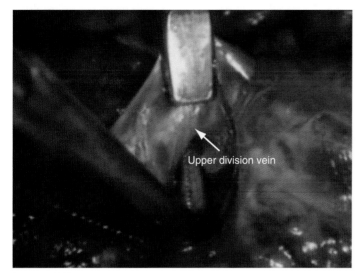

Figure 6-7

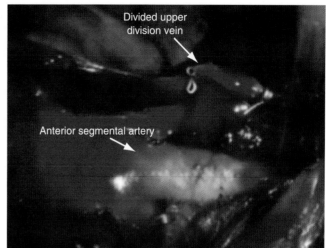

Figure 6-8

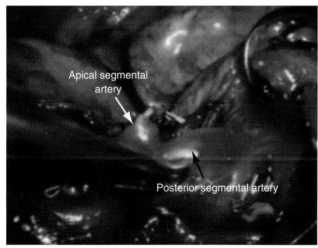

Figure 6-9

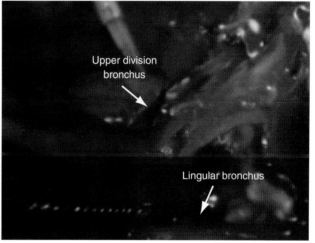

Figure 6-10

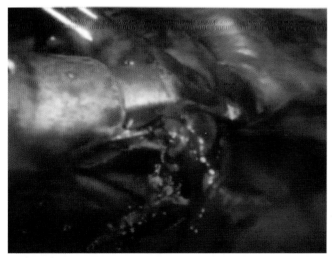

Figure 6-11

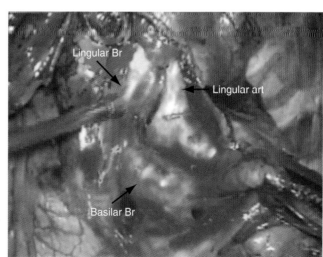

Figure 6-12

Step 4. Postoperative Care

- Postoperative patient management after segmentectomy is similar to that of patients undergoing lobectomy.
- Mediastinal lymph node sampling or dissection is performed when indicated following segmentectomy. The pleural space is usually drained by placing one chest tube through the accessory incision during thoracotomy or the camera port during thoracoscopy. When appropriate, patients are extubated in the operating room or in the intensive care/step-down unit.
- Patients are transferred to a step-down unit on postoperative day 1. Cardiac monitoring, radial artery pressure measurement, and continuous plethysmography are standard. Calcium-channel blockers and amiodarone are frequently used to treat atrial arrhythmias given the relatively high incidence of chronic obstructive pulmonary disease (COPD) and risk of bronchospasm. β-Blockers are administered if the patient has a history of β-blocker use. Pain control includes catheter-based intercostal nerve block and patient-controlled analgesia. Intravenous nonsteroidals, such as ketorolac tromethamine (Toradol), are used primarily in young patients with refractory pain or when narcotic agents are poorly tolerated. We limit Toradol use to 48 hours. Histamine$_2$ blockers are provided, and renal function is monitored closely when intravenous nonsteroidals are used. Chest tubes are removed when the 24-hour output is less than 150 mL and no air leak is present. The typical hospital stay is 3 to 5 days. Patients usually have follow-up about 3 weeks after discharge for wound check and plain-film reading. A chest CT is obtained at 3 months post resection.

Step 5. Pearls and Pitfalls

- Two rib spreaders may be inserted at right angles to maximize exposure during vertical axillary thoracotomy. Exposure can be augmented by partial third-rib resection for upper lobectomy and fourth-rib resection for lower lobectomy.
- Camera port placement during thoracoscopic segmentectomy should be placed no lower than the sixth interspace in morbidly obese patients to avoid poor visualization resulting from the relatively small intrathoracic volume.
- Early completion of the horizontal fissure can greatly facilitate exposure of the anterior segmental bronchovascular supply. The entire dissection must be performed along the anterior hilum.
- Division of the suprahilar tissue during thoracoscopic left upper division resection facilitates safe stapler application for division of the apical and posterior segmental arteries.
- Cephalad traction during upper division resection and lingulectomy improves visualization of the corresponding arteries and bronchi.
- Excision of periarterial and peribronchial lymph nodes facilitates stapler application.
- In patients with a poorly developed fissure, dissection should begin along the anterior hilum. This avoids the prolonged air leak associated with exploring the fissure.

- The right upper lobe posterior segmental artery may arise from the superior segmental artery in a small number of patients. Completion of the posterior aspect of the oblique fissure during superior segmentectomy may risk injury to the posterior segmental artery.
- Imprecise dissection anterior to the posterior segmental or superior segmental bronchi from the posterior hilum risks injury to the corresponding artery, which lies immediately anterior to its bronchus.
- The posterior segmental vein is at great risk of perforation when encircling the anterior segmental bronchus. The dissection must be limited to the bronchial wall to minimize this complication. Venous injury will require a posterior segmentectomy or complete lobectomy if the hemorrhage is poorly controlled.
- The apical and anterior segmental arteries should be identified to avoid sacrifice of the anterior segmental branch during apical segmentectomy.
- The stapler may "catch" along the port site and then release with subsequent impalement or avulsion of the pulmonary artery or its branches. This can be avoided by passing the endostapler beyond the target, opening the jaws, and then engaging the target bronchus or artery.
- Use of an "insulated" Bovie catheter extension is recommended during thoracoscopic dissection. Use of a "bare" catheter extension can result in thermal injury to adjacent structures.

Suggested Readings

Birdas TJ, Koehler RP, Colonias A, et al. Sublobar resection with brachytherapy versus lobectomy for stage Ib non–small cell lung cancer. Ann Thorac Surg 2006;81:434-438.

Ginsberg RJ, Burbinstein LV, for the Lung Cancer Study Group. Randomized trial of lobectomy vs. limited resection for T1N0 non–small cell lung cancer. Ann Thorac Surg 1995;60:615-623.

Harada H, Okada M, Sakamoto T, et al. Functional advantage after radical segmentectomy versus lobectomy for lung cancer. Ann Thorac Surg 2005;80:2041-2045.

Jensik RJ, Faber LP, Milloy FJ, Monson DO. Segmental resection for a lung cancer: A fifteen year experience. J Thorac Cardiovasc Surg 1973;66:563-572.

Landreneau RJ, Sugarbaker DJ, Mack MJ, et al. Wedge resection versus lobectomy for stage I (T1N0M0) non–small cell lung cancer. J Thorac Cardiovasc Surg 1997;113:691-700.

Okada M, Yoshikawa K, Hatta T, Tsubota N. Is segmentectomy with lymph node assessment an alternative to lobectomy for non–small cell lung cancer of 2 cm or smaller? Ann Thorac Surg 2001;71:956-961.

Pettiford BL, Schuchert MJ, Santos R, Landreneau RJ. Role of sublobar resection (segmentectomy and wedge resection) in the surgical management of non–small cell lung cancer. Thorac Surg Clin 2007;17:175-190.

Schuchert MJ, Pettiford BL, Keeley S, et al. Anatomic segmentectomy in the treatment of stage I non–small cell lung cancer (NSCLC). Ann Thorac Surg 2007;84:926-932; discussion 932-933.

Yoshikawa K, Tsubota N, Kodama K, et al. Prospective study of extended segmentectomy for small lung tumors: The final report. Ann Thorac Surg 2002;73:1055-1059.

CHAPTER 7

CARINAL RESECTIONS

David J. Finley and Valerie Rusch

Step 1. Surgical Anatomy

- Tracheal blood supply is segmental, requiring minimal circumferential dissection to reduce the risk of anastomotic strictures and dehiscence (Fig. 7-1).
- Detailed understanding of the surrounding vital structures is imperative for safe carinal resections (Fig. 7-2). The superior vena cava, vagus nerve, azygos vein, esophagus, and innominate artery are all adjacent to the trachea on the right. On the left, the recurrent laryngeal nerve and aortic arch are the two main structures within the dissection field.

Step 2. Preoperative Considerations

- The pulmonary and cardiac fitness of the patient must be determined. Complete pulmonary function tests, and possibly ventilation and perfusion scans, are necessary to determine whether the patient will tolerate the procedure and potential pulmonary parenchymal resection. It is prudent to obtain cardiac imaging (echocardiography, sestamibi and thallium stress tests, technetium-99m sestamibi [MIBI] scans, or stress echocardiography) for the older patient who may have co-morbid conditions.
- Computed tomography scan of the chest (with three-dimensional reconstruction if available) is obtained to delineate the extent of disease and help determine the type of resection required (carinal with or without pulmonary resection), the length of tracheal resection, and adjacent structures that might be involved.
- Positron emission tomography imaging should be used to determine whether extrathoracic disease is present, which would preclude the patient from being a surgical candidate.
- Epidural anesthesia for intraoperative and postoperative pain management may reduce postoperative pulmonary complications.
- The approach to the intraoperative management of the airway should be discussed between the anesthesiologist and the surgeon.
- Most carinal resections are best approached via a right posterolateral thoracotomy. A left posterolateral thoracotomy facilitates left pulmonary parenchymal resections. With disease that crosses the midline, a clamshell incision (bilateral anterior thoracotomies with transverse sternotomy) may be useful. Limited carinal resections can be performed via a median sternotomy.
- Bronchoscopy must be performed before resection to confirm location and extent of tumor.

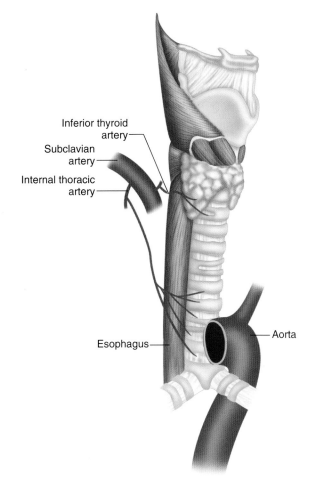

Figure 7-1

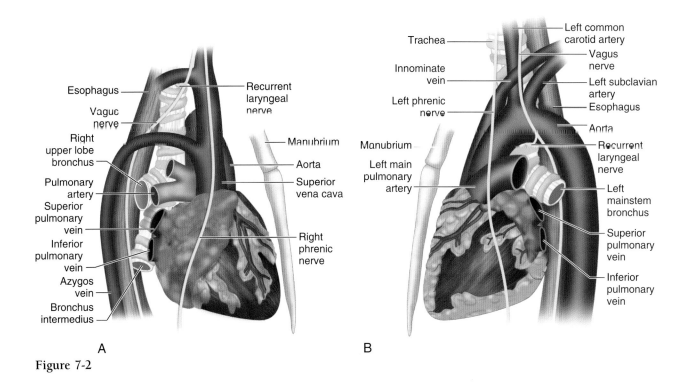

A

B

Figure 7-2

1. Incision

♦ Depending on the type of resection required, the patient may be in left lateral decubitus, right lateral decubitus, or supine position.
♦ A standard right posterolateral thoracotomy is performed, sparing the serratus anterior. Entry through the fourth interspace allows for exposure of the distal trachea and carina. Care should be taken to preserve the intercostal muscle to use as a muscle flap to protect the anastomosis.
♦ A clamshell incision, through either the third or fourth interspace, allows for the best exposure when performing a left carinal pneumonectomy. The incision should follow the inframammary folds and peak at the level of fourth interspace across the sternum.

2. Airway Management

♦ Single-lumen endotracheal intubation is performed using a full length endotracheal tube (ET), which is advanced into the left mainstem bronchus to isolate the right lung, if possible.
♦ Implement cross-field ventilation using sterile anesthesia tubing and a small-caliber re-reinforced ET (e.g., 6 French armored tube) into the left mainstem bronchus after transection and retraction of the ET tube.
♦ Complete resection of the carinal mass is undertaken. Anastomotic sutures are placed, moving the cross-field tube as necessary for exposure. Once complete, the ET tube is advanced back into the left mainstem bronchus.
♦ Alternatively, this may be accomplished with jet ventilation, using a small 8 French suction catheter for cross-field ventilation or advancing it through the retracted ET tube. The entire resection and anastomosis can be completed with minimal difficulty because the size of the jet ventilation catheter rarely interferes with your exposure (Fig. 7-3). Once complete, the ET tube is advanced below the anastomosis.

3. Simple Carinal Resection

♦ Tumor must involve less than a 1-cm section of the trachea, right mainstem bronchus, and left mainstem bronchus.
♦ Minimal lateral dissection of the trachea is undertaken. The azygos vein is transected, the pleura incised, and the anterior pretracheal fascial plane dissected to mobilize the proximal trachea. The lung is retracted anteriorly for exposure (Fig. 7-4). The subcarinal lymph nodes are excised. Circumferential dissection is required only at the level of the carina, with special care taken to identify and preserve the left recurrent laryngeal nerve. After lateral traction sutures are placed, the left mainstem bronchus distal to the lesion is transected. Margins should be assessed by frozen section.

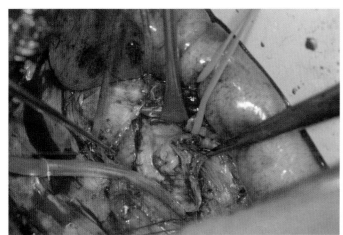

Figure 7-3

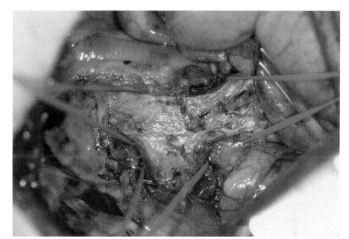

Figure 7-4

◆ A double-barrel anastomosis is often difficult to perform because of tension. Interrupted 3-0 polyglactin (Vicryl, Ethicon Inc., Somerville, NJ) or polydioxanone (PDS, Ethicon Inc.) sutures are placed between the left and right mainstem bronchus through the tracheal rings, recreating a carina. This so-called double barrel is then sutured to the distal trachea in an interrupted fashion with 3-0 or 4-0 suture, with the knots on the outside of the anastomosis (Fig. 7-5). A running 4-0 PDS suture can be used to approximate the posterior membranous wall, carefully avoiding tearing of this delicate tissue. A vascularized flap (intercostal muscle or pericardial fat pad) should be used to bolster the anastomosis, tacking the pedicle at numerous points around the anastomosis with partial-thickness bites into the wall of the airway.

4. Extended Carinal Resection

◆ This type of resection is required for most carinal tumors. The anastomosis can be completed in two ways, depending on the length of distal trachea resected.
◆ Left end-to-end with right end-to-side anastomosis is selected when only a small amount of distal trachea is resected (Fig. 7-6A). The anastomosis is first completed between the left mainstem bronchus and trachea. Two traction sutures, usually 3-0 PDS, are positioned on the left and right lateral walls of the left mainstem bronchus and distal trachea, one ring away from the transected edges. Interrupted 3-0 or 4-0 PDS sutures (depending on the size of the bronchial wall) are placed starting along the left lateral wall, placing the stitch to allow the knot to be outside the lumen. The posterior membrane is closed in a running fashion with 4-0 PDS suture. After the traction sutures are tied, the remainder of the sutures are secured from left lateral to anterior and then right lateral. The posterior membrane suture should be tied at the left lateral end and left loose until all the other anastomotic sutures are tied down.

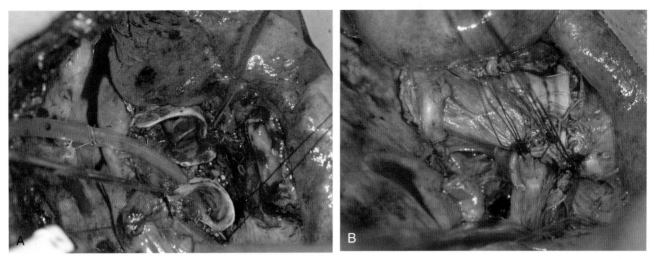

Figure 7-5

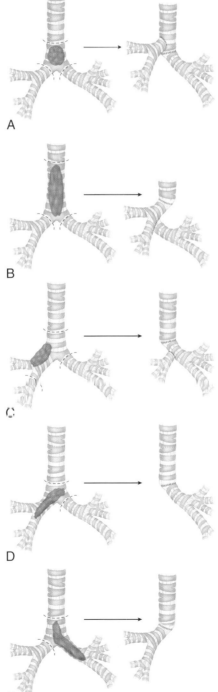

Figure 7-6

Finally, this suture is gently tightened and tied in place. One centimeter proximal to this anastomosis, an oval section of trachea is resected in the right lateral wall, completely within the cartilaginous rings. The right mainstem bronchus is then positioned over this opening, which may require a hilar release maneuver (transection of the inferior pulmonary ligament with circumferential opening of the pericardium around the pulmonary hilum; Fig. 7-7). Interrupted 3-0 or 4-0 sutures are used to complete this anastomosis as described earlier.

- When a significant portion of the distal trachea or left mainstem bronchus is resected, a right end-to-end with left end-to-side anastomosis is required. A hilar release maneuver is necessary to provide a tension-free anastomosis. The right mainstem bronchus is sutured to the distal trachea while cross-field ventilation to the left lung is performed. An oval orifice is created in the bronchus intermedius; the opening should be as long as the bronchus is wide. The anteroposterior diameter should be slightly smaller than the left mainstem bronchus, keeping the opening completely within the cartilaginous wall (see Fig. 7-6B).

5. Carinal Resection with Pulmonary Resection

- The tumor location may require resection of pulmonary parenchyma in addition to a tracheal and bronchial resection. This is usually seen with a right upper lobe tumor. Rarely is a carinal resection required for a similar tumor on the left given the length of the mainstem bronchus. Occasionally a carinal pneumonectomy is required to achieve adequate bronchial margins.
- These resections are approached via a right posterolateral thoracotomy. However, a left carinal pneumonectomy is best approached from the left.
- For a right upper lobectomy with carinal resection, hilar dissection and isolation of the vasculature are accomplished, confirming no involvement with tumor. The trachea and left mainstem bronchus are exposed to just beyond the tumor. Pulmonary artery and vein are ligated and transected. The bronchus intermedius is transected just distal to the right upper lobe orifice, ensuring adequate margins. If tumor extends to the middle lobe bronchus, sparing of the lower lobe is usually not possible. The trachea and left main bronchus are transected with small margins. An end-to-end anastomosis is completed between the trachea and left mainstem bronchus while ventilating only the left lung. Intrapericardial hilar release is required before an end-to-side bronchus intermedius to left mainstem bronchus anastomosis (see Fig. 7-6C). A vascular pedicle flap (intercostal muscle, pericardial fat pad, pleural flap) should be placed around both anastomoses.
- A right carinal pneumonectomy is simpler to perform because only an end-to-end anastomosis is required (see Fig. 7-6D). Care must be taken not to resect too much of the trachea or left mainstem bronchus; only a 4-cm distance can be bridged without undue tension when performing anastomosis of the left mainstem to the trachea.
- A left carinal pneumonectomy can be performed using a left thoracotomy, although access to the carina is limited by the aortic arch. Mobilization of the aorta, careful dissection of the recurrent laryngeal nerve with division of the vagus distal to the recurrent takeoff, transection of the ligamentum arteriosum, and cervical flexion can achieve adequate exposure (Fig. 7-8). Dissection of the carina, distal trachea, right mainstem bronchus, and pretracheal plane to determine resectability is mandatory before taking the hilar vessels. Traction sutures are placed on the trachea and right mainstem bronchus distal to the resection margin. The right mainstem is transected first to allow for cross-field ventilation of the right lung. Hilar structures are divided and the trachea is transected. Intermittent retraction of the aorta is required while placing anastomotic sutures. Once complete, the cross-field ventilation is removed, the ET is advanced into the right mainstem, and the traction sutures are tied before the remainder of the sutures (see Fig. 7-6E).

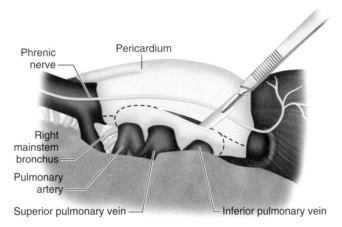

Phrenic nerve

Pericardium

Right mainstem bronchus

Pulmonary artery

Superior pulmonary vein

Inferior pulmonary vein

Figure 7-7

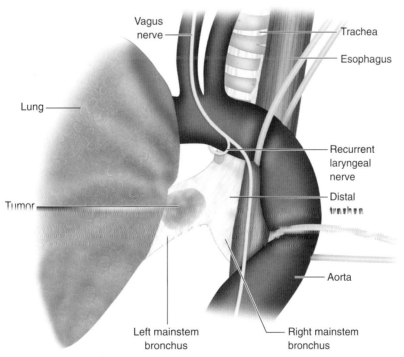

Vagus nerve

Trachea

Esophagus

Lung

Recurrent laryngeal nerve

Tumor

Distal trachea

Aorta

Left mainstem bronchus

Right mainstem bronchus

Figure 7-8

6. Carinal Resection for Recurrence or Stenosis

- Similar to a standard carinal resection, a recurrence after a left carinal pneumonectomy should be approached from the right. This allows for right hilar release and provides better exposure to the distal trachea. Hand or jet ventilation, along with gentle retraction of the lung, is necessary during dissection. Care must be taken to avoid injury to the left pulmonary artery while exposing the area for resection. Anastomosis is performed in the standard fashion.
- After a right carinal pneumonectomy, a short-segment resection can be undertaken via a right thoracotomy. This may be difficult to accomplish without tension on the new anastomosis with the inability to mobilize the left side.

Step 4. Postoperative Care

- Flexible bronchoscopy on completion of the resection is performed on all patients to assess the anastomosis as well as to suction out any secretions.
- Immediate extubation following carinal resection is feasible and desirable. Positive pressure ventilation will place more stress on a fresh anastomosis, and rigorous pulmonary physiotherapy cannot be accomplished in an intubated patient.
- Sometimes extubation is not possible, and in those situations, the ET should be placed away from the anastomosis with minimal air in the ET tube cuff. Flexible bronchoscopy should be performed to confirm position of the tube. If possible, the patient should be spontaneously breathing. As soon as it is safe, the patient should be extubated.
- Care in the intensive care unit is necessary for 24 to 48 hours after resection, providing a skilled nursing staff who understands the problems and complications associated with carinal resections. Humidified air, along with intensive chest physiotherapy, is instituted immediately. Airway problems arise quickly and must be urgently assessed and treated, including emergent intubation. Bronchoscopy is performed on patients with a change in respiratory status (wheezing, rhonchi) who are unable to clear secretions or when parenchymal collapse is noted on radiography.
- On completion of the resection, a heavy-gauge suture is placed to maintain slight neck flexion and to reduce any risk of hyperextension and anastomotic disruption (Fig. 7-9) This chin stitch remains in place for 5 to 7 days.

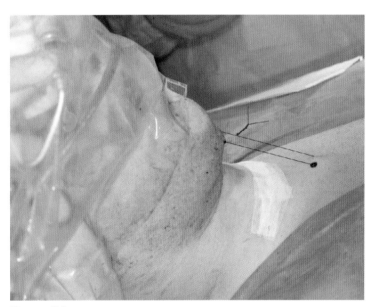

Figure 7-9

Step 5. Pearls and Pitfalls

- ◆ Tracheal blood supply is segmental and tenuous. Meticulous surgical technique, along with limiting circumferential dissection, will reduce the risk of ischemia at the anastomosis, resulting in fewer anastomotic complications, including dehiscence and stricture.
- ◆ Anastomotic tension will often lead to potentially life-threatening complications. No more than 4 cm can separate the left mainstem bronchus from the distal trachea after resection. Hilar release maneuvers, dissection of the pretracheal plane, and neck flexion will all help to reduce tension at the anastomosis but cannot replace appropriate preoperative or intra-operative decisions about the amount of trachea that can be resected safely. Especially with adenoid cystic carcinoma, it is better to have a positive margin and a tension-free anastomosis than a negative margin and a complication.
- ◆ Aggressive chest physiotherapy, early ambulation, and adequate pain control will minimize postoperative pulmonary complications—but not completely. Therefore, early bronchoscopy in patients with poor cough, inability to clear secretions, or changes in respiratory status will reduce the risk of reintubation and further complications in this group of patients.

Acknowledgment

The authors are grateful to Dr. Raja Flores for providing the intraoperative photos.

Suggested Readings

Dartevelle P, Macchiarini P. Carinal resection for bronchogenic cancer. Semin Thorac Cardiovasc Surg 1996;8:414-425.

de Perrot M, Fadel E, Mercier O, et al. Long-term results after carinal resection for carcinoma: Does the benefit warrant the risk? J Thorac Cardiovasc Surg 2006;131:81-89.

Macchiarini P, Altmayer M, Go T, et al. Technical innovations of carinal resection for non–small-cell lung cancer. Ann Thorac Surg 2006;82:1989-1997.

Mathisen DJ. Carinal reconstruction: Techniques and problems. Semin Thoracic Cardiovasc Surg 1996;8:403-413.

Mitchell JD, Mathisen DJ, Wright CD, et al. Clinical experience with carinal resection. J Thorac Cardiovasc Surg 1999;117:39-52.

Rea F, Marulli G, Schiavon M, et al. Tracheal sleeve pneumonectomy for non small cell lung cancer (NSCLC): Short and long-term results in a single institution. Lung Cancer 2008;61:202-208.

Regnard J-F, Perrotin C, Giovannetti R, et al. Resection for tumors with carinal involvement: Technical aspects, results, and prognostic factors. Ann Thorac Surg 2005;80:1841-1846.

Roviaro G, Vergani C, Maciocco M, et al. Tracheal sleeve pneumonectomy: Long-term outcome. Lung Cancer 2006;52:105-110.

Yamamoto K, Miyamoto Y, Ohsumi A, et al. Results of surgical resection for tracheobronchial cancer involving the tracheal carina. Gen Thorac Cardiovasc Surg 2007;55:231-239.

Yamamoto K, Miyamoto Y, Ohsumi A, et al. Surgical results of carinal reconstruction: An alternative technique for tumors involving the tracheal carina. Ann Thoracic Surg 2007;84:216-220.

CHAPTER 8

BRONCHIAL AND PULMONARY ARTERIAL SLEEVE RESECTION

Philippe G. Dartevelle and Bedrettin Yıldızeli

Surgeons began to develop an interest in preserving normal lung in an era when many parenchymal resections were done for tuberculosis (TB) or bronchiectasis and the complications and functional limitations of pneumonectomy became known. In 1947, Sir Clement Price Thomas gave a detailed account of sleeve lobectomy and the clinical observations that led to its development. The first sleeve lobectomy was done in 1947 for a "bronchial adenoma" of the right upper lobe in a Royal Air Force cadet. The patient went on to active flying duty, a status he could not have achieved had pneumonectomy been performed. In 1956, Allison reported the first case of bronchogenic carcinoma treated by right upper lobectomy sleeve resection of the right main bronchus as well as partial elliptical resection of the right main pulmonary artery (PA). By 1959, Johnston and Jones had already collected a series of 98 sleeve lobectomies for bronchogenic carcinoma, with an operative mortality of 8%. The procedure was at first considered solely for patients who, for lack of cardiopulmonary reserve, could not undergo pneumonectomy. However, by 1970, most of the sleeve lobectomies that Paulson and colleagues performed for bronchogenic cancer were in candidates with adequate cardiopulmonary reserve rather than in compromised patients only. The concept of sleeve resection was also almost immediately applied to resections of the PA.

The intervening four decades have added validity to the oncologic value of sleeve lobectomy, provided our understanding of and improved the bronchial anastomosis to prevent fistula formation, extended the concept to more peripheral pulmonary units, and advanced the functional studies of the reimplanted lobe. Time has not changed the basic concept or the indications for this procedure. In this millennium, it is very well shown that sleeve lobectomy offers better long-term survival and quality of life than does pneumonectomy and is more cost effective. On the other hand, the techniques we use for sleeve lobectomy help us to perform easier anastomosis for lung transplantation.

Step 1. Surgical Anatomy

1. Tracheobronchial Tree

♦ The trachea originates below the cricoid cartilage and extends from front to back to the carina, which is located at about the level of the fourth thoracic vertebra. At that point, the trachea bifurcates into the right and left mainstem bronchi. The right main bronchus is in direct line with the trachea, and its length from carina to upper lobe takeoff varies between 1.5 and 2.0 cm. Distal to the right upper lobe bronchus, the primary bronchus becomes the bronchus intermedius, which is about 2 cm long.

- The middle lobe bronchus arises from the anterior surface of the bronchus intermedius, almost in direct line with the origin of the superior segmental bronchus of the lower lobe, which arises from the posterior wall of the bronchus intermedius.
- The left main bronchus arises from the carina at a more oblique angle than the right main bronchus. It is 4 to 6 cm long and passes under the aortic arch to lie posteriorly in the left hilum. It then bifurcates to form the upper and lower lobe bronchi. The lower lobe bronchus gives off its first segmental bronchus, the superior segmental bronchus, posteriorly 0.5 cm from the left upper lobe orifice. The distal bronchial section after left upper lobe sleeve resection is often dictated by the level of the orifice of the bronchus to the apical segment of the left lower lobe because of the absence of bronchus intermedius.
- Care must be taken to preserve the left recurrent laryngeal nerve during bronchoplasties involving the proximal left main bronchus. The left recurrent laryngeal nerve originates close to the ligamentum arteriosum, where it courses from front to back around the aorta before ascending in the neck in the tracheoesophageal groove.

2. Blood Supply and Innervation of the Lower Trachea and Bronchi

- Bronchial arteries mostly arise separately from the anterolateral aspect of the descending thoracic aorta or from intercostal arteries located within 2 to 3 cm distal to the left subclavian artery. Most commonly, there are three bronchial arteries, two on the left side and one on the right side. Therefore, the right main bronchus is more susceptible to ischemia than its left counterpart.
- The bronchial arteries circulate posteriorly to the airway, where they lie on the membranous portion of mainstem bronchi and where they eventually divide to supply lobar and segmental bronchi. On the right side, the single bronchial artery runs parallel to the azygos vein, by which it is overlapped. Another important feature of the bronchial circulation system is the rich anastomotic network interconnecting it with the pulmonary arterial circulation. This network is significant at the level of the lobar or segmental bronchi, and the pulmonary circulation may account for up to 75% to 90% of the airway blood supply.
- Most of the venous drainage from the bronchial arterial system empties into the pulmonary veins; the rest empties into the bronchial veins located around the segmental and subsegmental bronchi. These bronchial veins subsequently empty into the azygos and hemiazygos systems.

3. Pulmonary Arterial System

- The main PA originates in the pericardial sac from the right ventricle, and its axis is oriented in an anteroposterior direction, slightly upward and to the left. Below the aortic arch, it bifurcates into the right and the left branches.
- The right PA runs horizontally to the right, behind the ascending aorta and the superior vena cava (SVC) and in front of the carina. Lateral to the SVC, the right PA lies in front of the right main bronchus, and it almost immediately gives rise to its first branch, to the right upper lobe. Shortly thereafter, the vessel curves inferiorly between the bronchus intermedius

posteriorly and superior pulmonary vein anteriorly. Subsequently, the interlobar PA turns posteriorly behind the origin of the middle lobe bronchus. In this portion, one or two ascending arteries originate posterior to the segment of the upper lobe and the middle lobe artery. The middle lobe artery arises from the anteromedial surface of the interlobar artery, and the ascending arteries originate posteromedially at a slightly lower level. Distal to the latter is the origin of the artery to the apical segment of the lower lobe, and, subsequently, the PA branches into the arteries to the basal pyramid.

♦ The left PA is shorter than its right counterpart; at its origin is the ligamentum arteriosum, and its relationship with the aortic arch continues posteriorly. Because the left PA curves around 60% to 75% of the circumference of the origin of the upper lobe bronchus, left upper lobe sleeve resection combined with resection of the PA is the most common type of bronchovasculoplasty. In fact, the PA abuts the superior, posterior, and inferior aspects of the upper lobe bronchus, leaving its anterior surface in contact with the superior pulmonary vein. The first branches, the apical and the anterior segmental arteries, arise anteriorly and superiorly to the upper lobe bronchus and posteriorly and superiorly to the superior pulmonary vein. Throughout its course around the upper lobe bronchus, the interlobar PA delivers branches to the upper lobe that are highly variable in number and location and are usually surrounded by lymph nodes. The most distal of these branches is the lingular artery, which usually arises distally or at approximately the same level as the artery that leads to the superior segment of the lower lobe. The lingular artery arises from the anteromedial surface of the interlobar PA, and the superior segmental artery originates posterolaterally. The PA axis is then oriented anteriorly, and the vessel branches into the arteries to the basal segments.

Step 2. Preoperative Considerations

1. Indications

♦ The term *sleeve lobectomy* refers to resection of a circumferential sleeve of mainstem bronchus contiguous with a pulmonary lobe, whereas *bronchial sleeve resection* is used to describe excision of the airway with sparing of parenchyma. At first conceived for patients unable to tolerate pneumonectomy, sleeve lobectomy has rapidly become an option for patients suitable for the more radical procedure. The former group of patients has been termed *compromised,* whereas the latter group with adequate cardiopulmonary reserve is named *deliberate* or *elective.* Bronchoplastic procedures have been reported being performed on 3% to 13% of the patients diagnosed with a resectable pulmonary malignant tumor. It is important to point out that this increased rate of sleeve lobectomy is achieved at the expense of a decreased incidence of pneumonectomy and not of lobectomy while the oncologic results remain unchanged. The indication for a sleeve resection for lung cancer is well established (Table 8-1): a tumor arising at the origin of a lobar bronchus precluding simple lobectomy but not infiltrating as far as to require pneumonectomy. As a general rule, all lobes and even segments of the lung on occasion may be involved with tumors that are amenable to some form of lung-sparing bronchoplastic procedure. Oncologically, the primary goal of surgery is complete resection of lung cancer with adequate resection margins free of tumor. This is all the more true for carcinoid tumors or benign lesions. Evidence has been obtained that there is little, if any, gain in extending the resection as far as pneumonectomy. These considerations apply also to patients with nodal involvement limited to hilar lymph nodes (N1). Reconstructive surgery of the PA has exactly the same indications.

♦ When considering surgical options and prognosis, it is useful to distinguish four anatomic situations in two groups of patients. The first and classic anatomic situation is a tumor found on bronchoscopy to arise in a lobar bronchus so as to preclude standard lobectomy. The second situation is where a carcinoma extrinsic to the airway may extend to the lobar

TABLE 8-1.	Indications for Sleeve Lobectomy

Compromised patients unable to tolerate pneumonectomy

Pulmonary malignant tumor

A routine procedure for proximally located tumors

Carcinoid tumors or benign lesions

Pulmonary hypertension

Benign or low-grade malignant tumors of the airway

Inflammatory strictures

Posttraumatic bronchial disruptions

Treatment of bronchial complications

Re-sleeve resection

bronchus. In the third situation, the bronchial margin may be found on frozen section to contain tumor. Finally, the fourth is where a lymph node with metastasis may adhere to the confluence of lobar and main bronchus and thus dictate resection of a sleeve of airway. Conversely, a metastatic node without adherence to the bronchus is not currently considered an indication for sleeve lobectomy.

◆ The success of elective sleeve lobectomy and the prognosis of the individual patient seem to depend greatly on the intraoperative diligence of the surgeon in assessing the extent of disease.

◆ A variety of benign or low-grade malignant tumors of the airway may necessitate sleeve lobectomy by their location within the airway.

◆ Inflammatory strictures requiring resection of the lung and adjacent main bronchus are rare and are almost always caused by TB. Resection cannot be recommended in the presence of active TB or when active disease remains after resection. Bronchial disruptions rarely require sleeve lobectomy.

◆ Besides all the above indications, we also consider sleeve lobectomy for patients who have pulmonary hypertension demonstrated by either echocardiography or right-sided heart catheterization. Sleeve lobectomy may also be performed for patients who have bronchial complications following lung surgery. In fact, "re-sleeve resection" for stenosis after sleeve right upper lobectomy has been reported.

2. Preoperative Evaluation

- Patients must be screened from a medical standpoint to be certain that they can tolerate thoracotomy.
- Physical examination, chest radiography, spirometry, arterial blood gases, and quantitative ventilation and perfusion scans are performed routinely to evaluate functional status. Patients at high risk for heart disease are screened by echocardiography, thallium stress testing, and, in some cases, selective coronary arteriography. Tumor spread to the airway may be evaluated by fiberoptic bronchoscopy, which plays a key role in selecting patients for sleeve lobectomy; patients who have submucosal invasion or extrinsic compression of a lobar orifice with a positive elective biopsy are good candidates for sleeve lobectomy. Mediastinal nodal status is investigated by computed tomography (CT) or positron emission tomography (PET) scan. In patients with non–small cell lung cancer (NSCLC), mediastinoscopy is usually performed when CT shows mediastinal nodes larger than 1.0 cm in diameter or when PET-CT scan shows mediastinal fixation; mediastinoscopy is not used in patients with carcinoid tumor. Investigations for extrathoracic metastases are performed routinely. The need for resection of the PA in carcinomas of the upper lobes is usually established at the time of thoracotomy; however, a pulmonary angiogram may be performed when the tumor is adherent to the main PA in a patient whose preoperative functional test results contraindicate pneumonectomy. In patients at high risk, a right-sided heart catheterization is performed before and after balloon occlusion of the relevant PA to detect pulmonary hypertension, precluding pneumonectomy.
- For patients who have tuberculous bronchostenosis, bronchoscopy is important to rule out active disease before a decision is made to perform resection. TB drug therapy is recommended for at least 6 months before resection, even when stenosis is thought to be due to TB.

Step 3. Operative Steps

- Certain principles are common to all bronchoplastic techniques. Single-lung ventilation is established through a double-lumen endotracheal tube (ET). A posterolateral thoracotomy is performed in the fifth intercostal space. On the right, for upper sleeve lobectomy, the arch of the azygos vein is divided, allowing excellent exposure of the main bronchus. No irreversible procedures are performed until resectability is confirmed. Delicacy in handling of tissues is imperative. Unnecessary dissection that may devascularize the bronchial blood supply is to be avoided. Clean, sharp lines of bronchial transection are important. Special concern should attend reoperation on a bronchus (as when prior lobectomy has been done) because previous dissection and scar can damage bronchial blood supply. Bronchial margins are examined microscopically intraoperatively to ensure the greatest chance for cure. Frozen sections are imperative. Once again, a balance must be struck between the need for clear surgical margins and concern about reconstructing the airway.
- A variety of suture materials have been used for bronchial anastomosis. Our preference has been 4-0 polydioxanone suture (PDS, Ethicon Inc., Somerville, NJ) for posterior anastomosis and 3-0 or 4-0 polyglactin suture (Vicryl, Ethicon) for anterior anastomosis. We also prefer using 2.5× magnification loupes with headlight. We also believe long (24-cm), heavy titanium Castro-Viejo needle holder (for PA sutures) and long (24-cm), fine-tooth forceps (for manipulating the bronchus) are necessary to perform an excellent sleeve lobectomy.
- Excessive tension is the enemy of successful bronchoplastic procedures. Resection of the entire left main bronchus, however, plus or minus the upper lobe, is likely to produce excessive tension. The same is true for the right main bronchus when the upper lobe and bronchus intermedius are included. When tension is a concern, division of the inferior pulmonary ligament and a U-shaped pericardial incision just below the inferior pulmonary vein will give added mobility to the bronchus.
- First, the lobar branches of the PA and the lobar vein are dissected to permit an assessment of tumor spread and resectability. Then, the lobar and main bronchi are dissected. Again, care is taken to preserve as much as possible of the bronchial vascular supply in the remaining lobes during mediastinal lymph node dissection. The hilar, carinal, paratracheal, esophageal, and inferior pulmonary ligament lymph nodes are routinely dissected. Circumferential bronchial resection is performed with a knife to obtain straight margins distant from the tumor (Fig. 8-1).

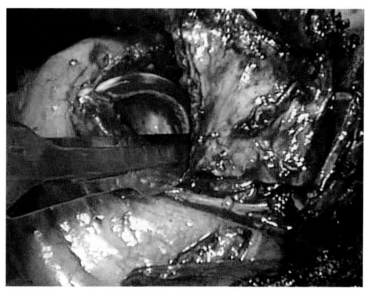

Figure 8-1

1. Anastomosis

- Although each surgeon has his or her surgical preference, open anastomotic technique is preferred, using a continuous suture for the posterior anastomosis and interrupted sutures for the anterior anastomosis, placed to allow the knots to be tied outside the bronchial lumen. Each suture is precisely placed through the full thickness of the bronchial wall, with minimal handling of the mucosa. Sutures are spaced proportionally with regard to different diameters of the two bronchial margins being approximated.

- The 4-0 PDS traction sutures placed in the midlateral wall of both ends of the airway allow for easy manipulation of the airway; assessment of tension; and, when tied together, reduction of tension on the individual anastomotic sutures. In most bronchoplasties, the length of resection is insufficient to produce significant anastomotic tension, so that traction sutures are chiefly for alignment. The traction sutures are placed full-thickness around a cartilaginous ring, at least one ring distant from the terminal ring where anastomotic sutures are placed. These sutures are used to test approximation of the two ends to determine whether any release maneuvers are necessary. For ease of identification, they are secured with clamps that are different from the clamps placed on the anastomotic sutures. Traction sutures should not be placed in the membranous wall because they may tear as they are tied.

- The first anastomotic suture is placed on the far (the deepest aspect, i.e., mediastinal) end of the cartilaginous portion for the back row (Fig. 8-2). The proximal part of this suture is secured with a clamp, and the anastomosis is started using a short, continuous running distal part of 4-0 PDS lying on one third of the cartilaginous airway wall. When the suture comes close to the second traction suture located on the pulmonary (distal) end of the cartilaginous portion, the suture is placed outside the lumen of the anastomosis. To complete the back row, the surgeon retracts each suture of the anastomosis with a nerve hook while the surgical assistant also retracts two traction sutures (Fig. 8-3). Initially, the mediastinal traction suture is tied extraluminally and also tied with the proximal end of the back row suture. Care must be taken to the alignment of the anastomosis. Then the pulmonary traction suture and the distal end of the 4-0 PDS are tied in the same fashion.

- When the back row has been completed (Fig. 8-4), the interrupted front-row sutures with 3-0 or 4-0 polyglactin are placed on the rest of the bronchial circumference and are left untied (Fig. 8-5). Each suture is secured with a clamp. The sutures are then tied, starting from either end of the cartilaginous portion and working toward the midline. The surgeon ties the suture on his or her side while the assistant approximates his or her side to relieve tension. The knots are placed outside the lumen. Placing and tying the sutures in this order allow compensation for even large-caliber discrepancies. This technique prevents torsion of the bronchial axis and gently stretches and dilates the circumference of the distal bronchus. The larger bronchial stump works as a stent, increasing the caliber of the anastomosis and minimizing secretion retention in the early postoperative course when edema at the site of the anastomosis is more likely to occur. The anastomosis is wrapped with a vascularized pedicle of autologous tissue, (i.e., mediastinal pleura, pericardial fat pad, or an intercostal muscle flap). After the last suture has been tied, the field is flooded with saline and the lung inflated to check for air leaks. The anastomosis should be airtight to a pressure of 35 to 40 cm of water. If any leaks are found, they must be repaired. The anastomosis is inspected with a flexible bronchoscope to identify any problems that are not apparent from the outside so that corrections can be made.

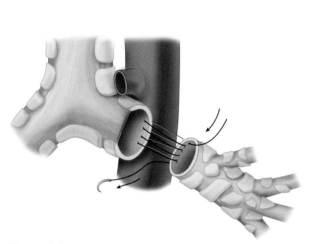

Figure 8-2

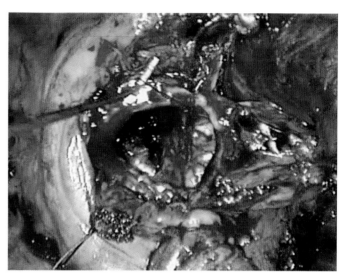

Figure 8-3

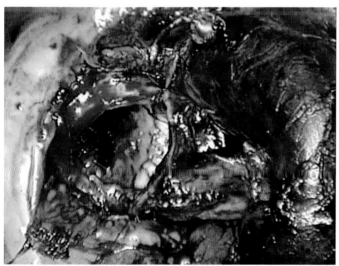

Figure 8-4

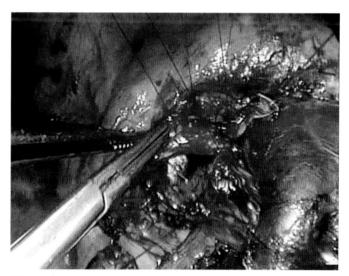

Figure 8-5

2. Special Circumstances

Size Discrepancies

- Often size discrepancies between the two ends of the airway to be joined are found. We believe this situation is best managed by careful spacing of sutures. Sutures should be placed closer together in the smaller end and farther apart in the larger end. This may lead to telescoping of the two ends, but it has not produced problems and, in fact, might be desirable. It is our belief that removing wedges, creating "pleats," or incising a bronchus are to be avoided.

3. Specific Bronchoplasties

Right Upper Lobe Bronchoplasty

- Right upper lobe sleeve resection is the most common of all bronchoplasties. Initial hilar dissection proceeds as in any right upper lobectomy until the bronchus is reached. The subcarinal space is dissected, and the bronchus is encircled by surgical tape at the levels of the right mainstem bronchus and bronchus intermedius. Proximal transection of the main bronchus is usually done first, any incomplete bronchial dissection completed, and the intermedius divided. Specimens for frozen sections are taken, as previously described. As noted, judgment must be exercised as to the extent of lymph node dissection.

Right Upper and Middle Lobe Bronchoplasty

- A right upper lobe tumor that involves the middle lobe parenchyma but spares the bronchus intermedius is best managed by right upper lobe bronchoplasty and standard in-continuity middle lobectomy. This avoids a major size discrepancy between the right main bronchus and the right lower lobe bronchus. It is important to preserve the peribronchial tissue around the bronchus intermedius and middle lobe bronchus.
- If it is necessary to remove the bronchus intermedius up to the right lower lobe bronchus, it is important to preserve as much of the right main bronchus as possible. Oblique transection of the right main bronchus sometimes facilitates anastomosis with the obliquity of division of the lower lobe bronchus that becomes necessary when the bronchus intermedius and middle lobe bronchus are removed. This is necessarily done at an angle to preserve the superior segmental bronchus of the lower lobe.
- These steps will minimize size discrepancy and reduce tension as well. When the entire right mainstem and bronchus intermedius are removed, it may be necessary to incise the pericardium beneath the inferior pulmonary vein to release the hilar structures and reduce anastomotic tension. The anastomosis is done as described for right upper lobe bronchoplasty.

Right Lower and Middle Lobe Bronchoplasty

◆ When a tumor of the right lower lobe extends proximally along the bronchus intermedius to compromise the point of the bronchial transection, it is possible to preserve the upper lobe. The lower and middle lobectomy proceeds as usual until only the bronchus remains. The bronchus is transected at the level of the right main bronchus and the origin of the right upper lobe bronchus. The upper lobe bronchus is properly aligned with the right mainstem bronchus. Size discrepancy is usually managed with careful placement and spacing of anastomotic sutures. Even though the right upper lobe originates perpendicular to the right main bronchus, rotating it 90 degrees aligns the bronchi without causing torsion or kinking of the major vessels. Alternatively, judicious trimming of both bronchial stumps, slightly on the oblique, can simplify alignment.

Left Upper Lobe Bronchoplasty

◆ Left upper lobe bronchoplasty is similar to right upper lobe bronchoplasty. The dissection is identical to a standard left upper lobectomy until the bronchus is reached.
◆ The PA is retracted, the mainstem bronchus is divided, and then the bronchus to the left lower lobe. In some cases, resection of the artery leads to a better exposure of the bronchial anastomosis. The bronchial ends are naturally in alignment.

Left Lower Lobe Bronchoplasty

◆ This procedure is similar to the procedure for right lower and middle lobe bronchoplasty. The lower lobe resection is carried out in standard fashion until the bronchus is reached. The bronchus to the left upper lobe is divided at its origin, the left main bronchus just proximal to the takeoff of the left upper lobe bronchus. Traction sutures are placed to ensure proper alignment. The remainder of the anastomosis is carried out as described previously.

4. Specific Types of Sleeve Lobectomies

◆ Patients who have an upper lobe tumor in the right lung that extends within 5 to 10 mm from the carina may undergo right sleeve upper lobectomy. In these patients, the main bronchus is transected at the level of the carina (Fig. 8-6) and the anastomosis performed between the tracheobronchial bifurcation and the bronchus intermedius. Because closing the main bronchus ostium at the level of the carina produces excessive suture tension, the sleeve lobectomy can be considered an alternative to sleeve pneumonectomy.

Right and Left Mainstem Bronchi

◆ Resection of the mainstem bronchi encompasses the same principles as the previously described procedures. The single most important difference is exposure of the left mainstem bronchus. If the resection requires removal of the proximal left mainstem bronchus, it may be necessary to mobilize the aortic arch for adequate exposure. The aorta is dissected circumferentially to allow passage of tapes for retraction to expose the bronchus fully. Care must be taken to avoid injury to intercostal vessels originating from the aorta. These can be difficult to repair. The recurrent laryngeal nerve must be protected from direct traction or injury because it passes beneath the aorta. It may be necessary to encircle the distal trachea and right mainstem bronchus with tapes for retraction. Resection of most or all of the left mainstem bronchus produces tension, which will require intrapericardial mobilization.

Segmental Bronchoplasty

◆ The most common of these operations involves resection of the superior segments of the lower lobes, the lingula, or the superior truncus of the left upper lobe. Once the dissected segment has been removed, the technique of anastomosis is the same as that described for lobar sleeve resection.

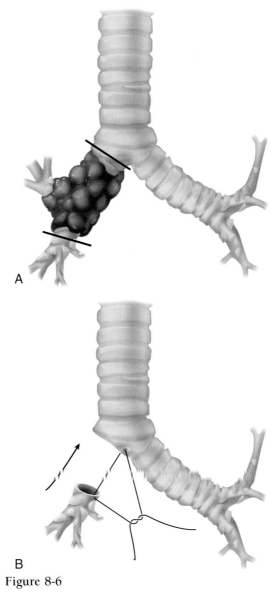

Figure 8-6

◆ Also, excision of the superior truncus of the left upper lobe for a carcinoid tumor, with pulmonary resection preserving the lingula, is performed. In this case, lingular segment is anastomosed "side-to-side" to the left lower lobe bronchus, and then this new orifice is anastomosed to the left mainstem bronchus as described earlier (Fig. 8-7).

◆ Although segmental bronchoplasties are fairly easy to do, the healing of the anastomosis is better than with sleeve lobectomies because there is less tension at the anastomosis and better blood supply from both pulmonary and systemic circulation and the site of the anastomosis is completely surrounded by lung tissue, which acts as a well-vascularized protecting flap. The negative pressure within the lung parenchyma also tends to pull the anastomosis in an outward direction, thus widening its diameter.

Wedge and Flap Reconstruction of the Bronchus

◆ Wedge resection of the main bronchus, instead of a full circumferential bronchial sleeve, has been reported infrequently as an alternative technique for preservation of lung tissue. In such cases, the wedge resection is carried out longitudinally along the bronchus and the bronchial defect is reapproximated transversely.

◆ In cases of flap bronchoplasties, a lobectomy and partial main bronchus wall resection is made in such a way that 2 to 3 cm of the unaffected lobar bronchus is preserved. This lobar remnant is spread out and used as a flap to cover the defect in the main bronchus.

◆ However, postoperative complications such as bronchostenosis, bronchial deformity, and pneumonia have been reported to be more common, especially after wedge bronchoplasties.

Bronchoplastic and Angioplastic Procedures

◆ When the tumor involves both the bronchus and the PA, consideration is given to sleeve resections of both the bronchus and PA to avoid pneumonectomy. Judgment must be exercised to determine whether such a procedure can be done without violating oncologic principles. Major complication has been related to the demands of the PA anastomosis. Just the right amount of tension is required to avoid kinking, twisting, or narrowing of the artery. It is imperative to interpose a viable tissue pedicle between the two suture lines to minimize the risk of bronchovascular fistula.

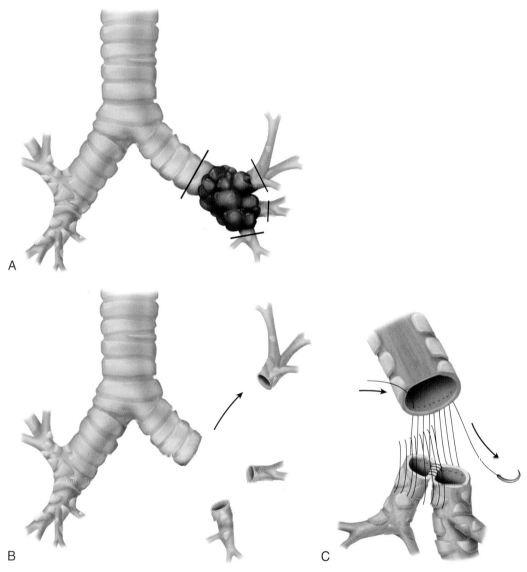

Figure 8-7

- When the point in the operation is reached for division of the artery and airway, proximal and distal control of the PA must be secured. Proximal occlusion requires a vascular clamp or a tourniquet, whereas distal control is achieved either with the use of vessel loops around the lower lobe pulmonary arterial trunk and its branches or by use of curved or straight bulldog artery clamps.
- We do not perform occlusion of the pulmonary veins. It is preferable to perform the arterial anastomosis first. Heparin 5000 units is administered intravenously before clamping. The PA is either divided to conduct a sleeve resection or part of the circumference is resected. A 6-0 continuous Prolene suture is preferred for the arterial anastomosis. Sleeve resection shortens the artery, avoids angulation, and is preferred over near-circumferential patching, particularly if a bronchial sleeve resection is combined with arterial resection.
- After lateral resection, transverse closure is considered to prevent kinking. For patch repair, autologous or bovine pericardium is available. Rendina and colleagues reported the use of a conduit made of autologous pericardium. Before tying the last suture, the proximal clamp is removed to flush any clots. The same is done with the distal clamp. If concern arises about the patency of the arterial anastomosis, pressures taken on either side of the anastomosis will show whether a significant gradient exists. The bronchoplasty is performed in exactly the same manner as described earlier. After completion, the reconstruction needs to be carefully inspected during inflation of the lung for angulation of the artery. A pedicled flap of pleura or pericardial fat is then passed around the anastomosis as a buttress and to separate the suture line from nearby vascular structures, thus preventing bronchovascular fistula. While the patient is hospitalized, subcutaneous heparin is administered at doses for prophylaxis of deep vein thrombosis. No additional anticoagulation is administered.

Step 4. Postoperative Care

- In most series, the reported operative mortality after sleeve resection is below 5% (Table 8-2). Most patients were extubated in the operating room after the procedure. When postoperative mechanical ventilation was necessary, a standard ET was substituted for the double-lumen tube.
- Careful attention should be given to postoperative pain relief, early ambulation, and relative fluid restriction supplement measures to encourage deep breathing and mobilization of respiratory secretions. Pain relief is achieved with epidural analgesia or patient-controlled analgesia.
- Patients are followed-up by routine chest radiographs and chest CT scans. Fiberoptic bronchoscopy is performed routinely before hospital discharge, 1 month after discharge, and when atelectasis or a persistent air leak indicates a need to look for anastomotic complications. Such a liberal use of bronchoscopy identifies not only many normal anastomoses but also the rare and unexpected problem that requires closer follow-up. Even when bronchoscopy is performed only selectively, it must be done when obvious problems are found, that is, atelectasis, pneumothorax, unexplained fever, or hypoxia, to rule out stricture and bronchial dehiscence. A stricture may be observed when pneumonia and sepsis are absent. Early narrowing of the anastomosis may be caused by mucosal swelling, which should improve with time. Bronchial stenosis may not be obvious during the initial hospitalization, and continued attention to new symptoms should extend over the first 3 months after operation. New onset of wheezing, pneumonia, or atelectasis in the reimplanted lobe should prompt a bronchoscopic examination. Strictures at the anastomosis that arise beyond 3 months may represent a local recurrence; a biopsy should be performed. Dilation of the anastomosis is best delayed for the first 3 weeks after the operation, but secretions should be removed aggressively and, if necessary, repeatedly. A stricture that recurs after dilation may require placement of a bronchial stent or a surgical attempt to reconstruct the anastomosis.

TABLE 8-2.	Operative Mortality and Survival Results After Bronchial Sleeve Resection					
AUTHOR	YEAR	NO. PATIENTS	COMPLICATIONS (%)	TECHNICAL COMPLICATIONS (%)	MORTALITY (%)	SURVIVAL (5 yr; %)
Kawahara	1994	112	NS	15.6	NS	NS
Van Schil	1996	145	18.6	NS	4.8	46
Gaissert	1996	72	11.0	1.3	4	42
Rea	1997	217	12.5	NS	6.2	49
Icard	1999	110	50.0	4.5	2.75	39
Kutlu	1999	100	12.0	2.0	2	49
Massard	1999	63	28.5	9.5	1.6	43
Suen	1999	77	41.3	3.8	5.2	37.5
Tronc	2000	184	14.1	3.2	1.6	52
Okada	2000	151	10.0	0	0	48
Lausberg	2000	81	NS	0	1.2	61.9
Rendina	2000	145	12.4	2.7	3	37.9
Tronc	2005	300			2.7	54
Nagayasu	2006	118			5.9	56
Yıldızeli	2007	218	22.9	3.6	4.1	53

- In most series, the incidence of anastomotic dehiscence with secondary bronchopleural fistula is below 5%. If a small fistula does develop, proper dependent drainage and cautious irrigation may lead to closure. When a dehiscence is discovered, its extent should be quantified. A partial dehiscence may be observed; however, an accompanying pneumothorax should be drained with a chest tube and every effort should be made to achieve complete expansion of the lung. If a fistula is large and is detected early, one may try to reconstruct the anastomosis. When discovered late or if the reimplanted lung is septic, completion pneumonectomy might need to be performed.
- Bronchovascular fistula is an almost lethal complication resulting from erosion of the adjacent PA into the bronchial tree across the anastomosis. This complication, which is rare (0%-1%) can be minimized by applying the principles for a healthy bronchial anastomosis, by avoiding suture material with hard knots or ends, and by using a pedicled flap around the completed anastomosis.

Step 5. Pearls and Pitfalls

- Intraoperative bronchoscopy should be used to check the anastomosis and clear the bronchial secretions.
- Be aware of arterial kinking.
- A flap is recommended to avoid the risk of PA ulceration by PDS.
- Postoperative bronchoscopic surveillance is recommended.
- Associated arterial sleeve resection is usually on the left side.
- Sleeve lobectomy can be performed for patients who are anatomically appropriate regardless of whether they would tolerate a larger resection. It is an alternative procedure to pneumonectomy and even to sleeve right pneumonectomy in selected patients. Sleeve lobectomy achieves local tumor control and is associated with acceptable rates of mortality and bronchial anastomotic complications.

Suggested Readings

Bueno R,Wain JC,Wright CD, et al. Bronchoplasty in the management of low-grade airway neoplasms and benign bronchial stenosis. Ann Thorac Surg 1996;62:824-829.

Fadel E, Yıldızeli B, Chapelier AR, et al. Sleeve lobectomy for bronchogenic cancers: Factors affecting survival. Ann Thorac Surg 2002;74(3):851-858.

Ferguson M, Lehman AG. Sleeve lobectomy or pneumonectomy: Optimal management strategy using decision analysis techniques. Ann Thorac Surg 2003;76:1782-1788.

Icard P, Regnard JF, Guibert L, et al. Survival and prognostic factors in patients undergoing parenchymal saving bronchoplastic operation for primary lung cancer: A series of 110 consecutive cases. Eur J Cardiothorac Surg 1999;15:426-432.

Martin-Ucar AE, Chaudhuri N, Edwards JG, et al. Can pneumonectomy for non–small cell lung cancer can be avoided? An audit of parenchymal sparing lung surgery. Eur J Cardiothorac Surg 2002;21:601-605.

Mathisen DJ, Grillo HC. Surgery of the Trachea and Bronchi. Hamilton, London: BC Decker; 2004:619-629.

Rendina EA, Venuta F. Reconstruction of the pulmonary artery. In Patterson GA, Cooper JD, Deslauriers J, et al, eds. Pearson's Thoracic and Esophageal Surgery, 3rd ed. Philadelphia: Elsevier; 2008:909-922.

Rendina EA, Venuta F, de Giacomo T, et al. Parenchymal-sparing operations for bronchogenic carcinoma. Surg Clin North Am 2002;82:589-609.

Ricci C, Rendina EA, Venuta F, et al. Reconstruction of the pulmonary artery in patients with lung cancer. Ann Thorac Surg 1994;57:627-633.

Tronc F, Gregoire J, Deslauriers J. Bronchoplasty. In Patterson GA, Cooper JD, Deslauriers J, et al, eds. Pearson's Thoracic and Esophageal Surgery, 3rd ed. Philadelphia: Elsevier; 2008:894-908.

Van Schil PE, Brutel de la Riviere A, Knaepen PJ, et al. Long-term survival after bronchial sleeve resection: Univariate and multivariate analyses. Ann Thorac Surg 1996;61:1087-1091.

Yıldızeli B, Fadel E, Mussot S, et al. Morbidity, mortality, and long-term survival after sleeve lobectomy for non–small cell lung cancer. Eur J Cardiothorac Surg 2007;31:95-102.

CHAPTER 9

TECHNIQUES FOR PARTIAL AND SLEEVE PULMONARY ARTERY RESECTION

Robert J. Cerfolio and Ayesha S. Bryant

Non–small cell lung cancer is the number one cause of cancer deaths worldwide. Surgical resection, which is offered for early-stage lung cancer, can be curative but is often associated with morbidity. Pneumonectomy, however, confers significantly greater morbidity and mortality rates and is also associated with a poorer quality of life. When possible, thoracic surgeons should perform lobectomy with sleeve resection of the bronchus or of the pulmonary artery (PA), or both, to avoid pneumonectomy. Knowledge of the anatomy of the tracheobronchial tree is essential to this technique.

Step 1. Surgical Anatomy

- The trachea originates below the cricoid cartilage and extends from front to back to the carina. The trachea then bifurcates into left and right mainstem bronchi, with length, depending on gender, ranging from 10 to 14 cm. The trachea and main bronchi have an anterior horseshoe-shaped cartilaginous portion comprised of 16 to 20 tracheal rings and a posterior membranous portion apposed against the upper esophagus and vertebral column. The membranous portion is more elastic and extensible in younger people and with age becomes more rigid, which is important to consider in deciding between sleeve lobectomy and pneumonectomy.
- The right main bronchus is in direct line with the trachea. The primary bronchus is distal to the right upper lobe bronchus and becomes the bronchus intermedius, about 2 cm long. Anterior to the bronchus intermedius is the middle lobe bronchus in direct line with the origin of the superior segmental bronchus of the lower lobe, arising from the posterior wall of the bronchus intermedius.
- The left main bronchus arises more obliquely from the carina than the right main bronchus and is longer, 4 to 6 cm long versus about 1.5 cm. It passes under the aortic arch posterior to the left hilum, where it bifurcates to form the upper and lower lobe bronchi. There is no bronchus intermedius on the left side, making sleeve resection on the left side more difficult.

Step 2. Preoperative Considerations

- If safe dissection of the pulmonary arterial branches cannot be performed but lobectomy can yield complete resection of all of the cancer, PA resection can be used. Indications for PA resection include localized tumors, strictures, impacted broncholiths, and traumatic damage to the mainstem bronchus. Whenever it is possible to achieve a margin-negative resection and yet preserve noncancerous, functioning pulmonary tissue, sleeve resection of the bronchus or of the PA should be employed, avoiding pneumonectomy. Compared with pneumonectomy, PA resection is associated with lower rates of morbidity and mortality, blood flow is unimpeded, and recurrence rate is uncompromised.
- Careful patient selection for this procedure is crucial. Preoperative tests should include a chest radiograph and conventional or computed tomography. Preoperative pulmonary function tests are of limited value. The main consideration in deciding to resect the mainstem bronchus should be based on the patient's overall cardiopulmonary status.

Step 3. Operative Steps

- The surgical approach is through a posterolateral thoracotomy, allowing access to the trachea, the mainstem bronchi, and the lung. Proximal control of the main PA is obtained extrapericardially. On the right side, proximal control is obtained posterior to the superior vena cava, and on the left side it is obtained just distal to the ligamentum arteriosum. Care is taken to avoid the left recurrent laryngeal nerve.
- The pulmonary vein of the lobe to be removed is encircled and then divided. A vascular stapler is used. Then about 500 units (we have not based the dose of heparin on the patient's weight) of intravenous (IV) heparin is given. Recently (i.e., in our last 15 procedures), we have not used any heparin. Approximately 1 minute later, a Satinsky clamp is placed on the proximal PA. It is positioned so that its handle is facing in the opposite direction of the Satinsky to be placed on the vein (Fig. 9-1). This allows more room for the operating surgeon. A Satinsky clamp is then placed on the remaining pulmonary vein(s). (See Figure 9-1, which shows a left upper lobectomy and a partial PA resection.) This clamp is positioned so that its handle faces opposite from the handle of the Satinsky on the artery as shown in Figure 9-1. A knife is used to cut out the part of the PA that has cancer invading its surface, and then the bronchus is cut as well. The lobe with the cancer is removed from the operative field. This opens up the entire surgical field and affords more room for the surgeon to work.

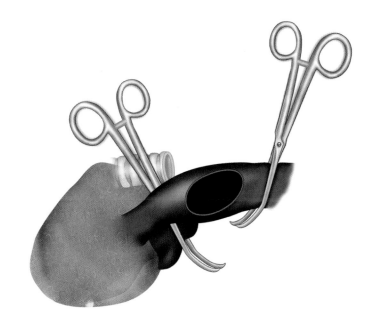

Figure 9-1

◆ At this time, separate frozen-section margins of the bronchus and the PA should be sent for evaluation. If sleeves of the bronchus and of the artery are both required, we prefer to perform the bronchus first, before the PA is sewn back together. We prefer the bronchus first, even though it prolongs PA clamp time slightly, so a freshly sewn PA is not retracted while the left upper lobe bronchial sleeve resection is being performed.

◆ The PA is now examined from inside to determine whether a partial or circumferential resection is needed. If removal of part of the PA narrows the lumen by more than 20% to 30% of its original size, then we prefer a circumferential resection. Another option is a patch angioplasty using a piece of bovine pericardium. If a circumferential resection is required, the PA is sewn back together using 5-0 Prolene (Ethicon, Somerville, NJ) (Fig. 9-2). Just before reestablishing PA continuity, the distal clamp is taken off the pulmonary vein before tying the arterial sutures to help "de-air" the pulmonary circuitry (Fig. 9-3). Then the proximal PA Satinsky clamp is removed to ensure hemostasis of the sewn PA. No further anticoagulation is used either in the operating room or postoperatively.

◆ The bronchus is closed with interrupted sutures and is covered with an intercostal muscle flap that is harvested before chest retraction, as we previously described in 2005. The muscle does not circumferentially wrap the anastomosis; rather, it goes around it about 180 degrees.

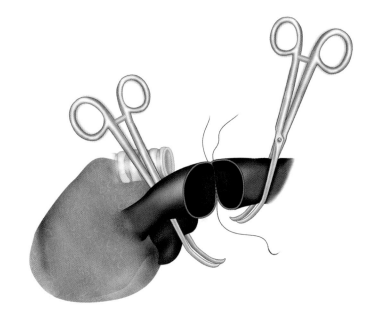

Figure 9-2

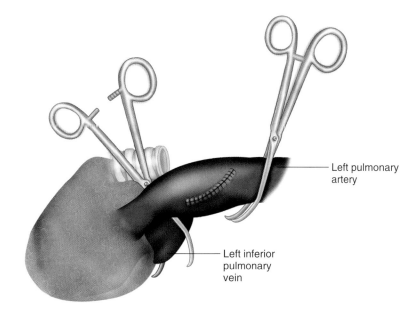

Left pulmonary
artery

Left inferior
pulmonary
vein

Figure 9-3

Step 4. Postoperative Care

- Patients are extubated in the operating room and sent directly to their hospital room. We do not routinely admit any patient to the intensive care unit. Chest tube output, urinary output, heart rate and rhythm, pulse, and oxygenation saturation are monitored. On postoperative day 1, ambulation is started four times daily, chest physical therapy is given every 6 to 8 hours, and a nebulizer treatment is given every 4 hours. The patient is encouraged to perform incentive spirometry every hour while awake. The patient's diet is advanced with aspiration precautions.
- On postoperative day 2, the IV line is usually "heplocked," and the epidural catheter is removed. The urinary catheter is also removed 8 hours after the epidural catheter is removed. Additionally on postoperative day 2, all medications are changed from the IV or intramuscular route to oral (including pain medication). Over the remainder of the patient's hospital course, the patient is encouraged to continue ambulation, perform incentive spirometry, and receive chest physiotherapy and nebulizer treatments. The last chest tube is removed when there is no air leak and no new or enhancing pneumothorax and the chest tube output is less than 450 mL for 24 hours. A pre–chest tube removal and 4-hour post–chest tube removal chest radiograph is obtained.
- On postoperative day 3, our social worker arranges for any home oxygen, post-discharge home health care needs, or other special needs. The nurses instruct the patient and family regarding home care. The patient is usually discharged on postoperative day 3 or 4, depending on his or her wishes and level of pain control.

Step 5. Pearls and Pitfalls

- This procedure carries less operative risk and improved postoperative quality of life.
- It is a more time-consuming and technically demanding procedure than pneumonectomy, but it is easier to do if one has proximal and distal control of the artery and uses the nonresected vein as distal control.
- The procedure is safe and allows precise assessment of the extent of diseased tissue for more complete excision.

Suggested Readings

Cerfolio RJ, Bryant AS, Yamamuro M. Intercostal muscle flap to buttress the bronchus at risk and the thoracic esophageal-gastric anastomosis. Ann Thorac Surg 2005;80:1017-1020.

Cerfolio RJ, Pickens A, Bass C, Katholi C. Fast-tracking pulmonary resections. J Thorac Cardiovasc Surg 2001;122:318-324.

Cerfolio RJ, Bryant AS. Surgical techniques and results for partial or circumferential sleeve resection of the pulmonary artery for patients with non-small cell lung cancer. Ann Thorac Surg 2007;83:1971-1977.

Cerfolio RJ, Deschamps C, Allen MS, et al. Mainstem bronchial sleeve resection with pulmonary preservation. Ann Thorac Surg 1996;61:1458-1463.

Rendina EA, De Giagomo T, Venuta F, et al. Lung conservation techniques: Bronchial sleeve resection and reconstruction of the PA. Semin Surg Oncol 2000;18:165-172.

Venuta F, Ciccone AM. Reconstruction of the pulmonary artery. Semin Thorac Cardiovasc Surg 2006;18:104-108.

CHAPTER 10

EXTRAPLEURAL PNEUMONECTOMY

Daniel L. Miller

Sarot first described the technique of extrapleural pneumonectomy (EPP) for the treatment of tuberculous empyema in 1949. Since the late 1970s, EPP has been performed almost exclusively for malignant pleural mesothelioma (MPM). Early series reported high perioperative morbidity and mortality rates. However, with improvements in patient selection, intraoperative management, and postoperative care, the morbidity, hospital stay, and mortality associated with EPP have been reduced substantially.

Step 1. Surgical Anatomy

- In traditional pneumonectomy, only the diseased lung is removed. In an EPP, the lung, parietal pleura, and a part of the diaphragm are removed.
- The anatomic location, extent, and histology subtype of MPM determine whether a patient should undergo an EPP.
- Several staging systems have been developed for MPM. The first and most widely used was developed by Butchart in 1976. In 1994, a tumor, node, metastasis (TNM)-based system was created by the International Mesothelioma Interest Group (IMIG). This system provides TNM descriptors and stage classifications. The most recent staging system (Brigham staging system) is based on analysis of more than 180 patients treated for MPM at the Dana-Farber Cancer Institute. This system considers resectability, tumor histology, and nodal status (Table 10-1).
- It is essential to accurately stage disease before performing an EPP. Only patients with early-stage resectable disease should undergo EPP; patients with nodal disease (mediastinal or extrapleural) are not candidates.

TABLE 10-1.	Revised Staging System for Malignant Pleural Mesothelioma
STAGE	**DEFINITION**
I	Disease completely resected within the parietal pleural capsule (pleura, lung, pericardium, diaphragm, or chest wall containing previous biopsy sites) without lymph node involvement
II	All of stage I with positive resection margins or intrapleural (N1 or N2) lymph node involvement
III	Local extension into the mediastinum, or chest wall, or through the diaphragm or peritoneum, or extrapleural or contralateral (N3) lymph node involvement
IV	Distant metastatic disease

From Sugarbaker DJ, Flores RM, Jaklitsch MT, et al. Resection margins, extrapleural nodal status, and cell type determine postoperative long-term survival in trimodality therapy of malignant pleural mesothelioma: Results in 183 patients. J Thorac Cardiovasc Surg 1999;117(1):54-63; discussion 63-65. Table II.

Step 2. Preoperative Considerations

- In MPM, after tumor stage, tumor histology is the single most important factor influencing survival. Epithelial cell type, the most common histology, confers the best prognosis; sarcomatous and mixed histologies are more aggressive; and desmoplastic MPM, the rarest subtype, is the deadliest. Most centers now operate only on patients with epithelial MPM because of the poor long-term survival after EPP for the other subtypes.
- Radiologic evaluation is essential to determine whether a patient with MPM has potentially resectable disease. Posteroanterior and lateral chest radiograph, computed tomography (CT) scan of the chest and upper abdomen, and magnetic resonance imaging (MRI) of the chest have been the most widely used modalities. CT scan provides an estimate of tumor burden and extent of tumor both locally and distantly. MRI can supplement the CT scan for detection of tumor extension into the mediastinum or the abdomen. More recently, positron emission tomography (PET) has been used to determine whether a patient has early resectable disease based on no evidence of contralateral disease or distant metastasis. Early results are promising.
- Other diagnostic modalities, such as minimally invasive procedures, also may be used to determine whether a patient can undergo an EPP. Transesophageal echocardiography can be used to assess mediastinal involvement, especially of the heart or vena cava, and to perform

BOX 10-1. Selection Criteria
1. Performance status 0-1
2. Predicted postoperative FEV_1 >1.0 L
3. Room air PaO_2 >65 mm Hg
4. Room air $PaCO_2$ <45 mm Hg
5. Ejection fraction >40%
6. Mean pulmonary artery pressure <30 mm Hg
7. Epithelial histology
8. No N2 or extrapleural lymph node involvement
9. No distant or contralateral disease
10. Ability to complete a trimodality treatment program

FEV_1, forced expiratory volume in the first second of expiration; $PaCO_2$, partial pressure of carbon dioxide, arterial; PaO_2, partial pressure of oxygen, arterial.

fine-needle aspiration of inferior mediastinal lymph nodes. Transthoracic needle aspiration via CT also can be performed to exclude extrapleural lymph node involvement (internal mammary lymph nodes). Mediastinoscopy is used frequently to determine nodal involvement if mediastinal lymph nodes (N2) are larger than 1.0 cm in diameter. Laparoscopic examination also can be used to identify transdiaphragmatic involvement that would preclude resection.

♦ For a patient to be considered for an EPP, the patient should have a normal performance status. Pulmonary function tests, especially forced expiratory volume in the first second of expiration (FEV_1) and forced vital capacity (FVC), are used to determine whether a patient can tolerate an EPP. For patients in whom a predicted postoperative FEV_1 is less than 1 L, a quantitative perfusion scan is useful to predict postoperative lung function after EPP. Arterial blood gases are obtained to rule out baseline hypoxia or hypercapnia. Two-dimensional dobutamine echocardiography is necessary to rule out ventricular dysfunction (ejection fraction <40%), significant coronary artery disease, and pulmonary hypertension (mean pulmonary artery pressure >30 mm Hg) that may increase perioperative risks. An agitated saline study also is performed to determine whether a patent foramen ovale is present that might result in a significant right-to-left shunt after EPP. Selection criteria are summarized in Box 10-1.

♦ Thoracoscopy has become the diagnostic procedure of choice, with a yield of greater than 95% for MPM. Talc pleurodesis (aerosolized 5 g) is usually performed at the time of the thoracoscopic pleural biopsy to prevent reaccumulation of a symptomatic pleural effusion. The talc pleurodesis facilitates extrapleural dissection at the time of EPP and also may prevent intraoperative spillage of malignant cells that could increase the risk of local recurrence. A single thoracoscopic access incision (Fig. 10-1A) is usually placed either in the fifth or eighth intercostal space. The eighth intercostal access incision is preferred because it can be incorporated into a utility thoracotomy incision, if necessary, at the time of EPP to facilitate resection and reconstruction of the diaphragm. The location of these incisions is important so that they can be incorporated into standard thoracotomy incisions at the time of the EPP.

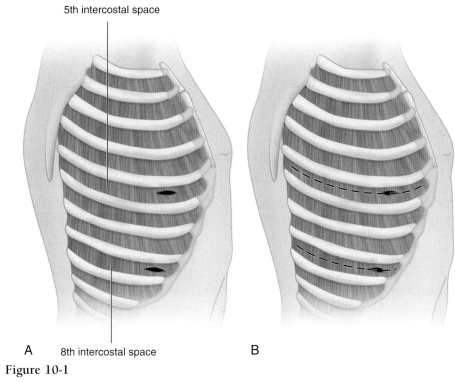

5th intercostal space

A   8th intercostal space

B

Figure 10-1

◆ To take full advantage of the extrapleural edema created by the talc, I have found that it is best to proceed with the EPP within 2 to 3 weeks after pleurodesis. This also allows time to complete the staging workup and to finalize the tissue diagnosis.

Step 3. Operative Steps

1. Right Extrapleural Pneumonectomy

◆ After induction of general anesthesia, a left-sided double-lumen endotracheal tube is placed and positioned fiberoptically. A nasogastric tube is placed to facilitate palpation of the esophagus during the posterior extrapleural dissection. Patients are monitored with an arterial line, continuous oximetry, central venous line, and urinary catheter. A thoracic epidural catheter is placed preoperatively and used for postoperative pain control. The patient is placed in the left lateral decubitus position.

◆ A standard posterolateral thoracotomy incision is carried out, making sure to incorporate all previous biopsy sites (see Fig. 10-1B). At the time of EPP, all previous incisions are excised to ensure removal of potential sites of mesothelioma implants.

◆ The serratus muscle is saved and retracted medially. The chest is entered, usually over the unresected sixth rib. The sixth rib may be removed to do a single thoracotomy incision approach. It is beneficial to use a second lower thoracotomy incision on the right to facilitate resection and reconstruction of the diaphragm.

◆ After division of the intercostal muscles, an extrapleural plane is developed superior and inferior to the thoracotomy incision. Great care is taken during the extrapleural dissection not to enter the pleural cavity to prevent spillage of malignant cells within the operative field. The superior component of the dissection is carried out first (Fig. 10-2). It is important not to injure the internal mammary artery and vein during the anterior dissection, which can lead to significant bleeding.

◆ Combined sharp and blunt dissection continues toward the apex of the thorax. Medially, the dissection is carried from the apex down to the azygos vein. The mediastinal pleura is then dissected free from the superior vena cava and azygos vein. The pericardium at the level of the azygos vein is opened to determine transpericardial or myocardial involvement; if no involvement is found, the pericardiotomy is extended anteriorly and inferiorly to encompass the tumor.

◆ Placement of the surgeon's left hand inside the pericardium helps determine the extent of pericardial resection. Intrapericardially, the pulmonary artery is dissected free as well as the superior and inferior vena cava and the superior and inferior pulmonary veins (Fig. 10-3). The dissection of the pericardium is completed at the pericardiopleural attachment overlying the junction of the inferior vena cava and the hepatic veins.

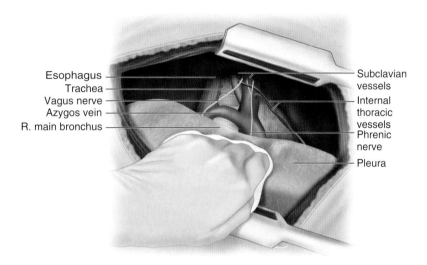

Esophagus
Trachea
Vagus nerve
Azygos vein
R. main bronchus

Subclavian vessels
Internal thoracic vessels
Phrenic nerve
Pleura

Figure 10-2

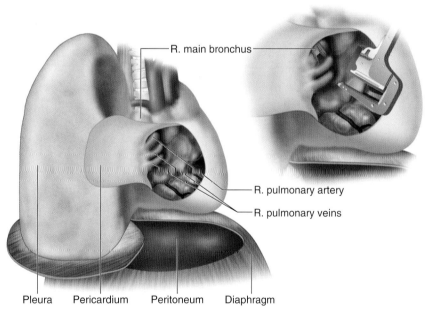

R. main bronchus

R. pulmonary artery

R. pulmonary veins

Pleura   Pericardium   Peritoneum   Diaphragm

Figure 10-3

◆ The diaphragm is excised starting at the anterior margin in a circumferential fashion working posteriorly (see Fig. 10-3). If possible, the peritoneum is not entered, preventing peritoneal seeding. Posteriorly, the peritoneum can be dissected free inferiorly with a sponge stick to separate it from the diaphragm (Fig. 10-4). However, if the tumor burden is too great to avoid entrance into the peritoneum, the abdominal cavity is entered to help facilitate dissection at the level of the inferior vena and hepatic veins. If necessary, a lower utility thoracotomy incision is used at this point to help with removal of the diaphragm. This second thoracotomy incision is usually placed at the site of the previous video-assisted thoracic surgery (VATS) access incision or chest tube site, which is excised to remove potential MPM implants. The diaphragm is divided over the inferior vena cava, and the dissection is carried posteriorly, leaving a rim of tissue, if not involved by tumor, to secure the diaphragmatic reconstruction patch. After this maneuver, the diaphragmatic dissection is completed. The lung is retracted medially, a complete mediastinal lymphadenectomy is carried out, and the thoracic duct is ligated to prevent a postoperative chylothorax.

◆ After completion of the en bloc dissection, 250 mg of Solu-Cortef is given intravenously. After approximately 10 minutes, the right pulmonary artery and the superior and inferior pulmonary veins are ligated and divided with endoscopic 45-mm vascular staplers intrapericardially (see Fig. 10-3). After the vessels are divided, the pericardium is opened posteriorly to the hilum, which completes the pericardial resection. The surgical specimen is then retracted anteriorly. The right mainstem bronchus is dissected free of peribronchial tissue and stapled with a 30- or 60-mm heavy wire stapler. The en bloc specimen containing the right lung, parietal pleura, pericardium, and diaphragm exhibits extensive growth over the entire pleural surface as well as the intrafissural surface.

◆ The specimen is removed and sent to the pathologist for inspection of resection margins, lymph node evaluation, and histologic identification of the tumor.

◆ After hemostasis is obtained, a tissue flap is developed to cover the bronchial stump. Options for tissue reinforcement include serratus muscle, intercostal muscle, thymic fat pad, or azygos vein. Pericardial fat is usually not available because of the extent of pericardium resected. Most commonly, a thymic fat pad is placed (Fig. 10-5) or, if this is not available, an azygos vein bivalved flap. The azygos vein is ligated and divided at the superior vena cava and only ligated, but not divided, at its origin near the spine and bivalved to create an azygos vein flap to cover the bronchial stump.

◆ The pericardium on the right side is always reconstructed with a patch to prevent cardiac herniation. This is done with supple bovine pericardium using running and interrupted 2-0 polypropylene sutures (see Fig. 10-5). The key to prevent tamponade physiology is to use a large patch. The patch should also be fenestrated. It is important not to make the patch too narrow at the level of the superior and inferior vena cava because you may impair venous return.

◆ The diaphragmatic defect is closed with a 2-mm soft tissue Gore-Tex patch (polytetrafluoroethylene) using interrupted and running 1-0 polypropylene sutures to help prevent patch dehiscence (see Fig. 10-5). If there is not enough diaphragmatic tissue remaining, then the sutures are placed around the ribs inferiorly. Medially, the diaphragmatic patch is sutured to the pericardial patch to prevent impaired venous return of the inferior vena cava. It is extremely important to make sure that the reconstruction patch of the diaphragm is placed

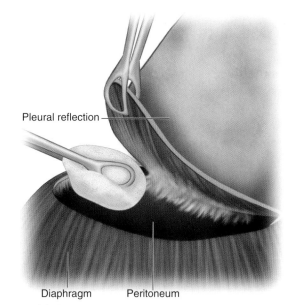

Figure 10-4

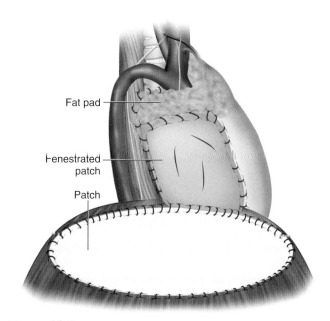

Figure 10-5

at or near the normal anatomic position to prevent intra-abdominal contents from migrating upward into the chest cavity, thus putting them at risk for injury during postoperative thoracic radiotherapy. By using the lower utility thoracotomy incision, excellent exposure can be obtained for placement of the diaphragmatic patch. While placing the patch anteriorly, a lighted retractor or disposable orthopedic light is used to ensure adequate bites of tissue are taken to help prevent dehiscence of the patch. Areas of gross disease that cannot be resected following EPP are outlined with metallic clips for subsequent boost doses of radiotherapy. The chest cavity is sprayed with a thrombin solution to augment hemostasis. A 32 French right-angle chest tube is placed and secured with a 0-silk purse-string suture and placed to gravity (water seal). The chest cavity is then closed in the usual fashion to ensure an airtight closure. A chest radiograph is obtained in the recovery room to check for position of the heart and the mediastinal structures. The chest tube is removed and the purse string is tied 24 hours later.

2. Left Extrapleural Pneumonectomy

♦ The technique for left EPP is similar to that described for a right EPP. During the dissection of the posterior aspect of the specimen, it is important to be in the correct plane in the periaortic region to avoid avulsion of intercostal vessels or injury to the aorta. It is also important to assess tumor involvement of the aorta at this time because direct aortic involvement precludes resection.

♦ The left main pulmonary artery is dissected and divided extrapericardially, if possible, using endoscopic vascular staplers to prevent impingement of the main pulmonary artery. The pulmonary veins are dissected free and stapled intrapericardially. The left mainstem bronchus is dissected free to the carina to ensure a short bronchial stump and is stapled with a 30- or 60-mm heavy wire stapler. The left bronchial stump is usually not reinforced. Initially I did not reconstruct the pericardium on the left side because the risk of herniation is low owing to the native position of the heart within the left hemithorax. Placement of a bovine pericardial patch allows near-normal position of the heart to minimize radiation exposure during adjuvant treatment, helps restore normal physiologic conditions, and prevents development of a constrictive peel that may form with maturing of the left postpneumonectomy pleural cavity.

♦ The diaphragmatic defect is reconstructed with a 2-mm soft tissue polytetrafluorethylene patch. Great care is taken in reconstruction of the esophageal hiatus. Too large an opening could result in intrathoracic herniation of the stomach or other viscera, and too tight an opening could result in postoperative dysphagia. Thus, the hiatus is reconstructed over a 50 Maloney dilator.

♦ When the graft is reconstructed at the hiatus, make sure not to leave an edge or shelf of graft at 90 degrees to the long axis of the esophagus, which may erode into the esophagus over time and cause perforation.

♦ If there is a paucity of tissue to anchor the patch at the hiatus, then smaller (3-0 or 4-0) polypropylene sutures are used to secure the patch to the periaortic tissue and/or pericardium or pericardial patch. The chest cavity is closed in routine fashion, and the chest tube is removed usually within 24 hours if the patient is hemodynamically stable.

Step 4. Postoperative Care

- The postoperative management of these patients is similar to patients undergoing a standard pneumonectomy. Yet, because of reconstruction of the pericardium, especially on the right, the patient is at risk of developing hypotension on arrival in the recovery room after being placed in the supine position. If this uncorrectable hypotension occurs, the patient may have too tight of a pericardial patch or a cardiac herniation secondary to dehiscence of a pericardial patch. The patient should be placed in the lateral position and taken to the operating room immediately for resuturing of the patch if disrupted or enlargement of the patch if it is constrictive.
- The most important issues in the postoperative period are pain control and minimization of intravascular volume changes. Pain control is vital to minimize postoperative atelectasis and pulmonary dysfunction of the remaining lung.
- Thoracic epidural catheters are used for 3 to 5 days postoperatively. The patients are enrolled in a pulmonary rehabilitation program, which starts on postoperative day 2. A negative fluid balance is maintained postoperatively to prevent postpneumonectomy pulmonary edema.
- Aggressive pulmonary toilet is also carried out to prevent this possible fatal complication. Atrial arrhythmias are treated aggressively to prevent cardiac dysfunction. The average hospital stay is usually 5 to 7 days.

Step 5. Pearls and Pitfalls

- Minimize blood loss with careful ongoing meticulous hemostasis.
- Prevent pleural spillage by avoiding entry into the pleural space.
- Prevent peritoneal entry to minimize tumor contamination of the abdomen.
- Use interrupted and running sutures to minimize the risk of patch dehiscence.
- Use a large pericardial patch to prevent tamponade.
- Place the diaphragmatic patch near normal position to prevent postoperative radiation injury to abdominal organs.
- Reinforce the bronchial stump (right) with viable tissue.
- Ligate the thoracic duct to prevent chylothorax.
- Use a utility thoracotomy incision inferiorly if necessary.
- Avoid too wide or too narrow a hiatal reconstruction.
- Poor fixation of a polytetrafluorethylene patch can lead to patch disruption and herniation of abdominal organs.
- Excessive bleeding before division of the pulmonary vessels increases the risk of postoperative complications such as postpneumonectomy pulmonary edema.
- Operative mortality has decreased significantly; however, postoperative morbidity is still a problem.
- The ideal treatment for MPM does not exist. Until it does, EPP, as a part of a trimodality treatment regimen, provides the best method of significant tumor reduction and survival benefit. This survival advantage can be achieved only by a low operative morbidity and mortality.

Suggested Readings

Butchart EG, Ashcroft T, Barnsley WC, et al. Pleuropneumectomy in the management of diffuse malignant mesothelioma of the pleura. Experience with 29 patients. Thorax 1976;31:15-24.

Gerbaudo VH, Sugarbaker DJ, Britz-Cunningham S, et al. Assessment of malignant pleural mesothelioma with (18)F-FDG dual-head gamma-camera coincidence imaging: Comparison with histopathology. J Nucl Med 2002;43:1144-1149.

Rusch VW. A proposed new international TNM staging system for malignant pleural mesothelioma: From the International Mesothelioma Interest Group. Chest 1995;108:1122-1128.

Rusch VW. Treatment of malignant pleural mesothelioma. Semin Resp Crit Care Med 1997;18:363-373.

Sarot IA. Extrapleural pneumonectomy and pleurectomy in pulmonary tuberculosis. Thorax 1949;4:173-179.

Sugarbaker DJ, Flores RM, Jaklitsch MT, et al. Resection margins, extrapleural nodal status, and cell type determine postoperative long-term survival in trimodality therapy of malignant pleural mesothelioma: Results in 183 patients. J Thorac Cardiovasc Surg 1999;117:54-65.

Sugarbaker DJ, Garcia JP. Multimodality therapy for malignant pleural mesothelioma. Chest 1997;112:272S-275S.

Sugarbaker DJ, Mentzer SJ, Strauss G. Extrapleural pneumonectomy in the treatment of malignant pleural mesothelioma. Ann Thorac Surg 1992;54:941-946.

Zellos L, Jaklitsch MT, Al-Mourgi MA, et al. Complications of extrapleural pneumonectomy. Semin Thorac Cardiovasc Surg 2007;19:355-359.

CHAPTER 11

TRACHEAL RESECTION AND RECONSTRUCTION

Moishe Liberman and Douglas J. Mathisen

Step 1. Surgical Anatomy

- ◆ Functionally, the trachea principally serves as a conduit for ventilation. Anatomically, it presents several unique features that partially account for the difficulty in its surgical management, including the following:
  - ▲ Unpaired nature
  - ▲ Unique structural rigidity
  - ▲ Short length
  - ▲ Relative lack of longitudinal elasticity
  - ▲ Proximity to major cardiovascular structures
  - ▲ Segmental blood supply
- ◆ The adult human trachea possesses the following anatomic features:
  - ▲ Average length is 11.8 cm (range, 10-13 cm) from the infracricoid level to the top of the carinal spur.
  - ▲ It has 18 to 22 cartilaginous rings.
  - ▲ There are approximately two rings per centimeter.
  - ▲ In an adult man, the internal diameter of the trachea measures about 2.3 cm laterally and 1.8 cm anteroposteriorly.
  - ▲ Measurements vary roughly in proportion to the size of the individual; therefore, they are usually smaller in women (13-27 mm in men; 10-23 mm in women).
  - ▲ The cross-sectional shape of the adult trachea is nearly elliptic.
  - ▲ In infants and children the trachea is more circular.
  - ▲ The trachea's configuration may change with disease.
  - ▲ The lower two thirds may be flattened in tracheomalacia or rigidly narrowed from side to side to produce a saber-sheath trachea.
  - ▲ The trachea becomes almost entirely mediastinal when the neck is flexed because the cricoid cartilage drops to the level of the thoracic inlet.
  - ▲ The trachea courses backward and downward at an angle from a nearly subcutaneous position at the infracricoid level to rest against the esophagus and vertebral column at the carina.
  - ▲ The larynx and the origin of the esophagus are intimately related anatomically at the cricopharyngeal level.
  - ▲ Below the cricoid, the posterior membranous wall of the trachea maintains a close spatial relationship to the esophagus.

▲ A distinct, easily separable plane between the trachea and esophagus is present below the cricoid level; however, a common blood supply is shared.

▲ Anteriorly, the thyroid isthmus passes over the trachea in the region of the second tracheal ring.

▲ The lateral lobes of the thyroid are closely applied to the trachea, and a common blood supply is shared from the branches of the inferior thyroid artery.

▲ Lying in the groove between trachea and esophagus are the recurrent laryngeal nerves: the left courses from beneath the arch of aorta and the right loops around subclavian artery and then approaches the groove. Therefore, the left recurrent laryngeal nerve has a longer course in proximity to the trachea than does the right.

▲ The recurrent nerves enter the larynx between the cricoid and thyroid cartilages just anterior to the inferior cornu of the thyroid cartilage.

▲ The blood supply of the human trachea is segmental, largely shared with the esophagus and derived principally from multiple branches of the inferior thyroid artery above and the bronchial arteries below.

▲ The arteries approach laterally, and fine branches pass anteriorly to the trachea and posteriorly to the esophagus.

▲ The inferior thyroid artery nourishes the upper trachea, usually through a pattern of three principal branches with fine subdivisions and extremely fine collateral vessels.

▲ The bronchial vessels nourish the lower trachea, carina, and mainstem bronchi.

▲ Occasionally, the internal mammary artery contributes to the distal blood supply.

▲ Excessive circumferential dissection with division of the lateral pedicles during an operative procedure can easily devascularize the trachea.

◆ The trachea lives in a crowded area surrounded by many important structures. Surrounding anatomy includes the following:

▲ The anterior pretracheal plane is made up of fibrofatty tissue, lymph nodes, and fine branches of the anterior jugular vein.

● This plane can be easily developed using blunt finger dissection through a cervical approach (similar to blunt, index-finger anterior tracheal dissection performed during mediastinoscopy).

▲ The innominate vein lies anteriorly, away from the trachea.

▲ The innominate artery crosses over the midtrachea obliquely from its point of origin on the aortic arch to the right side of the neck.

● In children, the innominate artery is higher and is encountered in the lower part of the neck.

● In some adults, the artery is unusually high and crosses the trachea at the base of the neck when slight cervical extension is present.

● Occasionally a tiny branch of this artery may be encountered stemming from the segment of the artery that crosses the trachea.

▲ At the level of the carina, the left main bronchus passes beneath the aortic arch and the right main bronchus beneath the azygos vein.

▲ The pulmonary artery lies just in front of the carina.

▲ On either side of the trachea lies fibrofatty tissue containing lymph node chains, and a large packet of nodes lies in the subcarinal space.

Step 2. Preoperative Considerations

◆ Patient should not require mechanical ventilation.
◆ Pulmonary function testing should be performed for patients with pulmonary disease.
◆ Patient should stop smoking.
◆ Nutritional optimization (malnourished) or weight loss (obesity) should be recommended.

- ◆ Appropriate staging tests should be completed when dealing with malignancy.
- ◆ If mediastinoscopy is required for staging purposes, it should be completed at the time of planned resection to aid in assessing the outer airway and in creating the pretracheal plane.
  - ▲ If mediastinoscopy is done during a separate operation before resection, mobility of the trachea will be compromised secondary to postoperative scarring.
- ◆ If neoadjuvant radiotherapy or prior mediastinal or cervical radiotherapy has been used, a pedicled muscle or omental flap to buttress the anastomosis should be planned to aid in anastomotic healing.
- ◆ Predictors of anastomotic complications following tracheal resections include the following:
  - ▲ Diabetes
  - ▲ Lengthy resection (>4 cm)
  - ▲ Laryngotracheal resection
  - ▲ Age 17 years or younger
  - ▲ Need for tracheostomy before operation
  - ▲ Steroid use

Step 3. Operative Steps

1. Anesthesia

- ◆ The airway must be under full control at all times during reconstructive surgery of the trachea to prevent hypoxia.
- ◆ The patient preferably should breathe spontaneously during the operation and always at its conclusion so that ventilatory support is not necessary postoperatively.
- ◆ Cardiopulmonary bypass has been used for tracheal resections; however, in our experience it is almost never necessary.
- ◆ Induction is carried out slowly and gently, especially in a patient with a highly obstructed airway.
- ◆ If a benign stenosis presents an airway diameter of less than 5 mm, dilatation is performed, and an endotracheal tube (ETT) is passed beyond the lesion to prevent arrhythmia caused by CO_2 buildup during the early stages of operation.
- ◆ Occasionally a nearly obstructing tumor requires prompt bronchoscopy with a ventilating bronchoscope shortly after induction, with subsequent intubation.
- ◆ Obstructing tumor may be cored out with the rigid bronchoscope aided by biopsy forceps. Frequent monitoring of blood gases and electrocardiography are essential.
- ◆ Bronchoscopic examination should be done by the surgeon and observed by the anesthesia provider, who must deal with this airway until surgical access distal to the lesion has been obtained.
- ◆ If tracheostomy is already present, induction is simplified. The anesthesiologist can ventilate and use inhalational agents by hooking the ventilator to the tracheostomy. Cross-field ventilation is used from the outset in these patients.
- ◆ In patients who are being ventilated above the lesion, initial dissection is always done carefully to avoid increasing the degree of obstruction by excessive tissue manipulation.
- ◆ In patients with critical airway stenoses, an inhalational induction technique should be employed to preserve spontaneous ventilation.
  - ▲ A slow inhalational induction is used if there is a high degree of obstruction.
  - ▲ This technique is preferable to paralysis of respiration, which may necessitate the urgent establishment of an airway.
- ◆ In patients with less critical airway stenoses, total intravenous anesthesia (TIVA) techniques (the use of IV agent[s] exclusively to provide a complete anesthetic) can be used.

▲ This allows for prompt reversal and spontaneous breathing following resection and reconstruction.

◆ The goal should be extubation at the end of the procedure for all patients undergoing tracheal resection.

◆ The area below the obstruction is isolated first so that transection of the trachea can be performed at any point and an airway can be introduced across the operative field if the degree of obstruction increases.

◆ Sterile anesthesia tubing, connectors, and ETTs are available on the operative field.

◆ At the time of tracheal division, the orotracheal tube is pulled back or removed and a sterile, cuffed, flexible, armored ETT is inserted into the distal airway across the operative field.

◆ Sterile connecting tubing is passed to the anesthesiologist to allow ventilation of the patient.

◆ This armored tube is removed whenever necessary for suctioning or placement of sutures.

◆ Toward completion of the operation, the original ETT is advanced into the distal airway and the anastomotic sutures tied.

▲ Before having the anesthesiologist pull the ETT back into the upper airway or larynx, we tie a red rubber catheter to the end of the tube and keep this in the operative field to assist in pulling the ETT back down into the field before tying down the anastomotic sutures.

◆ If transthoracic resection (via right thoracotomy) is performed close to the carina, the ETT is passed into the left main bronchus and that lung alone is ventilated.

▲ If the partial pressure of oxygen decreases toward unsatisfactory levels, a previously isolated right main pulmonary artery is temporarily clamped to eliminate the shunt through the right lung (rarely required).

◆ High-frequency ventilation is a useful adjunct, especially in complex carinal reconstruction.

2. Anatomic Mobilization

◆ The length of trachea that can be resected safely in an individual varies widely with age, posture, body habitus, extent of disease, and prior tracheal surgery.

◆ Attention must be paid to the lateral blood supply during tracheal mobilization.

◆ Mobilization of the proximal and distal segments should occur on the anterior and posterior portion of the airway.

◆ Use of blunt finger dissection on the anterior portion of the trachea moving downward toward the carina (mediastinoscopy plane) allows simple, safe anterior mobilization.

◆ Cervical flexion, combined with hilar and pericardial mobilization plus division of the pulmonary ligament, allows lengths of 5 to 6 cm of trachea to be removed by the transthoracic approach.

▲ Hilar release requires sternotomy or thoracotomy.

3. Surgical Approaches

◆ Lesions in the upper half of the trachea that are known to be benign are best approached cervically (Fig. 11-1). If a malignant lesion is present, one must be prepared for a cervicomediastinal and, possibly, a transthoracic approach. If a postoperative temporary tracheostomy stoma is required after a difficult tracheal anastomosis, the incision must be planned so that a stoma can be made away from the incision.

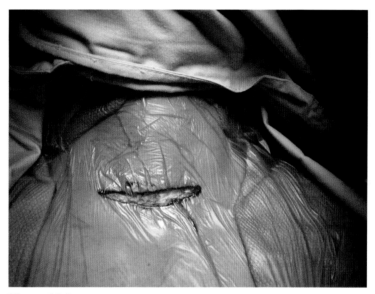

Figure 11-1

- If the initial dissection through the neck indicates need for further exposure, the upper sternum is split to a point just beyond the angle of Louis. Because the great vessels present anteriorly, division of more than the upper sternum is not helpful; division simply allows room to maneuver in managing the more distal trachea. Innominate vein division also does not add anything to the exposure.
- Rarely, this incision must be extended as a full sternotomy to permit additional mobilization of the intrathoracic trachea by freeing the hilus of the lung. Such an incision permits wide exposure of the entire trachea from cricoid to carina. This is almost never necessary in benign stenosis. If extirpative surgery and terminal tracheostomy are expected, the incision should avoid a vertical limb, even if sternal division is required.
- Neoplastic lesions of the lower half of the trachea are most easily approached directly through a high right posterolateral thoracotomy incision (third, fourth, or fifth interspace). Cervical flexion delivers sufficient trachea into the mediastinum so that lower tracheal tumors are usually approachable completely through the right side of the chest without a sternal component. Median sternotomy with dissection between the superior vena cava and aorta, and anterior and posterior pericardial division, provides access to the lower trachea and carina, but the exposure is poor for extensive dissection or complex reconstruction. It is possible to excise even low benign lesions from the anterior cervical approach.

4. Tracheal Resection

- For tracheal tumors, proximal and distal resection margins can be decided based on intra-operative flexible bronchoscopy through an ETT placed proximal to the tumor. A 25-gauge needle is passed through the anterior tracheal wall from the outside into the lumen while being visualized by the bronchoscope to decide the proximal and distal tracheal resection margins (Fig. 11-2). The area is marked from the outside with a fine suture in a ring of cartilage prior to removing the needle.
- Distal resection should always be performed first in order to pass the sterile ETT into the distal airway and allow ventilation during proximal resection.
- For benign stenoses, the resection is performed ring by ring, inspecting the internal airway diameter and assessing the ability of the airway to come together as well as the resulting tension.
    - ▲ It is always possible to remove more trachea; however, once a piece of airway is resected, it cannot be replaced
- In a long stenosis, if one is unsure where the distal margin will be, it is safest to transect the airway in the middle of the stenosis and then deal with the distal resection once the distal airway has been intubated through the field.
- Dissection should proceed from normal trachea to the scarred trachea. In tracheal stenosis, dissection is kept very close to the scarred area of trachea to avoid injury to the recurrent laryngeal nerves. No attempt is made to visualize the nerves; rather, dissection is kept as close to the airway as possible, allowing the nerves to fall away from the trachea as the scarred lateral tissue is dissected off of it.
- Attention must be paid not to damage the lateral blood supply of the area of trachea that is to remain. Circumferential dissection should be attempted only at the area of trachea to be resected and for a distance not exceeding 1 to 2 cm above and below the resection margins.
- The proximal and distal resection margins are cut sharply using a scalpel.
- In cases where the trachea is extremely calcified or too hard to cut using a scalpel secondary to fibrosis, parts of the resection margin can be cut with scissors, a drill, or small bone cutters.

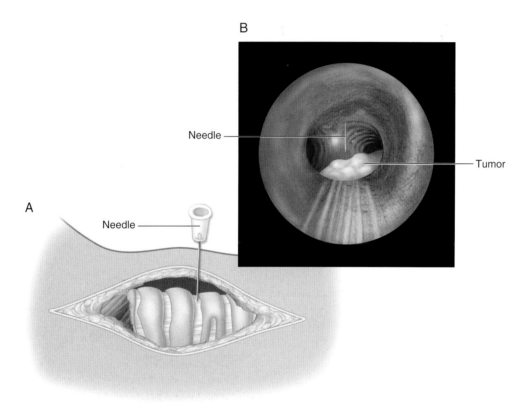

Figure 11-2

5. Resection and Reconstruction of the Upper Trachea

♦ The patient is positioned supine with an inflatable bag beneath the shoulders. This will permit neck extension during the mobilization and resection and also allows neck flexion (by letting the bag down) during tying of the knots for the anastomosis.

♦ A low cervical collar incision is used (see Fig. 11-1). The site of incision should be based on the expected area of resection estimated from preoperative bronchoscopy. The platysma is divided. Subplatysmal flaps are raised. The upper flap is raised with or without circumcising an existing tracheostomy incision or including it in the original incision. If the lesion is high, benign, and short, only a limited field is required.

♦ Dissection is confined chiefly to the midline, the upper subplatysmal flap being raised to the level of the cricoid and the lower to the sternal notch to allow dissection in the pretracheal plane as needed (Fig. 11-3).

♦ The strap muscles are divided in the midline.

♦ In the cervical trachea, the thyroid isthmus is divided in the midline, oversewn, and then retracted laterally.

♦ Dense scar is often present in association with benign stenosis, and dissection is performed close to the trachea to avoid damage to the recurrent nerves, especially near the cricoid.

♦ Isolation and visualization of the nerves are avoided because to do so increases the danger of injury. Freeing the trachea below the lesion early allows easy establishment of airway control (Fig. 11-4) and expedites dissection of a cicatrized segment from the esophagus.

♦ Mobilization is undertaken as required anterior and posterior to the trachea both proximally and distally. Horizontal mattress traction sutures of 2-0 Vicryl (Braided Polyglactin, Ethicon, Somerville, NJ) (surrounding one ring of trachea) are placed laterally at the 3- and 9-o'clock positions of the proximal and distal resection margins, one to two rings away from the site of the planned anastomosis (Fig. 11-5). Tentative approximation with traction sutures, while the neck is flexed by the anesthesiologist demonstrates whether approximation can be accomplished or whether further dissection is necessary.

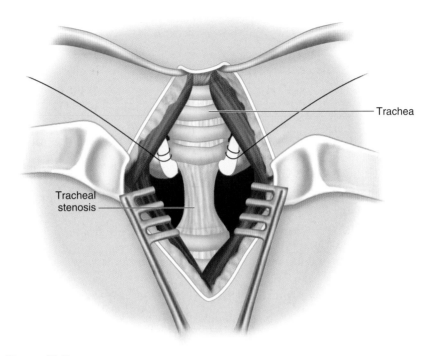

Figure 11-3

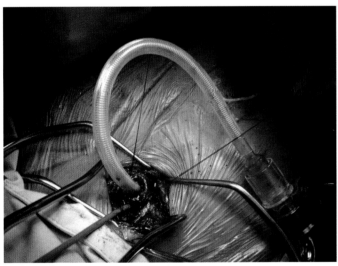

Figure 11-4

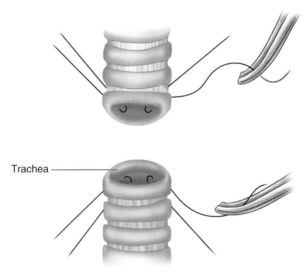

Figure 11-5

- A single layer of anastomotic sutures is placed in interrupted fashion so that the knots are tied on the outside (Fig. 11-6).
- Our preferred suture is 4-0 Vicryl.
- Interrupted, simple sutures are placed starting at the middle of the membranous wall.
- Sutures are placed 3 to 4 mm apart and 3 to 4 mm from the edge (membranous wall) or around or through one cartilaginous ring (cartilaginous trachea) (Fig. 11-7A)
- Sutures continue laterally until the corner is reached.
- The circumference is divided into four parts, and each quarter is completed separately (see Fig. 11-7B).
- The posterior quarters are completed first. The sutures are snapped with a hemostat, and each hemostat is sequentially clipped to the drapes around the anastomosis (Fig. 11-8).
- The ETT is pulled down through the anastomosis before tying down the lateral stay sutures by pulling on the red rubber catheter attached to the end of the tube. The suture holding the red rubber catheter to the tube is then cut and the catheter removed.
- The thyroid bag is let down by the anesthesiologist or circulating nurse.
- The neck is flexed by the anesthesiologist. Folded blankets are placed beneath the head to support it in the flexed position.
- The lateral stay sutures are tied to take tension off the anastomotic sutures.
- Tying of the sutures occurs in the opposite order from which they were inserted. This begins with the anterior sutures and finishes in the posterior midline.
- The posterior sutures become inaccessible to direct vision during tying and must not break.
- The anastomosis is tested under water by asking the anesthesiologist to let down the ETT cuff until a leak is heard, then occlude the patient's mouth and nose, and insufflate to 30 cm H_2O airway pressure while the surgeon inspects for bubbles at the anastomosis.
- The thyroid isthmus is reapproximated over cervical anastomoses.
- Strap muscles are reapproximated in the midline and can be used to cover the anastomosis, and the platysma and skin are then closed in the standard fashion.
- A "guardian" chin stitch of No. 2 Ti-Cron (braided polyester suture, Covidien, Mansfield, MA) is placed between the skin overlying the submental crease and the presternal skin.

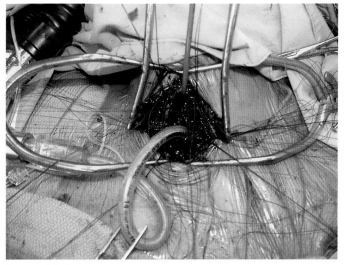

Figure 11-6

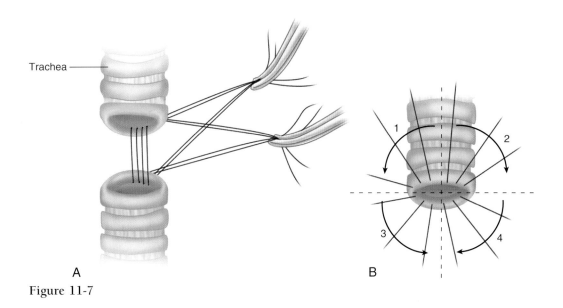

Trachea

A   B

Figure 11-7

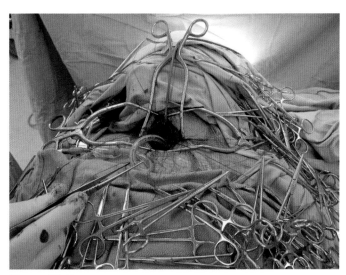

Figure 11-8

6. Subglottic Stenosis

- Subglottic stenosis occurs from prolonged oral intubation, erosion of tracheostomy through first tracheal ring, or as an idiopathic condition seen most commonly in young women. It can also occur secondary to trauma.
- To remove the area of stenosis, the anterior subglottic larynx is resected; and, in cases in which the stenosis is circumferential, the posterior cricoid lamina has traditionally been bared but preserved to protect the recurrent laryngeal nerves (Fig. 11-9).
- We use a modification of the standard technique of anterior cricoid resection to address this condition (tailored cricoplasty). Once the anterior cricoid is removed, a submucosal resection of thickened tissue is performed on the remaining cricoid (Fig. 11-10). The inner third to

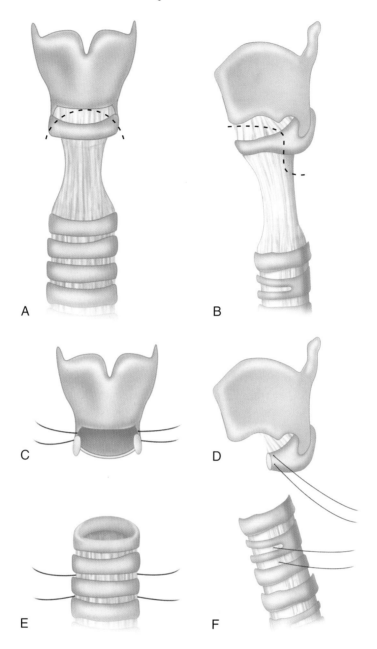

Figure 11-9

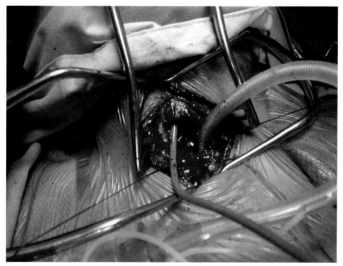

Figure 11-10

half of the cricoid cartilage is carefully removed (Fig. 11-11). The exposed cricoid cartilage is resurfaced by advancing the preserved mucosa over the cricoid with interrupted 5-0 chromic sutures (Fig. 11-12). This results in an additional horizontal enlargement of 4 to 5 mm in most patients (Fig. 11-13).

7. Reconstruction of the Lower Trachea

- ◆ Lower tracheal resection and reconstruction can be performed using an anterior approach (cervical incision with sternotomy or hemisternotomy) or via right thoracotomy.
- ◆ Following confirmation of the extent of an airway tumor, anatomic mobilization is usually accomplished before severing the trachea.
- ◆ If obstruction appears to be imminent during mobilization, the trachea is transected and distally intubated.
- ◆ If the line of transection is supracarinal, the left main bronchus is intubated.
- ◆ Access to the subcarinal lymph nodes and lower paratracheal nodes is excellent. However, one should rarely remove these nodes secondary to the blood supply they provide.
- ◆ The left recurrent nerve lies directly adjacent to the trachea and should be sacrificed deliberately only if required. Preoperative verification of a functioning right recurrent laryngeal nerve is required before sacrificing the left nerve.
- ◆ Cervical flexion by the anesthetist devolves a fair segment of trachea into the chest even in the lateral position, and this, in combination with release maneuvers permits end-to-end anastomosis.
- ◆ A pedicled flap should always be placed around intrathoracic anastomoses.
  - ▲ This typically consists of a carefully pedicled pericardial fat pad or pleura.
  - ▲ If intercostal muscle is used, care should be taken to ensure that the periosteum is not included because bone formation is deleterious to tracheal anastomotic healing.

8. Extensive Lesions

- ◆ One sees few benign lesions or potentially curable malignant lesions that require resection of lengths of trachea and still leave a functional larynx, in which end-to-end reconstruction may not be done by present methods. In these rare cases, one can carefully consider a prosthetic replacement or allograft.
- ◆ The best alternatives are T-tubes for benign lesions and irradiation for malignant lesions that are unresectable because of their length.

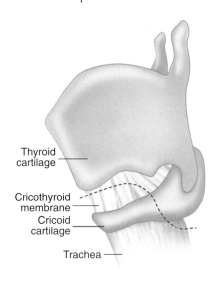

Thyroid cartilage

Cricothyroid membrane

Cricoid cartilage

Trachea

Figure 11-11

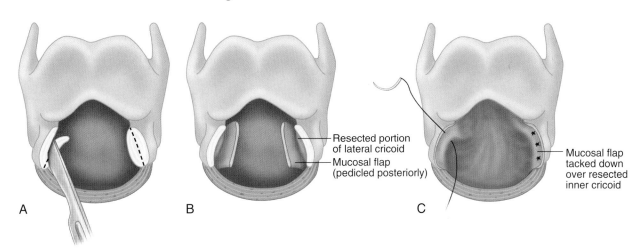

Resected portion of lateral cricoid

Mucosal flap (pedicled posteriorly)

Mucosal flap tacked down over resected inner cricoid

A   B   C

Figure 11-12

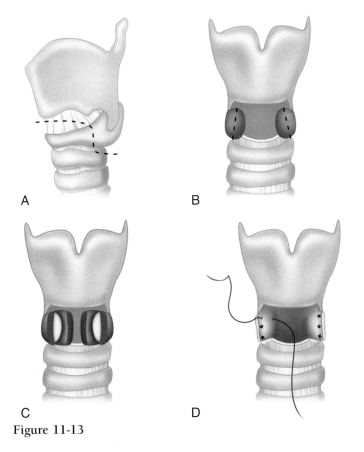

A   B

C   D

Figure 11-13

9. Tracheal-Release Maneuvers

- Neck flexion (Fig. 11-14)
- Blunt anterior mobilization using the surgeon's finger or a mediastinoscope (Fig. 11-15)
- Chin stitch placed at the end of the procedure reminds the patient to keep the neck flexed and avoid tension on the anastomosis (Fig. 11-16)
  - ▲ Stitch between submental crease and skin of the anterior chest wall.
  - ▲ Does not require the extreme situation described by others that consists of suturing the chin to the chest wall.
- Suprahyoid laryngeal release
- Mobilization of inferior pulmonary ligament
- Hilar release: U-shaped pericardial incision below the inferior pulmonary ligament
- Complete incision of pericardium around hilum (preserve a posteriorly based pedicle that includes the bronchial vessels and lymphatics)

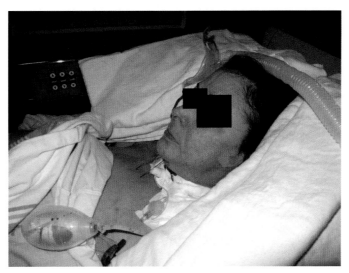

Figure 11-14

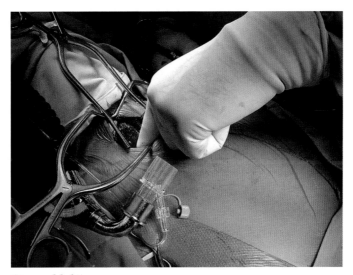

Figure 11-15

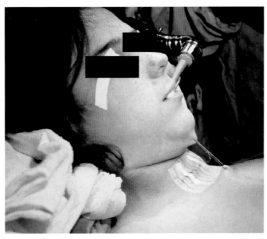

Figure 11-16

Step 4. Postoperative Care

- Every attempt should be made to extubate the patient in the operating room.
- Flexible bronchoscopy is performed in the operating room before extubation to clear secretions and blood as well as to assess the anastomosis.
- Tracheostomy is avoided after tracheal reconstruction to avoid drying of secretions or contamination of the anastomosis. On rare occasions, it may be necessary.
- Mechanism returns
- Aggressive pulmonary toilet (repeat flexible bronchoscopy may rarely be required)
- Incentive spirometry
- Aggressive chest physiotherapy
- To prevent postoperative laryngeal edema:
  - ▲ Provide racemic epinephrine.
  - ▲ Minimize intraoperative and postoperative IV fluids.
  - ▲ Elevate the head of the bed.
  - ▲ Minimize talking.
  - ▲ Provide 24 hours of IV steroids.
    - Decadron 10 mg IV in the operating room
    - Decadron 4 mg IV every 6 hours, three doses postoperatively
  - ▲ Maintain head in flexion.
  - ▲ Use chin stitch to remind the patient of the importance of head positioning (7 days).
- Flexible bronchoscopy in operating room under topical anesthesia at 7 days to ensure proper healing of anastomosis
  - ▲ If the patient is healing well, chin stitch is cut in the operating room.

Step 5. Pearls and Pitfalls

- Always avoid tension on anastomosis (use release maneuvers when necessary).
- Use sequential resection of tracheal rings (for benign lesions) to ensure that the anastomosis will come together without undue tension.
  - ▲ It is always possible to remove more trachea; however, once it is resected, it cannot be replaced.
  - ▲ Test the ability of the anastomosis to come together with lateral traction sutures on proximal and distal ends of resection while the anesthesiologist flexes the neck.
- Avoid lateral dissection of trachea to avoid devascularization.
- Sharp dissection close to the trachea to avoid recurrent laryngeal nerves
- Flex the neck before tying down the knots of the anastomosis.
- Use interrupted, absorbable suture.
- Place knots on the outside of anastomosis.
- One can use a pedicled, vascularized tissue flap to buttress the anastomosis.
  - ▲ Rotated strap muscle for cervical resection
  - ▲ Pericardial fat pad for mediastinal or carinal resection
  - ▲ Omentum for previously radiated resection
- Pitfalls—radiotherapy, steroids, quadriplegia

Suggested Readings

Ashiku SK, Kuzucu A, Grillo HC, et al. Idiopathic laryngotracheal stenosis: Effective definitive treatment with laryngotracheal resection. J Thorac Cardiovasc Surg 2004;127:99-107.

El-Baz N, Jensik R, Faber LP, et al. One-lung high-frequency ventilation for tracheoplasty and bronchoplasty. Ann Thorac Surg 1982;34:564-571.

Courand L, Brunteau A, Martigne C, et al. Prevention and treatment of complications and sequelae of tracheal resection and anastomosis. Int Surg 1982;67:235-239.

Donahue DM, Grillo HC, Wain JC, et al. Reoperative tracheal resection and reconstruction for unsuccessful repair of postintubation stenosis. J Thorac Cardiovasc Surg 1997;114:934-939.

Grillo HC. Circumferential resection and reconstruction of mediastinal and cervical trachea. Ann Surg 1965;162:374.

Grillo HC. Surgical approaches to the trachea. Surg Gynecol Obstet 1969;129:347.

Grillo HC. Surgery of the trachea. Curr Probl Surg 1970;7:3.

Grillo HC. Tracheal tumors: Surgical management. Ann Thorac Surg 1978;26:112.

Grillo HC. Carinal reconstruction. Ann Thorac Surg 1982;34:356.

Grillo HC. Primary reconstruction of airway resection of subglottic laryngeal and upper tracheal stenosis. Ann Thorac Surg 1982;33:3.

Grillo HC. Development of tracheal surgery: A historical review. I. Techniques of tracheal surgery. Ann Thorac Surg 2003;75:610.

Grillo HC, Donahue DM, Mathisen DJ, et al. Postintubation tracheal stenosis. Treatment and results. J Thorac Cardiovasc Surg 1995;109:486-493.

Grillo HC, Mathisen DJ. Primary tracheal tumors: Treatment and results. Ann Thorac Surg 1990;49:69-77.

Grillo HC, Mathisen DJ, Ashiku SK, et al. Successful treatment of idiopathic laryngotracheal stenosis by resection and primary anastomosis. Ann Otol Rhinol Laryngol 2003;112:798-800.

Grillo HC, Mathisen DJ, Wain JC. Laryngotracheal resection and reconstruction for subglottic stenosis. Ann Thorac Surg 1992;53:54-63.

Grillo HC, Zannini P, Michelassi F. Complications of tracheal reconstruction. Incidence, treatment and prevention. J Thorac Cardiovasc Surg 1986;91:322-328.

Mathisen DJ, Grillo HC, Wain JW, et al. Management of acquired nonmalignant tracheoesophageal fistula. Ann Thorac Surg 1991;52:759-765.

Wilson RS. Anesthetic management for tracheal reconstruction. In Grillo HC, Eschapasse H, eds. International Trends in General Thoracic Surgery, vol. 2. Philadelphia: WB Saunders; 1987:3.

CHAPTER 12

PANCOAST TUMORS

Frank C. Detterbeck

Step 1. Surgical Anatomy

◆ A Pancoast tumor is a lung cancer arising in the apex of the lung that involves structures of the apical chest wall.[1] In contrast to the original definition, involvement of the brachial plexus and the stellate ganglion is no longer absolutely required. This change has come from a more detailed understanding of the structures of the thoracic inlet, which is divided into several compartments (Table 12-1, Fig. 12-1). The many important structures coursing through this area makes the anatomy of this area complex (Fig. 12-2). Surgery for Pancoast tumors also requires a clear understanding of the posterior ribs and spine (Fig. 12-3).

Step 2. Preoperative Considerations

◆ There are so many different approaches to Pancoast tumors that choosing an incision is confusing. The traditional high posterolateral thoracotomy has some advantages but provides limited access to many structures of the thoracic inlet. Many variations of anterior approaches have been described. The incision in the neck can be either along the anterior border of the sternocleidomastoid muscle (SCM) or just above the clavicle. The incision continues down the midline and then extends laterally just below the clavicle with removal of the clavicle,[2] into the first intercostal space (ICS),[3] the second ICS,[4] the fourth ICS,[5] or hemiclamshell,[6] or simply into a full sternotomy. Furthermore, although it is ideal for a complete resection to be accomplished through one incision, one should not hesitate to use a combined anterior-posterior approach or an additional thoracotomy.

TABLE 12-1. Compartments of the Thoracic Inlet

COMPARTMENT	BOUNDARIES (ALONG FIRST RIB)	INCLUDED STRUCTURES
Anterior	Sternum to anterior edge of anterior scalene muscle	Sternocleidomastoid and omohyoid muscles, jugular and subclavian veins and branches
Middle	Anterior scalene muscle up to posterior border of middle scalene muscle	Anterior and middle scalene muscles, subclavian artery and branches, phrenic nerve, trunks of brachial plexus
Posterior	Behind middle scalene muscle	Posterior scalene muscle, posterior scapular artery, nerve roots of brachial plexus, long thoracic, spinal accessory nerves, sympathetic chain, stellate ganglion, neural foramina, vertebral bodies

From Detterbeck FC. Changes in the treatment of Pancoast tumors. Ann Thorac Surg 2003;75:1900-1907.

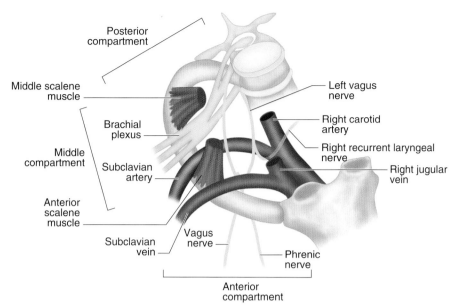

Figure 12-1

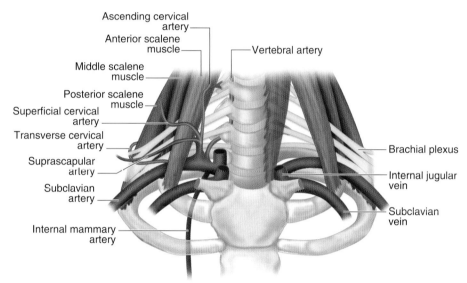

Figure 12-2

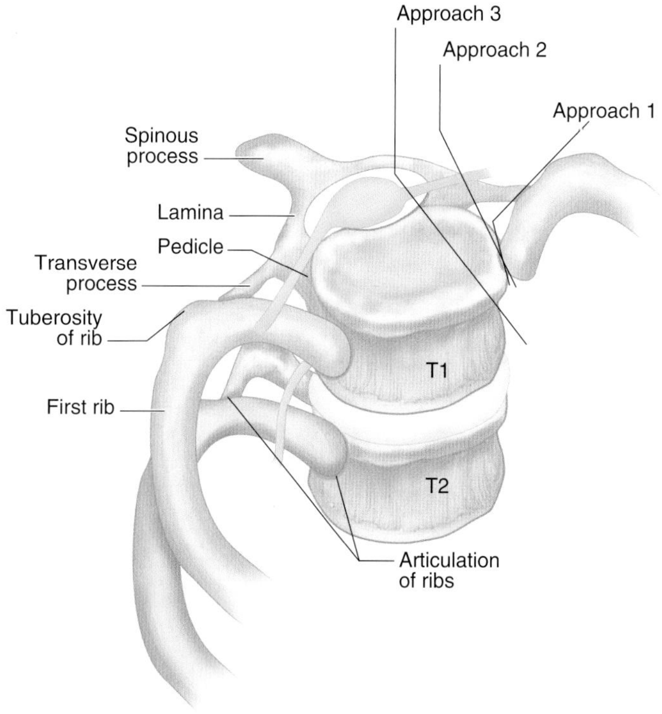

Figure 12-3

♦ The choice of incision is dictated by the characteristics of the tumor, which vary from patient to patient. The tumor location and resulting anatomic issues can be divided into several major categories, as described in this chapter.

1. Resection of the Anterior Chest Wall

Definition

♦ Tumors involving the anterior first rib from the manubrium up to and including insertion of the anterior scalene muscle

Recommended Incision

♦ Midline division of the manubrium is done with a lateral extension into the ICS below the tumor. The neck incision is generally made along the anterior border of the SCM because exposure of more lateral structures (i.e., the middle portion of the thoracic inlet) is not needed. The midline manubrial incision is useful because exposure of the innominate vein is usually required. The lateral extension of the incision allows lateral division of ribs and control of the axillary vessels for tumor resection together with the subclavian vein (or artery).

2. Access to Midline Structures

Definition

♦ Tumors involving a vertebral body, involving nerve roots as they exit the neural foramina, or requiring control of the innominate artery or vein

Recommended Incision

♦ Midline division of the manubrium, usually combined with an incision along the anterior border of the SCM, is recommended. (Alternatively, access to the innominate artery and vein can be achieved after resection of the clavicle and resection of the first rib starting right at the edge of the manubrium.)

3. Access to Lateral Structures

Definition

♦ Tumor involving the middle portion of thoracic inlet, lateral brachial plexus, lateral subclavian artery or vein

Recommended Incision

♦ Supraclavicular incision and partial sternotomy are recommended. (Alternatively, an incision along the anterior border of SCM extending to an infraclavicular incision with removal of the medial half of the clavicle can be used.)

4. Invasion of Posterior Chest Wall/Neural Foramina

Definition

♦ Tumor growing adjacent to or through the neural foramina

Recommended Incision

- Posterior approach, for example, a simple posterolateral (Shaw-Paulson) approach (either alone or a combined posterior and anterior approach)

5. Extensive Hilar Involvement

Definition

- Tumor extension to hilum or hilar node involvement (e.g., requiring a sleeve lobectomy)

Recommended Incision

- Midline division of the sternum, either with a lateral incision into the fourth ICS or a full sternotomy, is recommended. (Alternatively, a thoracotomy can be performed as a separate incision.)

Step 3. Operative Steps

1. Anterior Chest Wall Involvement

Superficial Structures

- An incision is made along the anterior border of the SCM (or modified with a supraclavicular incision) (Fig. 12-4).
- Attachment of strap muscles is divided (with or without omohyoid).
- Midline partial sternotomy is made through the manubrium.
- L-shaped extension is made into the second ICS (level modified as needed).
- Sternal attachments of the pectoralis major muscle are detached.
- Most of the pectoralis major muscle attachment to the clavicle is preserved.
- Pectoralis major muscle is divided between fibers.
- Internal mammary artery/vein (IMA/V) is divided (rarely, the proximal portion is dissected free and preserved).

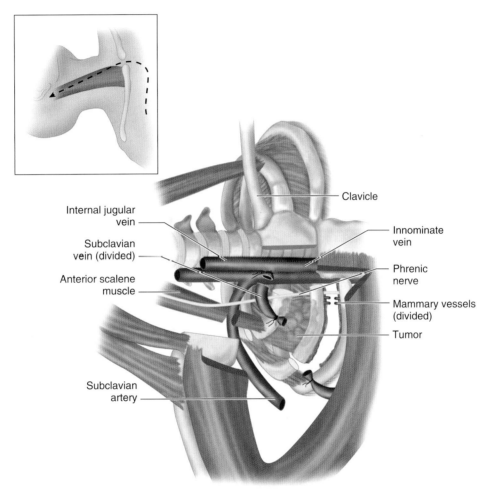

Internal jugular
vein

Subclavian
vein (divided)

Anterior scalene
muscle

Subclavian
artery

Clavicle

Innominate
vein

Phrenic
nerve

Mammary vessels
(divided)

Tumor

Figure 12-4

Mobilization of Bony Parts

◆ Costal cartilage of involved ribs is divided (see Fig. 12-4, inset).
◆ Manubrium/clavicle is raised by progressive dissection of ligamentous and muscular (subclavius) attachments on the undersurface of the clavicle.
◆ Axillary vessels are dissected free as they exit under the clavicle.
◆ After mobilization of manubrium/clavicle, the anterior scalene muscle is detached from the first rib (as needed).
◆ Lateral division of ribs is performed underneath mobilized pectoralis major/minor muscle (or through a small axillary incision as needed).

Deeper Dissection

◆ Internal jugular vein is dissected and divided if the tumor extends to the venous confluence (thoracic duct is ligated if the tumor is on the left side).
◆ Phrenic nerve is identified along the anterior scalene muscle in the neck and followed into the chest (Fig. 12-5).
◆ Innominate or subclavian vein or both are dissected medially.
◆ Axillary vein is ligated and subclavian vein is ligated medially (usually involved if there is anterior chest wall involvement).
◆ Vagus nerve is identified and generously dissected.
◆ Innominate or subclavian artery or both are dissected medially, as is the carotid artery.
◆ On the right side, the right recurrent nerve must be preserved as it loops under the proximal subclavian artery (unless involved).
◆ The IMA is divided at the origin (if needed).
◆ Vertebral artery is preserved (unless involved).
◆ Thyrocervical artery is exposed and preserved (unless involved).
◆ Use a proximal/distal clamp and divide the subclavian artery (if involved).
◆ Formal lobectomy is performed through an anterior chest wall opening.
◆ Resection of the involved anterior chest wall/thoracic inlet structures en bloc with upper lobe is performed (Fig. 12-6).
◆ Formal lymph node dissection or systematic sampling of hilar and mediastinal node stations (including station 7) is performed.

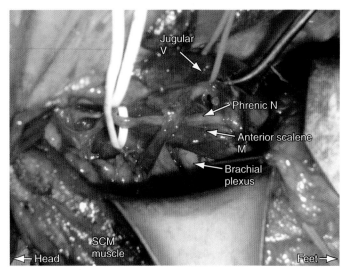

Figure 12-5

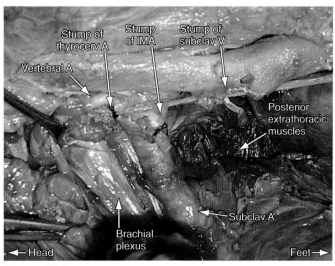

Figure 12-6

Reconstruction and Closure

- No reconstruction of the subclavian vein is necessary.
- Direct reanastomosis or interposition graft of subclavian artery (usually 6- or 8-mm polytetrafluoroethylene [PTFE]) is performed.
- Reattach the manubrium with three or four wires (or No. 5 heavy suture).
- Place a chest tube and a lateral subpectoral drain.
- Close pectoralis muscle fascia.

Key Points

- Cervical incision can be modified to supraclavicular incision if there is also involvement of the middle compartment; intercostal space incision is chosen based on the ribs involved.
- Midline division of manubrium usually is needed to expose the innominate vessels.
- Early division of costal cartilage is crucial to allow retraction of the manubrium/clavicle.
- Manubrium/clavicle can be retracted superiorly or inferiorly as needed.
- Dissection of innominate/subclavian vessels must be generous to provide retraction and easy exposure.
- Formal lobectomy is relatively easy if the second rib is resected, but it can be accomplished if only the first is resected.
- Usually, pure anterior thoracic inlet tumors have no brachial plexus involvement.

2. Access to Midline Structures

Superficial Structures

- Incision is made along the anterior border of the SCM (or modified to a supraclavicular incision) (see Fig. 12-4, inset).
- Attachment of strap muscles is divided (with or without omohyoid).
- A midline partial sternotomy through the manubrium is performed.
- L-shaped extension is continued into the second ICS (level modified as needed).
- IMA/V is divided (rarely, the proximal portion is dissected free and preserved).

Mobilization of Bony Parts

- Ribs must be divided on the anterior/medial side of the tumor before significant retraction is feasible.
- Anterior/medial division of ribs can be accomplished through an L-shaped lateral extension of the incision, through a small axillary incision, or through a previously performed posterior incision.
- Division of part of the intercostal muscle is needed to allow independent retraction of the manubrium/clavicle.
- Generally, lateral and downward retraction of the manubrium/clavicle is best.

Deeper Dissection

- Formal lobectomy with lymph node dissection or systematic sampling of hilar and mediastinal node is accomplished through partial sternotomy.
- Phrenic nerve is identified and dissected from the anterior scalene muscle into the chest.
- Innominate, subclavian, and internal jugular veins are dissected generously, and the thoracic duct is ligated if the tumor is on the left side.
- Innominate, carotid, and subclavian arteries are dissected generously.
- Vagus nerve is identified and generously dissected.
- Right recurrent nerve must be preserved as it loops under the proximal subclavian artery.
- Internal mammary artery is divided at its origin (if needed).
- Vertebral artery is preserved (unless involved) (Fig. 12-7).
- Medial portion of the lower brachial plexus is exposed posterior and superior to the subclavian artery.
- Divide ligamentous attachments of the head of rib to vertebral body and to transverse process (as dictated by bony involvement) (see Fig. 12-3)
- Retraction of mobilized ribs allows exposure of proximal upper thoracic nerve roots, which are divided at the level of the neural foramina as needed.
- Involved nerve roots are transected again lateral to the tumor.
- Trachea and esophagus can be retracted to the contralateral side (carefully protecting the left recurrent nerve) to expose the vertebral bodies for resection (if needed) (Fig. 12-8).
- Tumor with posterior rib involvement can be removed anteriorly en bloc with formally dissected lobe once the involved ribs and nerve roots have been divided medially and laterally.

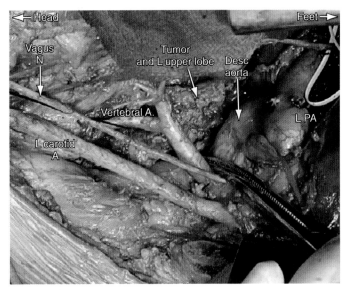

Figure 12-7

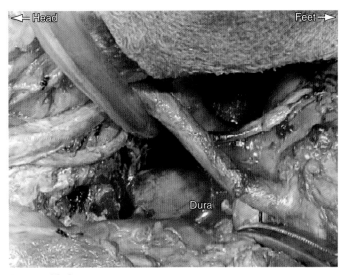

Figure 12-8

Reconstruction and Closure

◆ Reattach the manubrium/clavicle with three or four wires (or No. 5 heavy suture).

Key Points

◆ Early division of ribs is crucial to allow retraction of the manubrium/clavicle.
◆ Generous dissection of the innominate, subclavian, and carotid vessels (including on the contralateral side) provides mobility and prevents the need for division of the left innominate vein to improve retraction.
◆ Incision along the anterior border of the SCM provides excellent exposure of the vertebral bodies and attachments, but limits exposure of the brachial plexus lateral to the anterior scalene muscle.

3. Access to Lateral Structures

Superficial Structures

◆ Incision is made 2 cm above the medial half to two thirds of the clavicle, midline partial sternotomy through the manubrium, and L-shaped extension into the ICS (level modified as needed) (Fig. 12-9, inset).
◆ Attachment of strap muscles is divided (including the omohyoid).
◆ SCM muscle is divided.

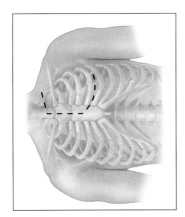

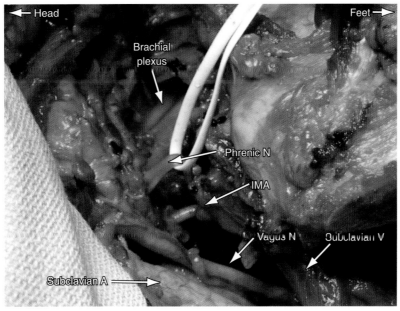

Figure 12-9

Mobilization of Bony Parts

♦ Ribs must be divided on the anterior/medial side of the tumor before significant retraction is feasible.
♦ Anterior/medial division of ribs is performed through an extension of the incision into the deltopectoral groove, through a lateral extension into an ICS, through a separate small axillary incision, or through a previously performed separate posterior incision.

Deeper Dissection

♦ Phrenic nerve is identified along the anterior scalene muscle (see Fig. 12-9).
♦ Anterior scalene muscle is divided.
♦ Generous dissection and mobilization of innominate and subclavian vessels, internal jugular vein, and carotid artery are undertaken.
♦ Vagus nerve is identified and generously dissected.
♦ Right recurrent nerve must be preserved as it loops under the proximal subclavian artery.
♦ Internal mammary artery is divided at origin.
♦ Vertebral artery is preserved (unless involved).
♦ Thyrocervical artery is exposed; the suprascapular branch crosses over the anterior scalene muscle and often must be divided.
♦ Next branches of the subclavian artery (costocervical trunk and transverse colli artery) are usually too lateral to be involved.
♦ Entire arch of subclavian artery is dissected (or resected if involved).
♦ Brachial plexus is exposed posterior and superior to the subclavian artery, and any involved nerve roots are divided medial and lateral to the tumor (Fig. 12-10).
♦ Medial scalene muscle behind the brachial plexus is divided if involved; posterior scalene muscle behind medial scalene muscle usually is not involved.
♦ Ribs are disarticulated from the vertebral bodies–transverse processes (or divided posteriorly) as dictated by tumor involvement.
♦ Formal lobectomy is done through an upper sternotomy and anterior intercostal incision, including lymph node dissection or systematic sampling of hilar and mediastinal node stations.
♦ En bloc removal of the upper lobe, the involved anterior chest wall, and thoracic inlet structures is performed (see Fig. 12-10).

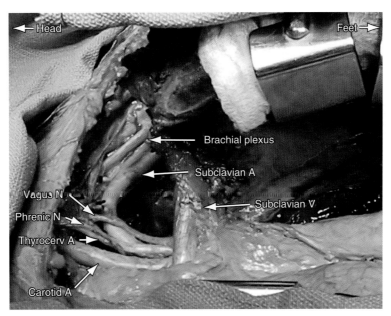

Figure 12-10

Reconstruction and Closure

♦ No reconstruction of the subclavian vein is necessary; direct reanastomosis or an interposition graft of subclavian artery can be used if resected.
♦ Reattach manubrium with three or four wires (or No. 5 heavy suture).
♦ Reattach SCM and strap muscles.

Key Points

♦ Early division of ribs is crucial to allow retraction of manubrium/clavicle.
♦ Usually, the jugular vein can be preserved if vessels are adequately mobilized.
♦ Extensive dissection of the phrenic nerve allows mobility and prevents nerve damage.
♦ Division of the anterior scalene muscle provides wide exposure to the arch of the subclavian artery and brachial plexus.

4. Alternative Approach to Lateral and Anterior Structures

Superficial Structures

♦ Incision is done along the anterior border of the SCM and extends laterally just below the clavicle (Fig. 12-11, inset).
♦ Divide SCM insertion onto clavicle and manubrium.
♦ Divide attachments of pectoralis major to clavicle.

Mobilization of Bony Parts

♦ Remove medial one half to two thirds of the clavicle (can be modified to simple division of the clavicle) (see Fig. 12-11).

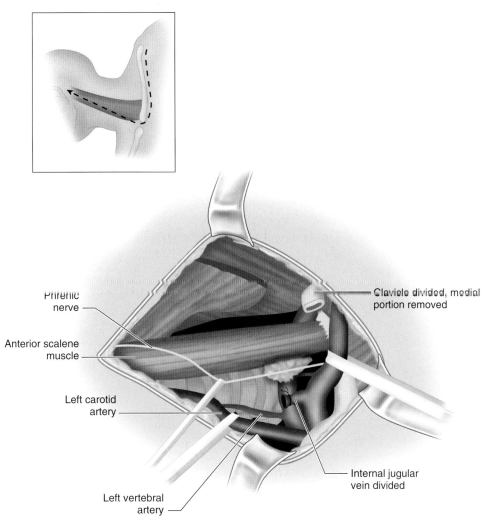

Phrenic
nerve

Anterior scalene
muscle

Left carotid
artery

Clavicle divided, medial
portion removed

Internal jugular
vein divided

Left vertebral
artery

Figure 12-11

Deeper Dissection

- Proceed as in "Access to Lateral Structures."

Reconstruction and Closure

- SCM is reattached to the pectoralis fascia.
- If the clavicle is merely divided, it can be reconstructed using plates and screws.

Key Points

- Removal of the clavicle results in moderate disability.
- Reconstruction of the clavicle is difficult.
- Exposure to lateral thoracic inlet, subclavian vessels, and brachial plexus is excellent.
- Exposure to medial innominate vein and subclavian artery is limited.
- Exposure of T2 or lower nerve root at the level of the foramen is limited unless anterior ribs are resected.
- Lobectomy is difficult and requires either removal of the upper anterior ribs or a separate thoracotomy.

5. Invasion of Posterior Chest Wall/Neural Foramina

Superficial Structures

- A posterolateral thoracotomy is performed, extending from the base of the neck around the tip of the scapula (halfway between the spinous processes and posterior edge of the scapula) (Fig. 12-12, inset)
- Divide trapezius and latissimus dorsi muscles.
- Divide rhomboid muscles; the serratus anterior muscle usually can be preserved.
- An incision in the fourth or fifth ICS, with digital exploration to define extent of chest wall involvement of tumor, is performed.

Mobilization of Bony Parts

- Laterally divide involved ribs at least 2 to 3 cm from the tumor (see Fig. 12-12).
- Ribs without neural foraminal involvement are mobilized by dividing ligamentous attachments between the rib and transverse processes.

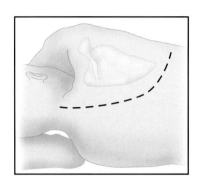

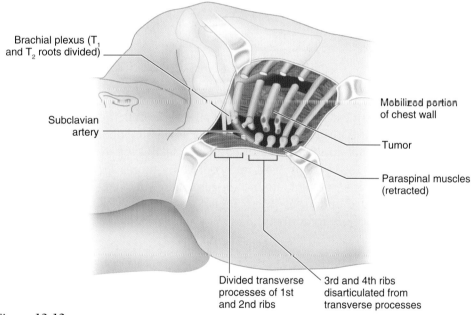

Brachial plexus (T₁
and T₂ roots divided)

Subclavian
artery

Divided transverse
processes of 1st
and 2nd ribs

3rd and 4th ribs
disarticulated from
transverse processes

Paraspinal muscles
(retracted)

Tumor

Mobilized portion
of chest wall

Figure 12-12

- Transverse processes and posterior laminae are divided as dictated by foraminal involvement.
- Final step is division of ligamentous attachments of head of ribs to vertebral bodies.
- If needed, a lateral partial vertebrectomy is performed instead.

Deeper Dissection

- After chest wall is mobilized, ligate and divide involved nerve roots medially.
- Divide nerve root attachments to brachial plexus laterally/superiorly.
- Inferior retraction of detached chest wall allows dissection of lobe/parietal pleura from the subclavian vessels.
- Proceed with standard lobectomy and mediastinal node sampling/dissection.

Reconstruction and Closure

- No reconstruction is needed for upper chest wall defects underneath the scapula.
- If ribs below the fourth rib are resected during reconstruction, nonabsorbable mesh is recommended to prevent subluxation of the tip of the scapula to the inside of remaining ribs.
- Mesh should be stretched taught with nonabsorbable sutures through the ends of divided ribs and transverse processes and around the remaining ribs.
- Drain is recommended underneath the scapula for 5 to 7 days.
- Closure of posterolateral thoracotomy incision is standard.

Key Points

- Formal lobectomy can be done either before or after the chest wall mobilization.
- Proximal exposure of the nerve roots is facilitated by division of posterior rib attachments or division of transverse processes.
- Exposure of subclavian vessels is limited and difficult until the tumor and ribs are mobilized out of the apex, making this incision a poor choice if there is subclavian vessel involvement.

6. Extensive Hilar Involvement

Superficial Structures

♦ Midline division of the sternum is done either with a lateral incision into the fourth ICS or with a full sternotomy.
♦ Neck incision is made along the anterior border of the SCM (or modified to the supraclavicular incision).
♦ Completion of dissection of superficial structures is as described in the section "Access to Midline Structures."

Mobilization of Bony Parts

♦ Ribs must be divided laterally to allow full retraction and exposure of the thoracic inlet.
♦ Often, lateral division of ribs can be accomplished from inside the thorax via the sternotomy incision.
♦ Approach to posterior upper ribs is as described in the section "Access to Midline Structures."

Deeper Dissection

♦ Mobilization of structures of the thoracic inlet is done as described in the section "Access to Midline Structures."
♦ Standard methods are used to accomplish a lobectomy or extended lobectomy via a sternotomy.

Reconstruction and Closure

♦ Standard sternotomy closure

Key Points

♦ Undue retraction of the upper chest wall can result in stretch injury to the brachial plexus.

Step 4. Postoperative Care

♦ Postoperative care is similar to that after a lobectomy in other circumstances. The amount of pain from anterior approaches is generally less than for a thoracotomy. A particular consideration is the risk of chylothorax. Injury to the phrenic or recurrent laryngeal nerves is also more common, and atelectasis or aspiration can complicate the course.

Step 5. Pearls and Pitfalls

♦ The bony structures complicate access to the thoracic inlet, and the number of major structures in a small space makes complete resection difficult. Most recurrences are local, often because of an incomplete resection stemming from limited experience and poor exposure. A full understanding of the anatomy and flexibility in the choice of incision, as well as a commitment to accomplish a complete resection, is crucial to achieve cure.

References

1. Detterbeck FC. Changes in the treatment of Pancoast tumors. Ann Thorac Surg 2003;75:1990-1997.
2. Dartevelle P, Chapelier A, Macchiarini P, et al. Anterior transcervical-thoracic approach for radical resection of lung tumors invading the thoracic inlet. J Thorac Cardiovasc Surg 1993;105:1025-1034.
3. Grunenwald D, Spaggiari L. Transmanubrial osteomuscular sparing approach for apical chest tumors. Ann Thorac Surg 1997;63:563-566.
4. Vanakesa T, Goldstraw P. Antero-superior approaches in the practice of thoracic surgery. Eur J Cardiothorac Surg 1999;15:774-780.
5. Masaoka A, Ito Y, Yasumitsu T. Anterior approach for tumor of the superior sulcus. J Thorac Cardiovasc Surg 1979;78:413-415.
6. Korst RJ, Burt ME. Cervicothoracic tumors: Results of resection by the "hemi-clamshell" approach. J Thorac Cardiovasc Surg 1998;115:286-295.

CHAPTER 13

RADIOFREQUENCY ABLATION

Michael S. Kent and Malcolm M. DeCamp

Step 1. Surgical Anatomy

- Surgical resection is the mainstay of treatment for patients with early-stage lung cancer.
- Radiofrequency ablation (RFA) is an appropriate alternative for patients who either refuse surgery or have a prohibitive risk for surgical resection. In our experience many patients who are considered "inoperable" on the basis of poor pulmonary function are acceptable candidates for a thoracoscopic wedge resection, a procedure that has a superior local control rate compared with RFA.
- Patients should be adequately staged before considering RFA. Those with suspected nodal involvement on the basis of computed tomography (CT) or positron emission tomography criteria should undergo invasive staging (either mediastinoscopy or endobronchial ultrasound) before RFA is offered to treat the primary lesion.
- Before RFA is done, tissue confirmation of malignancy is mandatory. A CT-guided needle biopsy can be scheduled at the same setting as the planned RFA. Ablation of pulmonary nodules without a tissue diagnosis will lead to unnecessary treatment of patients with benign disease.
- Characteristics of the primary tumor are critical for selecting patients for RFA. For example, tumors larger than 5 cm in diameter should not be treated with RFA given the high recurrence rate when tumors of this size are ablated. In addition, significant hemoptysis can occur after RFA in patients with central tumors.
- Patients with metastatic disease to the lungs can be considered for RFA, assuming they are not operative candidates and meet the accepted criteria for metastasectomy (e.g., good control of the primary tumor with limited disease in the chest). Patients with multiple pulmonary metastases should not be offered RFA unless all sites of disease are treatable.

Step 2. Preoperative Considerations

- RFA causes coagulative necrosis by heating tissue to a temperature of 60°C. RFA energy is produced by a generator, is dispersed through the active electrode of the RFA probe, and then travels to a "dispersive electrode" (the Bovie pad). The target tissue is heated as energy alternates between the probe and the dispersive electrode.

- ◆ Currently three probes are available for RFA of pulmonary lesions.
  - ▲ *Boston Scientific* (Natick, MA): This probe consists of expandable tines that assume an umbrella configuration. RFA energy is dispersed throughout the length of each tine. The tines can be expanded to a maximum length of 5 cm. Proper use of this probe will consist of deploying the probe into the center of the target lesion. The tines are then sequentially expanded so the entire volume of the lesion is treated (Fig. 13-1). This probe is impedance-based. Heating of the target tissue is maintained until the impedance measured across the probe rises to the appropriate level. Impedance, a measure of resistance to flow of RFA energy, will reach a plateau level as the tissue is coagulated and unable to maintain conduction.
  - ▲ *RITA* (Mountainview, CA): The design is similar to the Boston Scientific probe. However, the RITA probe is temperature-based. In this system, the tissue is considered ablated once it has been heated to a target temperature (usually 90°C) for a specified amount of time.
  - ▲ *Valley Laboratory* (Boulder City, CO): Unlike the Boston Scientific and RITA systems, this probe does not have expandable tines. Instead, the probe consists of either a single needle or an assembly of three needles that are placed within the tumor (Fig. 13-2). The distal 2.5 cm is uninsulated and represents the active portion of the electrode. The probe is continuously irrigated with ice water and is often referred to as a "cooltip" probe. Because the probe does not have tines, the distal end of the probe should be deployed to the depth of the target lesion. A 4.5-cm zone of ablation will extend around the probe. The Valley Lab probe is temperature-based.
- ◆ RFA is commonly used under CT guidance, although it can be used in the operating room through a thoracotomy.
- ◆ We have not found that RFA is appropriate to use during thoracoscopy. Tactile feedback is necessary to ensure that the probe is appropriately deployed within a collapsed lung. This can be quite difficult during a VATS procedure.

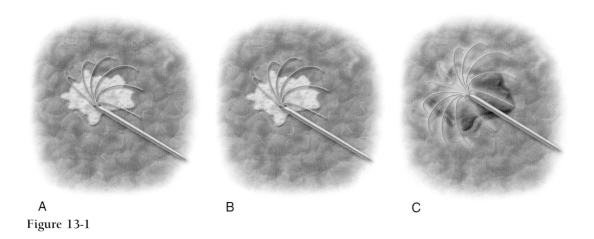

A   B   C

Figure 13-1

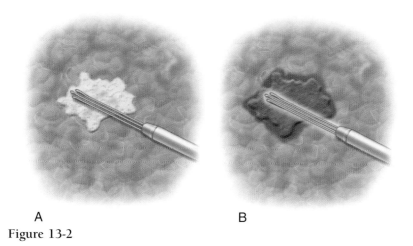

A   B

Figure 13-2

Step 3. Operative Steps

- We will describe the use of RFA under CT guidance.
- The procedure can be performed under conscious sedation or general anesthesia. General anesthesia should be considered if a longer procedure is anticipated (e.g., RFA is combined with a needle biopsy and placement of fiducial seeds for future stereotactic radiosurgery). General anesthesia may be necessary if the patient is unable to lie flat for the duration of the procedure. However, the use of positive-pressure ventilation likely increases the risk of procedure-related pneumothorax.
- The patient may be positioned prone, supine, or in a lateral position based on the location of the target lesion. The operator should remember that the clearance between the patient and the scanner is limited if the patient is in the lateral position (Fig. 13-3).
- We prefer to place the patient feet first into the scanner so that access to the airway is maintained. We do not routinely place an arterial line because this may inadvertently come out as the position of the patient within the scanner is adjusted.
- A pigtail catheter kit should be available for use. A small pneumothorax will make it much more difficult to place the probe properly. We have found that the probe will have a tendency to "bounce off" the visceral pleura if the lung is not expanded. In addition, the pneumothorax may expand during the treatment session, leading to a shift in the location of the lesion. For these reasons, we place a pigtail catheter even for a small pneumothorax.
- The depth from the skin to the target lesion is measured, and the RFA probe is deployed to this level. We typically perform an initial scan before the probe penetrates the pleura to ensure that the angle is appropriate.
- The probe tract can also be heated as the probe is removed to prevent seeding of the subcutaneous tissue with tumor cells.
- A posttreatment scan should also be taken to ensure that a pneumothorax has not developed. A small amount of parenchymal hemorrhage is often seen on this scan.
- Some staining of the endotracheal tube with blood is not uncommon after RFA treatment. A bronchoscope should be available for these situations.

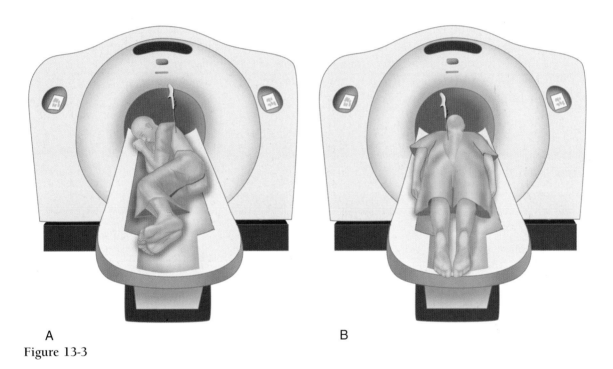

A

Figure 13-3

B

Step 4.   Postoperative Care

- ◆ A chest radiograph should be repeated 2 hours after the procedure. If no pneumothorax is present, or if it is stable, the patient may be discharged home
- ◆ Patients who require pigtail placement are admitted for observation. As for pulmonary resections, the catheter is placed to water seal if possible. On rare occasions the pigtail catheter is unable to control an air leak and a larger-bore chest tube is required.
- ◆ Chest pain and fever are not uncommon following RFA and should be discussed with the patient preoperatively.

Step 5. Pearls and Pitfalls

- ◆ If the target temperature cannot be reached, consider that one of the tines might be one of the following.
  - ▲ On a rib
  - ▲ In normal lung (which is difficult to heat because of air)
  - ▲ Near a blood vessel (which will serve as a heat sink)
  - ▲ Covered with an eschar
- ◆ Flushing the probe with water (to remove the eschar) or repositioning the probe may be useful. The operator may choose to delete temperature data from one of the tines and conclude the procedure if the target temperature has been reached with the other tines.
- ◆ Proper patient selection is critical. Central tumors or those adjacent to a major blood vessel should not be treated with RFA.
- ◆ Even a small pneumothorax should be evacuated before continuing with the RFA procedure.

Suggested Readings

Ambrogi M, Lucchi M, Dini P, et al. Percutaneous radiofrequency ablation of lung tumors: Results in the mid-term. Eur J Cardiothorac Surg 2006;30:177-183.

Dupuy D, DiPetrillo T, Gandhi S, et al. Radiofrequency ablation followed by conventional radiotherapy for medically inoperable stage I non–small cell lung cancer. Chest 2006;129:738-745.

Fernando H, de Hoyos A, Landreneau R, et al. Radiofrequency ablation for the treatment of non–small cell lung cancer in marginal surgical candidates. J Thorac Cardiovasc Surg 2005;129:639-644.

Herrera L, Fernando H, Perry Y, et al. Radiofrequency ablation of pulmonary malignant tumors in nonsurgical candidates. J Thorac Cardiovasc Surg 2003;125:929-937.

Pennathur A, Luketich J, Abbas G, et al. Radiofrequency ablation for the treatment of stage I non–small cell lung cancer in high-risk patients. J Thorac Cardiovasc Surg 2007;134:857-864.

Sano Y, Kanazawa S, Gobara H, et al. Feasibility of percutaneous radiofrequency ablation for intrathoracic malignancies: A large single-center experience. Cancer 2007;109:1397-1405.

Thanos L, Mylona S, Pomoni M, et al. Percutaneous radiofrequency thermal ablation of primary and metastatic lung tumors. Eur J Cardiothorac Surg 2006;30:797-800.

Thoracic Benign

CHAPTER 14

GIANT BULLOUS EMPHYSEMA

Aaron D. Fain and Joseph B. Zwischenberger

Step 1. Surgical Anatomy

- A resurgence in the surgical treatment of giant bullous emphysema has been due mainly to an increased understanding of the pathophysiology. Patients undergoing surgery have improved clinical symptoms, exercise tolerance, radiographic evidence of pulmonary function, and quality of life postoperatively. A major goal of this type of surgery is the sparing of underlying compressed lung tissue, which might be able to reexpand after removal of the bullae. Knowledge of lung anatomy is essential, especially when deciding between open versus video-assisted thoracoscopic surgery (VATS) techniques.
- A classification schema based on the number of bullae present and on the quality of the surrounding pulmonary parenchyma has been developed. Groups I and II recover best following surgical intervention, whereas surgery for groups III and IV is controversial.

Step 2. Preoperative Considerations

1. Clinical Presentations

- Patients likely to see the most benefit from surgery generally have moderate to severe dyspnea as well as clearly defined normal lung tissue distinct from a single large bulla. A single large, isolated bulla has the best success after surgery compared with surgery concerning many smaller bullae. By performing a resection, the compressed normal lung tissue should be able to expand fully, and oxygenation should improve. Some larger bullae can be asymptomatic; these patients should be followed up for observation before surgery is performed (see "Surgery in Nondyspneic Patients"). Surgery is also indicated for debilitating symptoms associated with a bulla, such as dyspnea, pneumothorax, empyema, or massive hemoptysis. Conversely, patients who do not quit smoking or those who have other symptoms, such as chronic bronchitis, bronchospasm, or recurrent infections, have a lower chance for a sustained benefit following surgery.
- The decision for bullectomy is always predicated on a thorough assessment of risk and benefit. The most benefit will be seen with successful reduction of the compressive bulla on adjacent pulmonary parenchyma, greater concordance between the ventilation-perfusion ($\dot{V}/\dot{Q}$) ratio, and a reduction of dead space when dealing with cases involving communications between the bronchial terminals. The primary complaint for giant bullous emphysema is almost always dyspnea. Therefore, quantifying the patient's degree of dyspnea both preoperatively and postoperatively helps to predict and verify surgical success. The modified scale created by the Medical Research Council of Great Britain (Table 14-1) can be used to quantify dyspnea.

TABLE 14-1.	Modified Medical Research Council Dyspnea Scale
GRADE	**DESCRIPTION**
0	Not troubled with breathlessness except with strenuous exercise
1	Troubled by shortness of breath when hurrying on the level or walking up a slight hill
2	Walks slower than people of the same age on the level because of breathlessness or has to stop for breath when walking at own pace on the level
3	Stops for breath after walking about 100 yards after a few minutes on the level
4	Too breathless to leave the house or breathless when dressing or undressing

From Mahler DA, Wells CK. Evaluation of clinical methods for rating dyspnea. Chest 1988;93:580-586.

2. Preoperative Preparation

◆ Chest computed tomography (CT) scanning is mandatory in determining the extent of surgical resection and provides the best dimensional assessment and extent of the dominant bulla. A chest CT can also be used during expiration (dynamic CT) for clarification of multiple issues with regard to the surgery. Pulmonary angiograms can also be helpful in determining the amount of compression (Fig. 14-1). A good way to address the gained reperfusion after surgery is to perform both presurgical and postsurgical quantitative $\dot{V}/\dot{Q}$ scanning. This test helps to demonstrate the amount of perfused lung parenchyma garnered after resection.

◆ The primary goal for all patients before surgery is smoking cessation; however, we are often conflicted in the clinic regarding smoking cessation. Ultimately, the patient benefits from smoking cessation, and we have professionals dedicated to this cause. However, most patients prefer to continue to smoke in the weeks before surgery. Surprisingly, the literature supports this practice.

◆ Pulmonary function (spirometry, blood gas analysis, perfusion, and ventilation scintigraphy) testing should be gathered on all candidates for surgery. Bronchoscopy should be performed to exclude obstructive lesions. Outpatient pulmonary rehabilitation and education concerning methods for coughing, deep breathing, incentive spirometry, and chest physiotherapy should be required for all appropriate surgical candidates. Cardiac assessment should be considered, with electrocardiogram and echocardiography with concurrent measurement of pulmonary pressure.

◆ Before beginning an operation, a thoracic epidural catheter should be inserted, with continuous administration of epidural narcotics perioperatively. During this procedure, the surgeon must be present because of the chance of an ipsilateral or contralateral pneumothorax that requires rapid decompression. Patients are ventilated and anesthesia is maintained with a double-lumen endotracheal tube so that the lung being operated on can be collapsed if the situation is warranted. To avoid the potentially life-threatening situation created by excessive positive pressure, namely, a tension pneumothorax, one must keep tidal volumes low and maintain a low inspiratory pressure. By allowing for long expiratory phases, trapped air in the bullae and compressed tissue is given a chance to escape. Postoperatively, assisted ventilation is discontinued when the patient regains consciousness and body temperature has returned to normal.

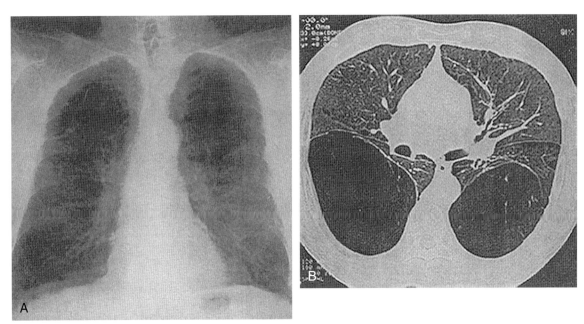

Figure 14-1
(From Dartevelle P, Macchiarini P, Chapelier A. Operative technique of bullectomy. Chest Surg Clin North Am 1995;5:735-749.)

3. Surgery in Nondyspneic Patients

◆ Although the primary symptom of giant bullous emphysema is dyspnea, surgery for complications in nondyspneic patients can be warranted in special circumstances. One instance is for the presence of carcinoma in the bulla. Carcinoma can be observed by particular radiographic patterns of neoplasm development, such as nodular opacity within or adjacent to the bulla; partial or diffuse thickening of the bulla wall; and, finally, secondary signs of the bulla, such as a changed diameter, fluid retention, or pneumothorax. Rarely, bullae become infected. The first choice should be conservative management with antibiotic treatment for a minimum of 6 weeks but is often not sufficient because of poor communication between the infected bulla and bronchial tree. If the patient does not improve, drainage via the modified Monaldi procedure should be considered. Hemoptysis can occur as the result of an eroded artery, although this is less common than an infection. Because of the rarity of this condition, lesions in other lung zones that could account for the bleeding should be suspected and ruled out before surgery.

Step 3. Operative Steps

1. Open Bullectomy

◆ Choice of thoracic incisions depends on the unilateral or bilateral nature of the bullous disease and severity of the respiratory insufficiency. The open thoracotomy is used most often in patients who have large bullae compressing underlying normal lung parenchyma. If the bullae involve only one hemithorax, the patient is positioned for a standard posterolateral or lateral thoracotomy. For bilateral disease, the surgeon can use a median sternotomy or anterior bithoracotomy with or without transverse sternotomy. Bilateral resections can be accomplished in either a one- or two-stage procedure. Most surgeons use either muscle-sparing thoracotomy or VATS.
◆ The main objective of bullectomy is to resect as much diseased lung as possible while avoiding functional tissue reduction that may preclude adequate gas exchange or reexpansion of the residual lung. Before bullectomy, all parietal pleura adhesions are freed. Bulla walls are opened longitudinally (Fig. 14-2A) and explored from within to excise the trabeculae and

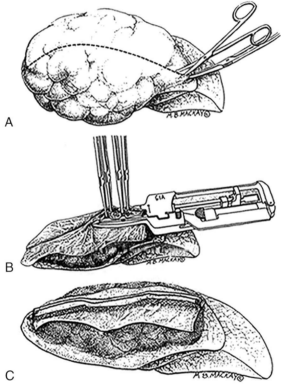

A

B

C

Figure 14-2
(From Deslauriers J, LeBlanc P, McClish A. General
Thoracic Surgery, 3rd ed. Philadelphia: Williams &
Wilkins; 1989:741.)

vessels present at its base. Using long forceps, the visceral pleura is grasped at the reflection of near-normal parenchyma within the cyst cavity (see Fig. 14-2B). The stretched apron of visceral pleura is then reflected over the surface of the interior of the cavity that has been opened (see Fig. 14-2C). The stapler is applied to the base of the bulla until it seals the cavity. All staple lines should be inspected carefully underwater for air leaks. Many use hemostatic, biocompatible glue to aid control of air leaks and bovine pericardial strips to buttress the staple lines. Chest tubes are placed and pleurodesis can be performed. If reexpansion of the residual lung is incomplete or there is not enough lung to fill completely the pleural cavity, the pleural space can be reduced by dissecting a parietal pleura tent from the apex to the lower border of the incision.

2. Axillary Thoracotomy

♦ Axillary thoracotomy is best used for bullae located in either apex of the upper lobes of young patients whose chest cage is not rigid. Muscle-sparing incision is placed over the third or fourth intercostal space. Opening and close times are shorter than for the posterolateral thoracotomy and less painful.

3. Posterolateral Thoracotomy

♦ Posterolateral thoracotomy is the most frequently used approach for operations involving the lung or posterior mediastinum and is the approach of choice for pulmonary resection. It provides excellent exposure of the pleural cavity and all surfaces of the parenchyma, permitting bullectomy of posteriorly located bullae. An incision is made in the submammary fold and continued posteriorly along the ribs and upward as far as the spine of the scapula, resulting in a division of the trapezius, rhomboideus, latissimus dorsi, and serratus anterior muscles. It is, however, associated with severe postoperative pain, which often leads to ineffective coughing, ineffectual physiotherapy, limited shoulder mobility, delayed ambulation, and, consequently, increased postoperative morbidity.

4. Modified Posterolateral Thoracotomy

◆ A modified posterolateral thoracotomy combines the advantage of excellent exposure with complete muscle sparing of the serratus anterior. It is easy to perform, and initial incision is performed through the fifth intercostal space. This technique is often applied for wedge resections, lobectomies, and pneumonectomies. A drawback to its application is its difficulty for use in muscular patients and the time required for the initial muscle dissection and delay of entry into the thorax.

5. Median Sternotomy

◆ The median sternotomy offers simultaneous exposure of both pleural cavities, and the incisional discomforts and ventilatory restriction are less severe compared with thoracotomy. Patient is in decubitus dorsalis position, which has a physiologic advantage in patients with severe pulmonary insufficiency. A vertical inline incision is made along the sternum, and the sternum is then divided. Whereas the anterior aspects of the lung are easily visualized, the posterior aspects of the lungs are difficult to expose. This can become an issue in patients with diffusely emphysematous lungs or posterior adhesions. This procedure is applied for heart transplant, corrective surgery for congenital heart defects, and coronary artery bypass surgery.

6. Video-Assisted Thoracic Surgery

- This term refers to all procedures performed with the thoracoscope. Deflation of the ipsilateral lung can be regulated by the double-lumen endobronchial tube. The patient population best suited for this type of procedure is those at high risk with marginal pulmonary function.
- The goal is to obliterate the bulla with avoidance of air leaks. This procedure can be accomplished in a vast assortment of ways. Some surgeons prefer to use an argon-beam coagulator. When used at low power, the beam will cause the wall of the bulla to shrivel without actually entering into the bulla. The base of the shrunken bulla can be found and stapled to prevent air leaks. To help reinforce the staple line, a piece of bovine pericardium, polytetrafluoroethylene strips, or even the walls of the bulla themselves can be used for buttressing. This type of procedure helps prevent air leaks and is useful for smaller bullae. All bullectomy procedures require very low pressure chest tube suctioning with little (10 mm H_2O) or no (water seal) suction to control the inevitable air leak.
- The VATS is performed with the patient in the lateral decubitus position or in the supine position with arms moved over the head. A disadvantage with the lateral decubitus position is that the patient must be turned to operate on the other side. At about the fifth intercostal space above the anterior superior iliac spine, the initial trocar incision (10 mm in diameter) is made for the video thoracoscope (Fig. 14-3). Two additional incisions (15 mm) are made to form a triangle: one for a grasping instrument and the other for stapler placement. The grasping instrument incision is located anterior and superior to the first incision, which is aligned just posterior to the lateral border of the pectoralis major muscle. The final port is made anterior to the first incision at the same level.
- Another technique utilizes the Ligasure vessel sealing system (Valley Lab, Boulder, CO). With this method, the bulla is excised (see Fig. 14-3A) to the level of near normal parenchyma (see Fig. 14-3B). After complete excision of the bulla, the cut surface is approximated and clamped with forceps (see Fig. 14-3C), and the cut surface is sealed at 1-cm intervals with the Ligasure system.
- VATS often duplicates the open approach. One technique available, especially for small bullae, is the loop ligation approach (Fig. 14-4). In this approach, the bulla is stabbed using the tip of the electrocautery tool, causing it to collapse. To free the shrunken bulla, twist it to its base until normal lung tissue is reached. At this point, apply the endoloop to the shrunken bulla. The preformed loop is tightened using a knot advancer, and additional loops are applied as needed.

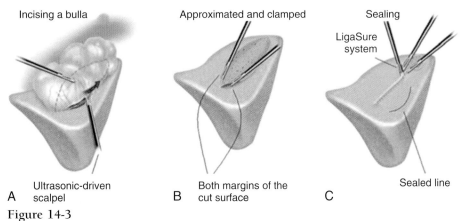

Figure 14-3
(From Shigemura N, Akashi A, Nakagiri T. New operative method for a giant bulla: Sutureless and stapleless thoracoscopic surgery using the Ligasure system. Eur J Cardiothorac Surg 2002;22:646-648.)

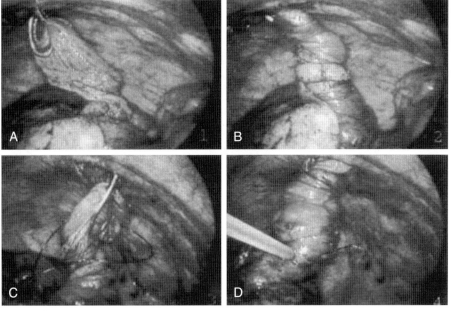

Figure 14-4

Step 4. Postoperative Steps

♦ Extubation should be performed before leaving the operating room. Tracheobronchial toilet care must be managed aggressively to avoid any major complications. To ensure adequate obliteration of the pleural space, a daily chest radiograph should be performed for several days following the surgery. Positive-pressure ventilation should be avoided postoperatively because of the high risk of aggravating air leaks. Managing the residual intrathoracic space and persistent air leaks are among the most challenging postoperative problems and are beyond the scope of this chapter.

♦ Inadequate postoperative pain control can often lead to problems such as poor inspiratory effort and secretion retention. Analgesia is given immediately postoperatively, either continuous morphine or fentanyl epidural infusion. Another important aspect of postoperative care is chest physiotherapy. A low-level, supervised exercise program is encouraged. Remove the chest tube within 24 hours of documented cessation of air leaks.

Step 5. Pearls and Pitfalls

♦ A variety of pulmonary complications can arise after surgery, including pneumonia, respiratory failure requiring use of a ventilator, and prolonged air leaks.

♦ Some patients have trouble weaning off the ventilator, which can be mitigated with early tracheotomy.

♦ Other complications include wound infections and empyema.

Suggested Readings

Dartevelle P, Macchiarini P, Chapelier A. Operative technique of bullectomy. Chest Surg Clin North Am 1995;5:735-749.

Deslauriers J, Gregoire J, LeBlanc P. Bullous and bleb diseases of the lung. In Shields TW, ed. General Thoracic Surgery, 6th ed. Philadelphia: Williams & Wilkins; 2004:1168-1186.

DeVries WC, Wolfe WG. The management of spontaneous pneumothorax and bullous emphysema. Surg Clin North Am 1980;60:851-866.

Divisi D, Battaglia C, Di Francescantonio W, et al. Giant bullous emphysema resection by VATS. Analysis of laser and stapler techniques. Eur J Cardiothorac Surg 2002;22:990-994.

Gamlie Z, Krasna MJ. Operative techniques for lung volume reduction surgery. Chest Surg Clin North Am 2003;13:687-700.

Greenberg JA, Singhal S, Kaiser LR. Giant bullous lung disease: Evaluation, selection, techniques, and outcomes. Chest Surg Clin N Am 2003;13:631-649.

Hugh-Jones P, Lambert AV. A simple standard exercise test and its use for measuring exertion dyspnea. BMJ 1952;12:65-71.

Liu HP, Chang CH, Lin PJ, et al. Emphysema surgery—loop ligation approach. Eur J Cardiothorac Surg 1999;16(suppl 1):S40-S43.

Mahler DA, Wells CK. Evaluation of clinical methods for rating dyspnea. Chest 1988;93:580-586.

Shigemura N, Akashi A, Nakagiri T. New operative method for a giant bulla: Sutureless and stapleless thoracoscopic surgery using the Ligasure system. Eur J Cardiothorac Surg 2002;22:646-648.

Shigemura N, Akashi A, Nakagiri T, et al. A new tissue-sealing technique using the Ligasure system for nonanatomical pulmonary resection: Preliminary results of sutureless and stapleless thoracoscopic surgery. Ann Thorac Surg 2004;77:1415-1419.

Taniguchi Y, Fujioka S, Adachi Y, et al. Video-assisted thoracoscopic bullectomy for an infectious giant bulla with the concomitant use of the perioperative intracavity fluid suction. J Thorac Cardiovasc Surg 2009;137:249-251.

Ueda K, Tanaka T, Jinbo M, et al. Sutureless pneumostasis using polyglycolic acid mesh as artificial pleura during video-assisted major pulmonary resection. Ann Thorac Surg 2007;84:1858-1861.

Wu YC, Chu Y, Liu YH, et al. Thoracoscopic ipsilateral approach for contralateral bullous lesion in patients with bilateral spontaneous pneumothorax. Ann Thorac Surg 2003;76:1665-1667.

Yamada S, Yoshino K, Inoue H. Resection and stapling technique for wide-based giant bullae in video-assisted thoracic surgery using a new end-stapler. Gen Thorac Cardiovasc Surg 2008;56:306-308.

CHAPTER 15

Surgical Management of Empyema

Mitchell J. Magee and Joshua R. Sonett

Step 1. Surgical Anatomy

- A thorough understanding of normal pulmonary hilar and mediastinal anatomy from the thoracic inlet to the diaphragm, which may be significantly altered in the presence of empyema, is essential for effective, safe surgical management.
- Pulmonary volume loss with elevation of the hemidiaphragm and mediastinal shift often occurs and should be considered when any intervention is planned.
- The phrenic and vagus nerves and esophagus should be identified and protected because they can be tethered and retracted with a fibrothorax.

Step 2. Preoperative Considerations

- A simple exudative parapneumonic effusion can progress to a complicated effusion with loculation and empyema thoracis. The stage of progression or chronicity is important to determine because it often influences treatment decisions.
- A thorough history and physical examination and a chest computed tomography (CT) scan are usually sufficient for treatment planning. Any history of antibiotic use, blood and pleural fluid cultures, and other pleural fluid characteristics can be useful if available. Characteristic symptoms include fever, chills, dyspnea, and pleuritic chest pain.
- The CT scan can be helpful in characterizing the parapneumonic effusion (e.g., pleural thickening, loculation, fluid complexity, pulmonary consolidation) and identifying concomitant chest pathology (e.g., adenopathy, pulmonary lesions, and esophageal pathology).
- Purulent pleural fluid should be managed initially with a large-bore chest tube. Intrapleural fibrinolytic agents such as tissue plasminogen activator can be used to enhance the effectiveness of tube drainage and avoid the need for surgery, with some reports demonstrating benefit.
- If the lung fails to fully reexpand or clinical signs and symptoms of infection persist, then operative intervention is warranted, with the primary goal to establish more complete drainage of infection and complete lung expansion (decortication).

Step 3. Operative Steps

♦ General anesthesia is used with provision for single-lung ventilation; the patient is placed in a full lateral decubitus position.

♦ One or two 5-mm thoracoports should be placed initially within the free pleural space, preferably within the effusion or empyema cavity. The free fluid is evacuated to allow inspection of the space with the 5-mm, 30-degree thoracoscope.

♦ Thoracoscopic assessment of the empyema cavity and the surrounding free or loculated pleural space will determine whether any of the drainage and decortication can be done effectively using a video-assisted thoracic surgery (VATS) technique and, if open thoracotomy is required, to select the best location for the thoracotomy incision (Fig. 15-1).

♦ A thick visceral and parietal pleural lining of the empyema cavity, typical of a chronic process, usually mandates open thoracotomy for safe, effective complete decortication of the lung, diaphragm, and mediastinum.

♦ Complete mobilization of the lung with lysis of chest wall adhesions should be performed initially; the lung should be mobilized completely to the hilum circumferentially, carefully identifying and preserving the phrenic and vagus nerves and esophagus (Fig. 15-2).

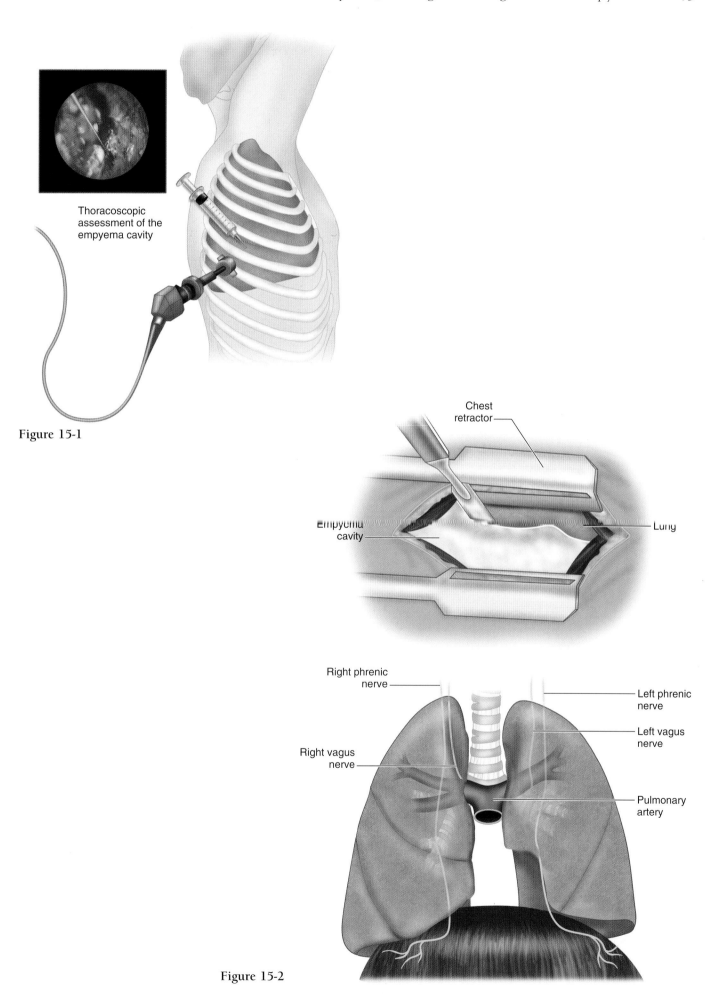

Thoracoscopic
assessment of the
empyema cavity

Figure 15-1

Chest
retractor

Empyema
cavity

Lung

Right phrenic
nerve

Left phrenic
nerve

Left vagus
nerve

Right vagus
nerve

Pulmonary
artery

Figure 15-2

- ◆ Decortication of the lung is best performed with the lung ventilated. The initial plane of decortication is best developed by sharp dissection with a scalpel. Decortication is then facilitated, within that sharply developed plane, by a Kittner dissector on the interface of lung and thickened visceral pleural fibrous "peel." Gentle retraction of the lung parenchyma with sponge sticks further facilitates the dissection (Fig. 15-3).
- ◆ After the lung is completely decorticated, including the fissures superficially, attention turns to the parietal pleural and diaphragmatic surfaces. Generous chest wall decortication will enhance pleural adhesions and avoid development of a restrictive fibrothorax.
- ◆ Careful decortication of the diaphragm should be performed medially to avoid injury to the phrenic nerve where it enters the chest (Fig. 15-4).

Step 4. Postoperative Considerations

- ◆ Two large-bore chest tubes should be placed at the completion of the procedure, one anterior into the apex and one posterior over the diaphragm, and placed on suction for the first 24 hours following surgery. Consider leaving the patient intubated and ventilated postoperatively for 12 to 24 hours to encourage complete lung expansion and pleurodesis that promotes closure of air leaks. Remove chest tubes when there is cessation of air leak and minimal pleural drainage.

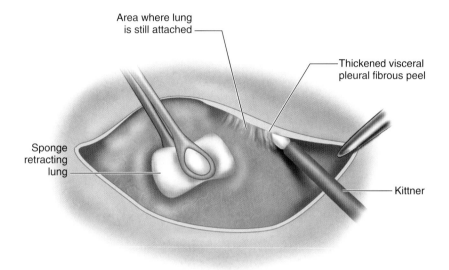

Area where lung
is still attached

Thickened visceral
pleural fibrous peel

Sponge
retracting
lung

Kittner

Figure 15-3

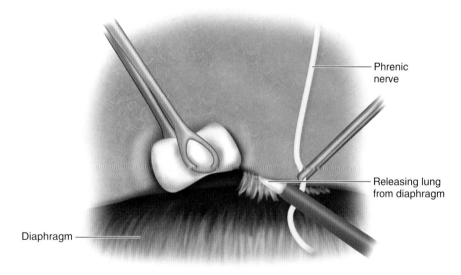

Phrenic
nerve

Releasing lung
from diaphragm

Diaphragm

Figure 15-4

Step 5. Pearls and Pitfalls

- Rule out carcinoma and mesothelioma before completing lung decortication.
- Routinely obtain cultures and histopathology of resected thickened pleural peel to identify unsuspected pathology.
- Protect the phrenic and vagus nerves, esophagus, pulmonary vasculature, and membranous bronchus.
- Lap pads should be used generously during the decortication procedure to tamponade chest wall and lung bleeding sites.
- Avoid excessive lung parenchymal rents that result from inappropriately deep dissection planes that result in large air leaks.
- Do not attempt repair of lengthy visceral pleural surface rents and avoid lung resection; ensuring complete lung expansion and pleural apposition will foster pleurodesis and usually seal even moderately large air leaks in a few days.

Suggested Readings

Chapman SJ, Davies RJ. Recent advances in parapneumonic effusions and empyema. Curr Opin Pulm Med 2004;10:299-304.
Colice GL, Curtis A, Deslauriers J, et al. Medical and surgical treatment of parapneumonic effusions: An evidence-based guideline. Chest 2000;118:1158-1171.
Light RW. Parapneumonic effusions and empyema. Proc Am Thorac Soc 2006;3:75-80.

CHAPTER 16

Lung Volume Reduction Surgery: Open Technique

Joseph M. Kinner, Brannon R. Hyde, and Joseph B. Zwischenberger

Step 1. Clinical Anatomy

- A thorough understanding of the key anatomic structures of the thoracic cavity, particularly the lungs, is essential for successful lung volume reduction surgery (LVRS).

Step 2. Preoperative Considerations

- Emphysema is an irreversible and progressive lung disease that results in the enlargement and destruction of terminal air spaces. LVRS is a procedure that removes the most diseased portions of the lung and provides emphysema patients an opportunity for a better quality of life.
- LVRS removes the nonfunctional, hyperinflated lung parenchyma and allows the remaining healthy lung tissue to expand and regain function. LVRS improves lung elasticity and chest-wall mechanics while increasing diaphragm contractility. After volume reduction, ventilation and perfusion in healthy lung tissue increase, allowing for both functional and symptomatic improvements.
- In response to concerns about the safety and effectiveness of LVRS, the National Heart Lung and Blood Institute and the Center for Medicare and Medicaid Services conducted the National Emphysema Treatment Trial (NETT). The study was designed to clarify the short- and long-term risks and benefits of LVRS by comparing medical treatment to LVRS in patients with severe emphysema. The 5-year study concluded that select patient groups experienced improved quality of life and increased exercise capacity after surgery. Patients with primarily upper lobe disease and low exercise capacity are considered preferred candidates for LVRS, and patients with diffuse or non–upper lobe emphysema and high exercise capacity are generally considered poor operative candidates because of their increased operative risk with minimal functional improvement. The only true predictor of operative mortality during LVRS has been shown to be the presence of non–upper lobe emphysema.

- LVRS requires strict patient selection guidelines to minimize morbidity and mortality. Candidates undergo a thorough preoperative evaluation, including chest radiograph, chest computed tomography (CT), echocardiogram, cardiac catheterization, pulmonary function tests, and arterial blood gas measurements.
- Cessation of smoking for a minimum of 6 months and completion of 6 to 10 weeks of preoperative pulmonary rehabilitation are considered absolute requirements before patients are allowed to undergo LVRS.
- Anesthetic considerations for LVRS are based on the goals of rapid emergence from anesthesia and immediate postoperative extubation. Rapid extubation after LVRS minimizes the potential for staple-line air leak secondary to positive-pressure ventilation. Thus, short-acting anesthetic agents along with optimal intraoperative and postoperative pain control are essential to regaining prompt spontaneous ventilation. Furthermore, optimal pain control is achieved through a preoperatively inserted thoracic epidural catheter. LVRS is successfully performed with a double-lumen endotracheal tube and either total intravenous anesthesia or inhalational agents.

Step 3. Operative Steps

1. Incision

- A median sternotomy incision is used to gain adequate exposure to both lung fields for bilateral LVRS. A midline vertical incision begins at the suprasternal notch and extends inferiorly to a position just below the xiphoid process (Fig. 16-1A).
- Alternatively, sequential muscle-sparing thoracotomies could be done at separate sessions if the disease predominates one hemithorax.

2. Exposure

- While dividing the sternum, ventilation should be discontinued to minimize the incidence of lung tissue injury. Sternal division is accomplished with a sternal saw through the midline of the sternal body and manubrium. This process can occur from either a sternal notch–down or xiphoid-up approach, depending on the surgeon's preference. Bleeding from the periosteum is controlled using electrocautery. After bleeding is controlled, sternal edges are retracted with a sternal spreader placed low in the incision. Generally, 8 to 10 cm of retraction will provide adequate exposure to complete resection of both the right and left lung (see Fig. 16-1B).

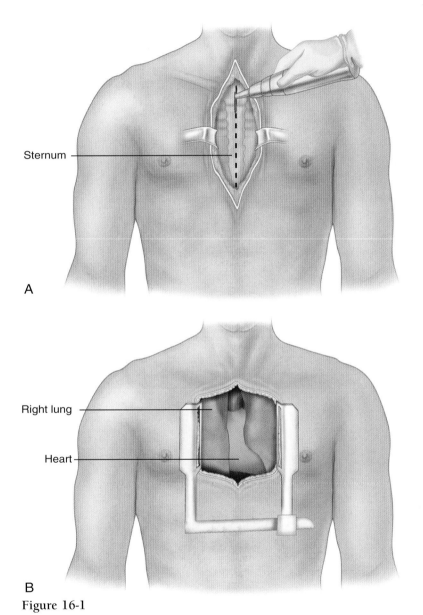

Sternum

A

Right lung

Heart

B

Figure 16-1

3. Resection

◆ Based on preoperative imaging studies (usually CT scan), the worst lung undergoes resection first. Using single-lung ventilation, the anesthesiologist should deflate the lung undergoing resection. On deflation, adhesions should be dissected.

◆ Bimanual palpation or finger pinch can demonstrate the transition between severely to less severely affected lung tissue. The area of lung that is more severely affected is isolated and held in a gastrointestinal clamp (Fig. 16-2). Using a linear GIA stapler, at least 20% to 30% of lung volume should be excised with a continuous staple line (Fig. 16-3). Almost all of upper lobe can be removed, but diseased tissue may still be present. Multiple techniques are used, but resection generally starts in the front of the upper lobe and progresses straight to the back of the lung. An inverted U-shaped technique has also been popular. Staple lines are buttressed with bovine pericardial strips in an attempt to minimize the severity and incidence of air leak (Fig. 16-4). Using low-volume ventilation, staple lines are examined for leak by filling the pleural cavity with saline (Fig. 16-5) to 10 cm H_2O for 3 to 5 seconds. The lung is then inflated to 20 cm H_2O for 3 to 5 seconds. If no bubbles are seen, the chest can then be closed.

◆ If an entire lobe requires resection, consider a lobectomy where control of the vessels and bronchus are more secure.

◆ After staple-line examination, two chest tubes are inserted through the anterior abdominal fascia. The first is placed toward the lung apex, and the second runs along the diaphragm. Chest tubes are initially set to water seal while in the operating room.

◆ After completion of the first lung, the second lung is deflated and resected using similar technique.

4. Closure

◆ Sternal closure is completed with at least five peristernal sutures using No. 5 stainless steel wire. An alternating peristernal and trans-sternal technique is also acceptable. The manubrium is approximated with 2 to 3 trans-sternal No. 5 stainless steel wires. The pectoral fascia and linea alba are closed with running polyglycolic acid suture. Using running absorbable suture, the subcutaneous tissue is closed. The skin is closed according to surgeon's preference.

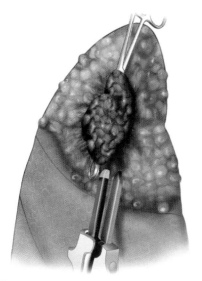

Figure 16-2

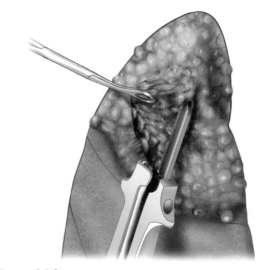

Figure 16-3

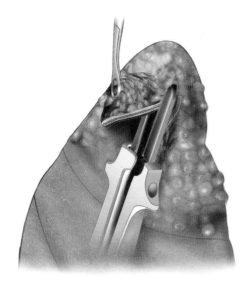

Figure 16-4

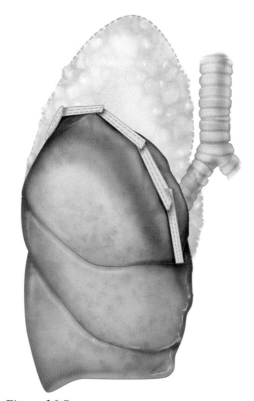

Figure 16-5

5. Prevention of Air Leaks

- Prolonged postoperative air leaks are an extremely common complication of LVRS. In an effort to reduce the incidence and severity of these air leaks, multiple buttressing materials and sealants are now being used intraoperatively to reinforce staple lines. Common buttressing materials include bovine pericardium strips and expandable polytetrafluoroethylene. These materials can also be combined with sealants such as fibrin glue and applied to the lung parenchyma.

Step 4. Postoperative Care

- After completion of the procedure, immediate extubation in the operating room with emergence of spontaneous ventilation allows for decreased incidence and severity of postoperative air leak.
- An immediate postoperative chest radiograph and electrocardiogram allow for early detection of complications and aid in chest tube management. Intensive care unit monitoring of vital signs, serum electrolytes, and urine output can optimize postoperative care.
- Patients generally leave the operating room with two chest tubes in each pleural space set to water seal. Changes in chest tube management are dictated by the severity of ongoing air leaks and the occurrence of pneumothorax. Negative pressure should be implemented in the presence of uncontrolled air leak or progressive pneumothorax.
- Optimal pain control is vital to patient recovery and can prevent hypoventilation, hypoxia, and respiratory failure secondary to pain in the chest wall.
- Early mobilization along with aggressive chest physiotherapy accelerates patient recovery and decreases pulmonary complications. Common postoperative complications include persistent air leak, pneumothorax, pneumonia, arrhythmias, panic attacks, and gastrointestinal complications.

Step 5. Pearls and Pitfalls

- ◆ Extremely rigorous patient selection and preoperative pulmonary rehabilitation are vital for LVRS. LVRS can produce functional and symptomatic improvements, but it is not a cure for severe emphysema. Rather it is a palliative treatment option that needs to be considered in a select group of patients.
- ◆ LVRS improves exercise capacity, lung function, quality of life, and dyspnea. These improvements are greatest in patients with upper lobe emphysema and a relatively low baseline exercise capacity. Ideal characteristics for LVRS are a heterogeneous disease distribution with clearly defined areas of diseased lung in the upper lung fields.

Selected Readings

Brister NW, Barnette RE, Kim V, et al. Anesthetic considerations in candidates for lung volume reduction surgery. Proc Am Thorac Soc 2008;5:432-437.

Daniel TM, Chan BB, Bhaskar V, et al. Lung volume reduction surgery: Case selection, operative technique, and clinical results. Ann Surg 1996;223:526-531; discussion 532-533.

Deslauriers J, LeBlanc P. Emphysema of the lung and lung volume reduction operations. In Shields TW, ed. General Thoracic Surgery, 6th ed. Philadelphia: Lippincott Williams & Wilkins; 2005:1187-1218.

Fishman A, Martinez F, Naunheim K, et al. National Emphysema Treatment Trial Research Group. A randomized trial comparing lung-volume-reduction surgery with medical therapy for severe emphysema. N Engl J Med 2003;348:2059-2073.

Fry WA. Thoracic incisions. In Shields TW, ed. General Thoracic Surgery, 6th ed. Philadelphia: Lippincott Williams & Wilkins; 2005:411-419

Losanoff JE, Collier AD, Wagner-Mann CC, et al. Biomechanical comparison of median sternotomy closures. Ann Thorac Surg 2004;77:203-209.

Naunheim KS, Wood DE, Krasna MJ, et al; National Emphysema Treatment Trial Research Group. Predictors of operative mortality and cardiopulmonary morbidity in the National Emphysema Treatment Trial. J Thorac Cardiovasc Surg 2006;131:43-53.

Sharafkhaneh A, Falk JA, Minai OA, et al. Overview of the perioperative management of lung volume reduction surgery patients. Proc Am Thorac Soc 2008;5:438-441.

Smythe WR, Reznik SI, Putnam JB. Lung (including pulmonary embolism and thoracic outlet syndrome). In Townsend CM Jr, ed. Sabiston Textbook of Surgery: The Biological Basis of Modern Surgical Practice, 18th ed. Philadelphia: Saunders; 2008:1698-1748.

CHAPTER 17

LUNG VOLUME REDUCTION SURGERY: THORACOSCOPIC

Jonathan G. Hobbs, Brannon R. Hyde, and Joseph B. Zwischenberger

Step 1. Surgical Anatomy

- Understanding the anatomy of the thoracic cavity, particularly the lung, is important for the successful completion of a lung volume reduction surgery (LVRS). Figure 17-1 demonstrates key anatomic structures that must be considered before performing a thoracoscopic LVRS.

Step 2. Preoperative Considerations

- LVRS is a treatment option for patients suffering from moderate to end-stage emphysema and serves as a bridge toward lung transplantation by improving pulmonary function. This procedure is designed to address physiologic manifestations through palliation of the symptoms by removing or plicating damaged areas of lung tissue to permit elastic recoil improvement and a reduction in residual volume. The thoracoscopic LVRS procedure helps minimize surgical trauma and significantly decreases wound infection and breakdown.
- Patient screening is paramount to optimizing the benefit of this procedure through identification of patients who have failed medical therapy and have an acceptable surgical risk.
- Screening should include an extensive history and physical examination, pulmonary function tests, and imaging studies or radiographic observation (radiographs and computed tomography [CT] scans).
- Distinguishing emphysema from intrinsic airway disease or chronic bronchitis is crucial in patient selection. A diagnosis of emphysema is made in patients with increased total lung capacity and residual volume, severely reduced expiratory airflow, and decreased diffusion capacity.
- Surgery should be performed after the greatest benefit is obtained from preoperative therapy.
- Surgical targets of the long are established preoperatively, and areas most severely affected by emphysema are identified through CT or lung scintigraphy (Fig. 17-2).
- The National Emphysema Treatment Trial (NETT Trial) mandated a stapled bilateral approach to LVRS unless contraindicated.

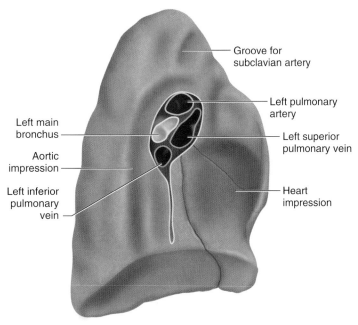

Figure 17-1

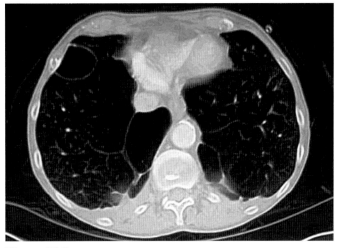

Figure 17-2

◆ Indications for unilateral LVRS include unilateral or asymmetric emphysema, contralateral pleurodesis, or thoracotomy (Table 17-1).
◆ A thoracic epidural catheter is placed and tested before inducing general anesthesia for postoperative analgesia.
◆ After general tracheal anesthetic, flexible bronchoscopy is performed with a single-lumen endotracheal tube, which allows for assessment, clearance, and culture of secretions and possible endobronchial malignancies.
◆ Patient is then reintubated with a double-lumen endotracheal tube for split-lung ventilation.
◆ Bilateral LVRS can be performed with the patient placed in a supine position with arms over head and secured to the operating table. Support may be added beneath the patient's spine, shoulders, and hips.
◆ Alternatively the patient can be placed in the lateral decubitus position, alternating for the bilateral procedure under one anesthetic. Ensure that the chest drains in the first pleural space remain unobstructed during contralateral procedure.
◆ Unilateral LVRS is best performed with patient in the lateral decubitus position.
◆ Presence of posterior pleural adhesions or resecting portions of the lower lobe requires the lateral decubitus position.
◆ A wide area of the chest is prepped for surgical incision. For alternating bilateral procedures, the patient needs to be reprepped and draped.

Step 3. Operative Steps

1. Port Placement

◆ Camera, stapler, and instrument ports are positioned along the thoracic cavity; specific positions can vary depending on individual surgeon's preference.
◆ Patient in supine position
  ▲ *Camera port:* Sixth intercostal space at the anterior axillary line
  ▲ *Stapling port:* Fourth intercostal space at the midclavicular line
  ▲ *Instrument port:* Third intercostal space at midclavicular line
  ▲ An additional port may be desired and placed at the surgeon's discretion.
◆ Patient in lateral decubitus position
◆ A 30-degree thoracoscope is placed in the eighth intercostal space in the posterior axillary line (some surgeons may prefer a 0-degree thoracoscope in the midaxillary line.)
◆ Two to three ports are placed carefully to facilitate the arrangement of the stapler, resection instrument (or plication instrument), and target areas of lung in a straight line.
◆ For upper lobe and superior lower lobe resections and plications, ports are placed in the fifth intercostal space at the anterior axillary line, in the fourth intercostal space posterior to the spine of the scapula, and in the eighth or ninth intercostal space at the surgeon's preference (Fig. 17-3).

TABLE 17-1.	Common Inclusion and Exclusion Criteria for Lung Volume Reduction Surgery

Inclusion Criteria

Radiographic evidence of emphysema, especially involving upper lobes
Hyperinflation
FEV_1 >20 and <45% predicted (post-bronchodilator)
DL_{CO} >20% predicted
Severe dyspnea
Restricted activities of daily living
Decreased quality of life
Abstinence from tobacco

Exclusion Criteria

Active smoking
Bronchiectasis
Pulmonary nodule requiring evaluation
Excessive daily sputum production
Previous thoracotomy
Obvious pleural disease
Active or induceable coronary ischemia
Pulmonary hypertension
Depressed LVEF(<45%)
Obesity
Systemic steroids ≥20 mg prednisone/d

DL_{CO}, diffusion capacity for carbon monoxide; LVEF, left ventricular ejection fraction.
From DeCamp MM Jr, McKenna RJ Jr, Deschamps CC, et al. Lung volume reduction surgery: Technique, operative mortality, and morbidity. Proc Am Thorac Soc 2008;5:443.

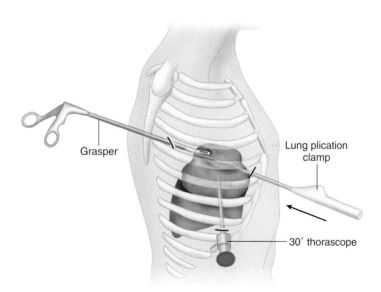

Figure 17-3

2. Intrathoracic Preparation

- Target lung is collapsed and the inferior pulmonary ligament is divided and adhesions are dissected, ensuring avoidance of air leaks.
- It is important to map a staple line before resection.

3A. Resection

- The lung with greater emphysema damage, as diagnosed by the image study, is reduced first.
- Lung is grasped anteriorly, and a linear cutting stapler is placed in the inferior stapling port.
- Because severely emphysemic tissue can tear through at the staple line during reinflation, some surgeons may want to reinforce the staple line using bovine pericardium, Gore-Tex strips, biologic glue, autologous tissues, or polytetrafluoroethylene (PTFE) (>95% in NETT Trial were buttressed).
- Orientation for stapling begins inferiorly and progresses superiorly toward and around the apex, continuing toward the posterior aspect of the lobe.
- Avoid over-resection and stapling too close to the hilum.
- Once resection is completed, the chest is partially filled with warm saline and the lung gently inflated to 10 cm H_2O for 3 to 5 seconds. The lung is then inflated to 20 cm H_2O for 3 to 5 seconds. If no bubbles are seen, the chest can then be closed.
- At completion of the procedure, the lung will assume a more normal size.

3B. Plication

- Alternatively to resection, a plication technique for LRVS achieves the volume reduction while maintaining the visceral pleura.
- A knifeless Endo 60 stapler (U.S. Surgical Corp., Norwalk, CT) and modified lung grasper (Microsurge, Needham, MA) are positioned to avoid unnecessary tension in the staple line.
- Grasp the peripheral edge of the targeted lung area with thoracoscopic ring forceps 4 cm from the pleural edge.
- Use a modified lung plication clamp to fold the lung 180 degrees, forming four layers of visceral pleura to support the staple (Fig. 17-4).
- The knifeless stapler is inserted in the port previously housing the ring forceps, opposite the plication clamp, and placed on the folded portion of the lung.
- Close stapler and remove plication lung clamp. Fire stapler.
- Examine staple for alignment and hemostasis.
- For upper-lobe plication, continue the procedure stepwise from the apex inferiorly toward the fissure.
- Reinflate the lung to evaluate the plicated area and ensure adequate volume reduction. Commonly, 2 cm of space remains between the inflated lung and the chest wall.
- Chest tubes are placed before contralateral lung plication, if indicated.
- An alternate plication technique involves stapling across the lung's apex, folding the lung at the staple line, and restapling across the fold line to achieve the proper reduction in volume.

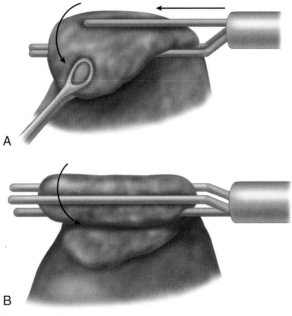

A

B

Figure 17 4

4. Chest Tubes

- One or two 28 French chest tubes are positioned anteriorly and posteriorly to the apex of the lung, paying attention to contralateral hemothorax.
- Chest tubes may be placed on -20 cm H_2O suction. Some surgeons may prefer water-sealed tubes with no pressure.

Step 4. Postoperative Care

- Patients require attentive postoperative care.
- Extubation occurs in the operating suite after completion of the procedure to reduce the effects of positive pressure on suture lines.
- Pain is managed by local anesthetic via the epidural.
- Epidural-induced hypotension may be treated with fluids. In some patients, vasoconstrictors have been associated with mesenteric ischemia.
- Patients are mobilized early.
- Aggressive pulmonary toilet is initiated.
- Pleural drainage should continue 3 to 5 days after the procedure.

Step 5. Pearls and Pitfalls

- Single-stage positioning allows the surgeon to move between pleural sacs more quickly in bilateral LVRS.
- It is paramount to select the target area accurately to minimize the resection or plication of properly functioning lung tissue.

Suggested Readings

Gilroy AM, MacPherson BR, Ross LM, eds. Atlas of Anatomy. New York: Thieme, 2008.

Ginsburg ME. Surgery for emphysema. In Kaiser LR, Kron IL, Spray TL, eds. Mastery of Cardiothoracic Surgery, 2nd ed. Philadelphia: Lippincott Williams & Wilkins, 2006:204-212.

Klena JW, Saari AF, Peterson DO, et al. Combined video-assisted thoracoscopic lung volume reduction surgery and lobectomy in a high-risk patient. Ann Thorac Surg 2003;76:2079-2080.

Daniel TM, Chan BK, Bhaskar V, et al. Lung volume reduction surgery: Case selection, operative technique, and clinical results. Ann Surg 1996;223:526-533.

DeCamp MM, McKenna RJ, Deschamps CC, Krasna MJ. Lung volume reduction surgery: Technique, operative mortality, and morbidity. Proc Am Thorac Soc 2008;5:442-446.

Maxfield RA. New and emerging minimally invasive techniques for lung volume reduction. Chest 2004;125:777-783.

Swanson SJ, Mentzer SJ, DeCamp MM Jr, et al. No-cut thoracoscopic lung plication: A new technique for lung volume reduction surgery. J Am Coll Surg 1997;185:25-32.

CHAPTER 18

Surgical Management of Bronchopleural Fistula

Mark S. Allen

Step 1. Surgical Anatomy

- Bronchopleural fistulae are more common after a right pneumonectomy than after a left pneumonectomy because the right main bronchus extends into the pleural space, whereas the aortic arch and the mediastinal tissues cover the left main bronchus (Fig. 18-1).
- A falling air-fluid level is usually diagnostic of fistula. A fall of more than 1.5 ribs is significant and should raise the suspicion of a bronchopleural fistula (Figs. 18-2 and 18-3).

Step 2. Preoperative Considerations

- It is important to protect the remaining lung by placing the patient with the operative side down so the infected fluid does not drain via the bronchus into the remaining lung.
- Antibiotics should be started and the fluid drained out of the space using a chest tube if the fluid has not already been coughed out by the patient.
- Nutritional status is an important consideration in this group of patients. Often they are debilitated from the chronic infection. Nutritional supplements should be considered in all patients.

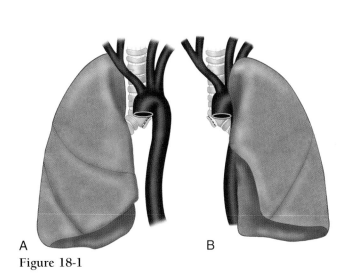

A   B

Figure 18-1

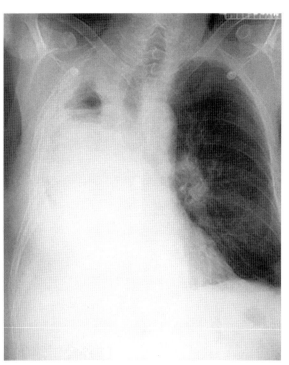

Figure 18-2

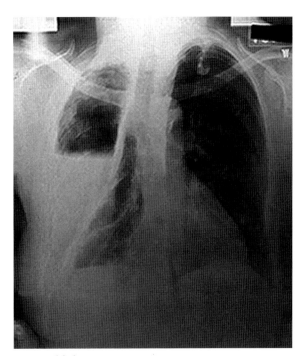

Figure 18-3

Step 3. Operative Steps

- Operative repair is usually necessary and requires careful airway management. A double-lumen tube or a single-lumen tube with a bronchial blocker can be used to protect the remaining lung when the patient is placed in the lateral decubitus position (Fig. 18-4).
- The prior thoracotomy is reopened, and the infected material is débrided. Once the chest cavity is clean, the bronchial stump is identified (pressurizing the airway with saline in the cavity will cause bubbles to come from the hole in the airway and facilitate identifying the stump) and its edges dissected (Fig. 18-5).
- The edges of the bronchial stump are then reapproximated with sutures; 3-0 monofilament sutures work best (Fig. 18-6).
- A muscle is harvested from the chest wall in preparation for its transfer into the chest (Fig. 18-7).

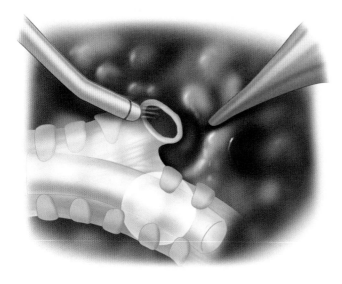

Figure 18-4

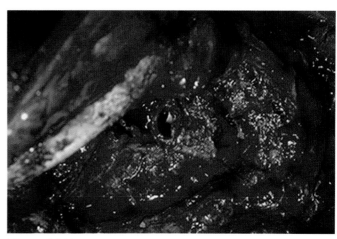

Figure 18-5

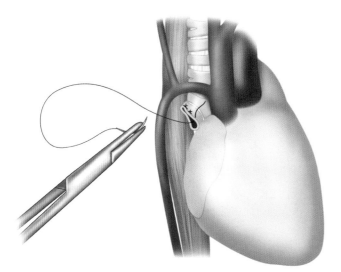

Figure 18-6

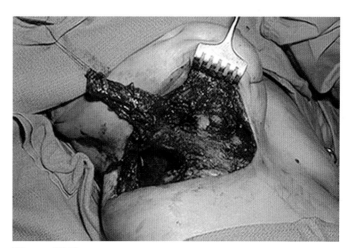

Figure 18-7

- Once the stump has been closed, it is covered with a muscle flap that is transposed into the chest through a partially removed rib (Figs. 18-8 and 18-9).
- The chest cavity is then packed open with gauze soaked in modified diaminobenzidine (DAB) solution (Fig. 18-10).
- This dressing is changed in the operating room every other day until the chest cavity is covered with clean granulation tissue. This usually takes about 5 to 10 trips to the operating room. Occasionally, with sedation, patients can tolerate the dressing changes on the floor (Fig. 18-11).

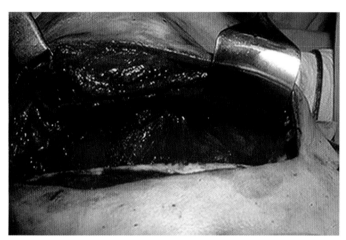

Figure 18-8

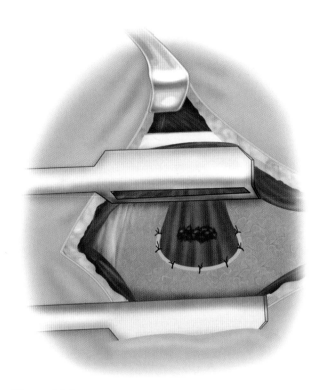

Figure 18-9

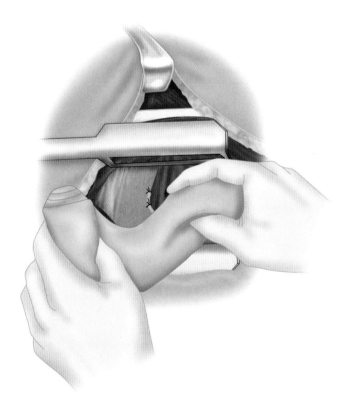

Figure 18-10

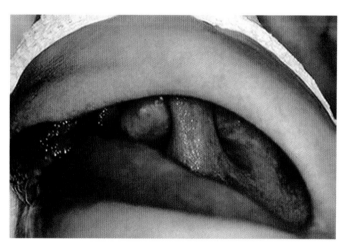

Figure 18-11

♦ Once clean, the edges of the incision are resected back to new tissue, the chest cavity is filled with modified DAB solution, and the incision is closed in watertight layers. A bit more of DAB solution is added just before the final closure so there is no air left in the cavity (Fig. 18-12).

Step 4. Postoperative Care

♦ The chest is wrapped with a 6-in. elastic bandage to allow the soft tissue to adhere to the chest wall and prevent a "seroma." Periodic chest radiographs are obtained to ensure that no air is in the cavity.
♦ Skin sutures are removed after 2 weeks. The elastic wrap is kept on for 2 months (Fig. 18-13).

Step 5. Pearls and Pitfalls

♦ Preserving the function of the remaining lung is the key to success. If patients require mechanical ventilation, it is difficult to keep the bronchial stump closed against the positive pressure.
♦ Nutritional support cannot be overemphasized. Patients are often nutritionally depleted, and the frequent trips to the operating room with the necessary "nothing by mouth" status after midnight can cause them to fall further behind.
♦ As always, prevention is best.
  ▲ There should be no long bronchial stumps.
  ▲ Do not devascularize the peribronchial tissues.
  ▲ Minimize positive-pressure ventilation after a pneumonectomy.
  ▲ A prophylactic muscle flap should be considered in high-risk patients, such as those who have pneumonectomy, who are post radiation therapy, or who are immunosuppressed.

Suggested Readings

Deschamps C, Bernard A, Nichols FC, et al. Empyema and bronchopleural fistula after pneumonectomy: Factors affecting incidence. Ann Thorac Surg 2001;72:243-248.
Zaheer S, Allen MS, Cassivi SD, et al. Postpneumonectomy empyema: Results after the Clagett procedure. Ann Thorac Surg 2006;82:279-287.

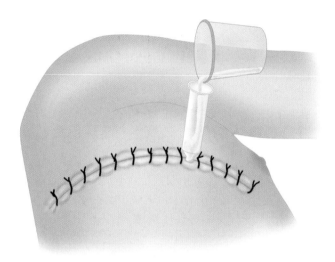

Figure 18-12

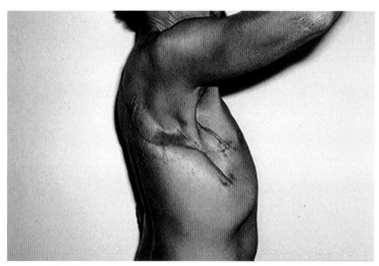

Figure 18-13

CHAPTER 19

DIAPHRAGMATIC EVENTRATION AND PARALYSIS

Li Guang Hu, Liu Wei, and Jean Deslauriers

Diaphragmatic eventration (Box 19-1) is an anomaly that can be defined as a permanent elevation of part or of an entire hemidiaphragm without loss in the continuity in the pleuroperitoneal layers. It is characterized by normal peripheral muscular insertions of the diaphragm but marked decrease in muscular fibers in the eventrated part, which has the appearance of a thin, translucent membrane. It is generally thought that diaphragmatic eventration is a congenital anomaly resulting from an incomplete migration of myoblasts during the fourth week of embryologic development. It has a marked left-sided predominance and does not generally result in paradoxical diaphragmatic motion.

Diaphragmatic paralysis is usually an acquired disorder in which the diaphragm, even if somewhat atrophic, is still muscular. It may manifest in childhood or adulthood and can be associated with phrenic nerve involvement. In many cases, especially in the adult, the exact cause of diaphragmatic paralysis will remain unexplained despite extensive investigation and follow-up.

Diaphragmatic herniation, with or without a hernia sac, involves the loss of continuity in one or more of the layers constituting the diaphragm.

Step 1. Surgical Anatomy

- The mature diaphragm is a dome-shaped muscle that is anchored to the bony structures of the thorax and is considered the most important inspiratory muscle. When it contracts, the dome moves inferiorly and becomes flattened, thus decreasing the intrathoracic pressure and allowing air to be taken into the lungs. The muscular parts that originate from the lower six ribs bilaterally, the posterior aspect of the xiphoid, and the external and internal arcuate ligaments unite at the central tendon. As such, the diaphragm should be viewed as a single muscular unit with two halves.
- The diaphragm receives its motor supply through the phrenic nerves, which are formed at the lateral border of the anterior scalenus muscles, chiefly from the C4 nerve roots but with contributions from the C3 and C5 nerve roots. From there, the phrenic nerves enter the superior mediastinum between the ipsilateral subclavian artery and innominate vein and pass anterior to the pulmonary hilum along the pericardium. It is at that level that they are most susceptible to surgical injury, which may result in complete paralysis and eventual muscular

BOX 19-1. Terminology

Eventration

Congenital in origin

Can be total or partial (anterior, posterolateral, medial)

Characterized by normal muscular insertions and thin membranous abnormal eventrated area

Predominantly left-sided

Paralysis

Nearly always acquired

Characterized by atrophic muscle

Can occur with or without phrenic nerve involvement

Hernia

Involves loss of continuity of one or more of the layers constituting the diaphragm

atrophy of the corresponding half of the diaphragm. The right phrenic nerve reaches the diaphragm lateral to the inferior vena cava, and the left phrenic nerve joins the diaphragm lateral to the left border of the heart. They both divide into several terminal branches whose anatomy delineates safe areas in the diaphragm where incisions can be made without creating loss of diaphragmatic function.

◆ Arterial supply to the diaphragm is through the pericardiophrenic and intercostal arteries; venous drainage is through the right and left inferior phrenic veins, which drain medially into the inferior vena cava.

Step 2. Preoperative Considerations

◆ In the adult population, symptoms related to an elevated diaphragm are predominantly respiratory, mainly dyspnea, cough, and retrosternal discomfort. The diagnosis can usually be made on standard posteroanterior chest films (Fig. 19-1A) which show a diaphragm in higher position than normal, forming a round, unbroken line arching from the mediastinum to the costal arch laterally. Often the mediastinum will be shifted toward the unaffected side. If there is diaphragmatic paralysis, paradoxical motion can be observed on fluoroscopic examination. Although seldom done, diagnostic pneumoperitoneum might be useful to distinguish between an elevated diaphragm and frank herniation (see Fig. 19-1B). Computed tomography (CT) scanning and ultrasonography are not particularly helpful in differentiating between an elevated diaphragm and true herniation, but magnetic resonance imaging (MRI) allows one to acquire high-quality images in several planes, which provides a better evaluation of the entire diaphragm.

◆ The most important preoperative considerations (Box 19-2) in patients with an elevated hemidiaphragm are to rule out a diaphragmatic hernia or thoracic (pulmonary or mediastinal) malignancy affecting the phrenic nerve, to document by pulmonary function studies and exercise testing the respiratory consequences of the elevated diaphragm, and finally to establish clearly the indication for surgery. This should be done with the understanding that most cases of eventration diagnosed in adults should be treated conservatively unless severe dyspnea that interferes with normal activities, orthopnea, or gastrointestinal symptoms are clearly related to the high position of the diaphragm. Indications for surgery in adults are thus uncommon, and the surgeon must be cautious before recommending plication for respiratory or digestive symptoms thought to be secondary to an elevation of the diaphragm.

Step 3. Operative Steps

◆ The objective of the procedure of diaphragmatic plication is to immobilize the diaphragm in a lower, relatively flat position (see Fig. 19-1C) to reduce lung and mediastinal compression. This can be done through an open posterolateral approach, video-assisted techniques, or a laparoscopic abdominal approach. For all these procedures, gastric decompression with a nasogastric tube is mandatory.

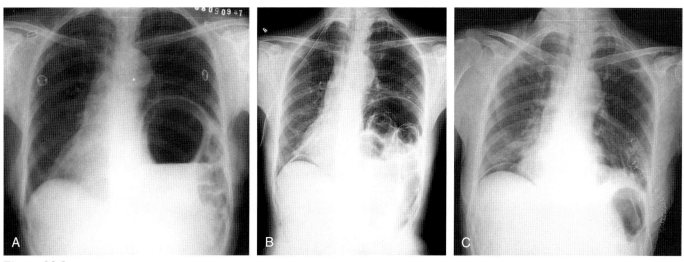

Figure 19-1

BOX 19-2. Important Preoperative Considerations in Patients with Diaphragmatic Eventration and Paralysis

Rule out a diaphragmatic hernia
Rule out a thoracic malignancy affecting the phrenic nerve
Document the respiratory consequences of the elevated diaphragm
Establish a clear indication for surgical repair

1. Open Posterolateral Approach

♦ The operation is carried out through a seventh interspace posterolateral thoracotomy. The lung and mediastinum are first examined to rule out unsuspected pathological processes, and the diaphragm is then plicated in successive layers until it becomes taut. This should be done with heavy interrupted silk sutures often reinforced with Teflon pledgets to prevent tearing. The direction of the plication is determined by the axis of the eventration, which is generally transverse rather than anteroposterior.

♦ In the "flag" plication technique, two Babcock clamps are used to raise the eventrated diaphragm, and the created fold is fixed at its base with U-shaped heavy silk sutures (Fig. 19-2A). This plicated area is then folded and resutured close to the intercostal insertion of the diaphragm by one or several rows of additional stitches (see Fig. 19-2B).

♦ In the "accordion" plication technique, the eventrated diaphragm is pulled in a radial direction, and folds are created by placing full-thickness sutures in the anterolateral to posteromedial direction (Fig. 19-3A). In this manner, the diaphragm can be plicated with as many rows of sutures as necessary to tighten it (see Fig. 19-3B).

♦ Other techniques that can be carried out through an open thoracotomy include mechanical stapling of the base of the eventration, incising the eventration and folding it onto one side, or plicating the fold with U-shaped sutures placed over one or two right-angle clamps. With this last technique, the created semilunar fold is laid down and sutured again to reinforce the thinnest portion of the eventration, usually its anterior part.

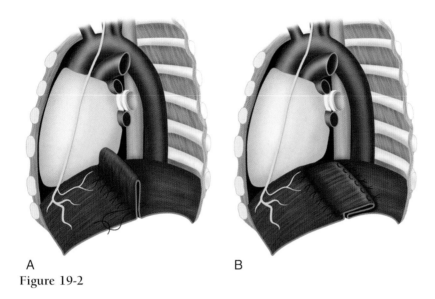

A   B

Figure 19-2

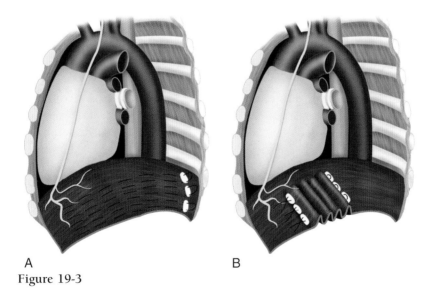

A   B

Figure 19-3

2. Plication by Minimally Invasive Thoracoscopic Technique

◆ This procedure, originally described by Mouroux, is carried out through two 5-mm thoracoports and a mini-thoracotomy made over the ninth intercostal space for the suturing of the diaphragm (Fig. 19-4A). The eventrated diaphragm is first pushed down toward the abdomen (see Fig. 19-4B), and the created transverse fold is closed with a back and forth continuous suture beginning at the periphery of the diaphragm down to the cardiophrenic angle (see Fig. 19-4C).This is followed by a second row of continuous suture burying the first suture line (see Fig. 19-4D). It is to be noted that the presence of extended pleuropulmonary adhesions is generally considered a contraindication to videothoracoscopic plication.

3. Laparoscopic Plication

◆ This technique for left-sided eventrations, which was described by Hüttl, is done with the patient in a 30-degree reverse Trendelenburg position where the surgeon is positioned between the legs of the patient. The redundant diaphragm is pulled down and plicated with 12 to 15 U-type sutures inserted from the left dorsal portion of the diaphragm to its ventral medial portion.

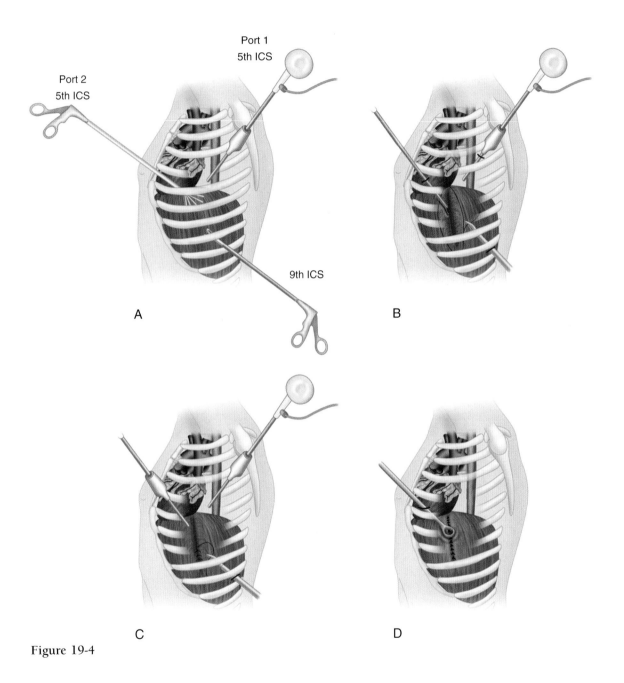

Port 1
5th ICS

Port 2
5th ICS

9th ICS

A

B

C

D

Figure 19-4

Step 4. Postoperative Care

◆ The postoperative care of these patients is usually fairly straightforward with placement of one chest tube, which is removed within 48 to 72 hours of the operation, and a nasogastric tube, which is kept in place until abdominal peristalsis has resumed (normally within 24 hours).

Step 5. Pearls and Pitfalls

◆ In adults, diaphragmatic eventration rarely requires surgical correction, except when respiratory or digestive symptoms are clearly related to the abnormality and other causes of elevated hemidiaphragm have been ruled out. In selected patients, however, there is evidence that diaphragmatic plication will provide substantial and long-lasting benefits in terms of improving symptoms and lung function. The possibility of performing these operations by less invasive techniques, such as video-assisted thoracoscopy, may lead to new interests in these disorders and their surgical treatment.

Suggested Readings

Graham DR, Kaplan D, Evans CC, et al. Diaphragmatic plication for unilateral diaphragmatic paralysis: A 10-year experience. Ann Thor Surg 1990;49:248-252.

Hüttl TP, Wichmann MW, Reichart B, et al. Laparoscopic diaphragmatic plication. Surg Endosc 2004;18:547-557.

Lai DTM, Paterson HS. Mini-thoracotomy for diaphragmatic plication with thoracoscopic assistance. Ann Thorac Surg 1999;68:2364-2365.

Mcnamara JJ, Paulson DL, Urschel HC, et al. Eventration of diaphragm. Surgery 1968;64:1013-1021.

Merendino KA, Johnson RJ, Skinner HH, et al. The intradiaphragmatic distribution of the phrenic nerve with particular reference to the placement of diaphragmatic incisions and controlled segmental paralysis. Surgery 1956;39:189-198.

Mouroux J, Padovani B, Poirier NC, et al. Technique for the repair of diaphragmatic eventration. Ann Thorac Surg 1996;62:905-907.

Mouroux J, Venissac N, Leo L, et al. Surgical treatment of diaphragmatic eventration using video-assisted thoracic surgery: A prospective study. Ann Thorac Surg 2005;79:308-312.

Piehler JM, Pairolero PC, Gracey DR, et al. Unexplained diaphragmatic paralysis. J Thorac Cardiovasc Surg 1982;64:861-864.

Schumpelik V, Steinan G, Schlüper I, Preschner A. Surgical embryology and anatomy of the diaphragm with surgical applications. Surg Clin North Am 2000;80:213-239.

Thomas TV. Congenital eventration of the diaphragm. Ann Thorac Surg 1970;10:180-192.

Wright CD, Williams JG, Ogilvie CM, et al. Results of diaphragmatic plication for unilateral paralysis. J Thorac Cardiovasc Surg 1985;90:195-198.

20

CHEST WALL RESECTION

Mark S. Allen

Step 1. Surgical Anatomy

- An understanding of the chest wall anatomy is important to plan and execute a resection of the chest wall. The intercostal artery, vein, and nerve run just inferior to the edge of the rib.
- The bony structure of the chest covers the lungs and portions of the upper abdomen. The diaphragm attaches to the ribs at various levels.
  - ▲ Bony structure of the chest superimposed on the underlying organs is shown in Figure 20-1.
- The muscles of the chest wall are important to plan the incision and use for reconstruction. Chest wall muscles that can be used for coverage include the latissimus dorsi, serratus anterior, pectoralis major, and rectus abdominis.
  - ▲ Latissimus dorsi muscle showing attachments and vascular supply is shown in Figure 20-2.
  - ▲ Pectoralis major muscle showing attachments and vascular supply is shown in Figure 20-3.

Step 2. Preoperative Considerations

- After a history and physical, the major consideration concerns the location of the mass. What is the size of the mass? Large tumors (i.e., >5 cm) should have an incisional biopsy rather than an excisional biopsy. Where is the mass located? Is it near the diaphragm, vertebral bodies, brachial plexus, or other vital structures?

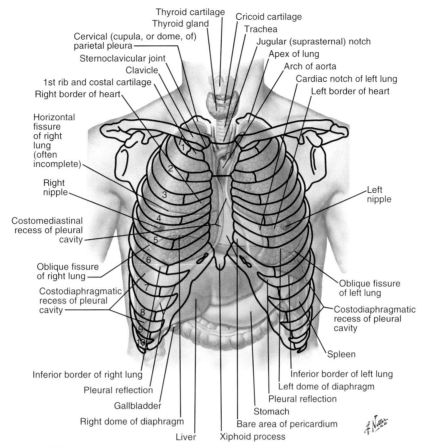

Figure 20-1
(From Netter FH. Atlas of Human Anatomy, 2nd ed. 1997, plate 184.
Netter Illustration Collection at www.netterimages.com. Copyright Elsevier
Inc. All rights reserved.)

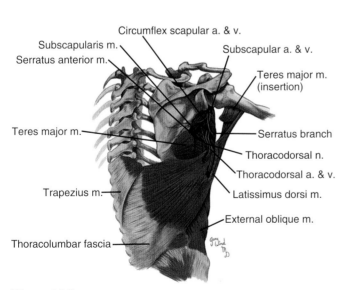

Figure 20-2
(From Netter FH. Atlas of Human Anatomy, 2nd ed. 1997,
plate 98. Netter Illustration Collection at www.netterimages.
com. Copyright Elsevier Inc. All rights reserved.)

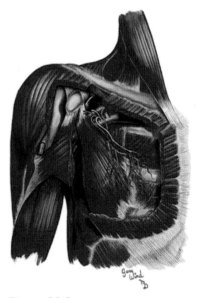

Figure 20-3
(From Netter FH. Atlas of Human
Anatomy, 2nd ed. 1997, plate 9.1.
Netter Illustration Collection at
www.netterimages.com. Copyright
Elsevier Inc. All rights reserved.)

▲ Example showing a chest wall tumor located low on the chest and likely involving the diaphragm is shown in Figure 20-4.

◆ Preoperative evaluation should include pulmonary function testing, which will be impaired by resecting part of the chest wall.

◆ Preoperative chemotherapy or radiation therapy or both should be considered.

Step 3.   Operative Steps

1. Incision

◆ Placement of the incision is very important. Usually an incision over the mass is acceptable, but occasionally other factors are more important. All incisional biopsy sites should be removed. Consideration for reconstruction should also be taken into account so that muscles that might be needed for reconstruction are not devascularized by the incision.

◆ Obviously the mass should not be entered anytime during the resection. If the mass is not palpable, it can be difficult to locate precisely on the chest wall; however, by correlating the preoperative computed tomography (CT) scan, a general approximation can be made. The chest cavity can be entered away from the mass, and then palpation of the mass from inside the chest can guide excision of the chest wall. Some have used video-assisted thoracic surgery (VATS) to visualize the mass directly and to guide placement of the incision for resection.

2. Resection

◆ Resection should be performed with 4-cm margins, if possible.

◆ When resecting ribs, removing a 1-cm piece on each end of the rib makes exposure easier because the ends of the cut rib are not hitting each other.

◆ When the tumor is near the articulation with the vertebral body, the rib should be disarticulated from the vertebral body. Exposure to perform this can be facilitated by removing the transverse process of the vertebral body. Neurosurgical assistance should be available in most instances.

   ▲ Chondrosarcoma that was near the articulation of the vertebral body is shown in Figure 20-5.

   ▲ Photo of the chest wall after the tumor has been resected showing the vertebral bodies is seen in Figure 20-6.

◆ If the tumor involves the diaphragm, this also can be resected as needed. Reconstruction of the diaphragm is accomplished by either artificial material or repositioning the attachment point of the diaphragm.

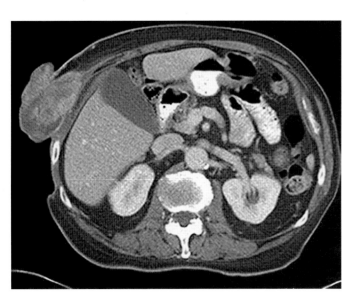

Figure 20-4

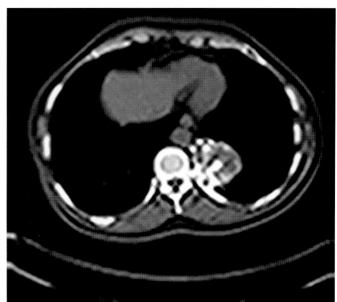

Figure 20-5

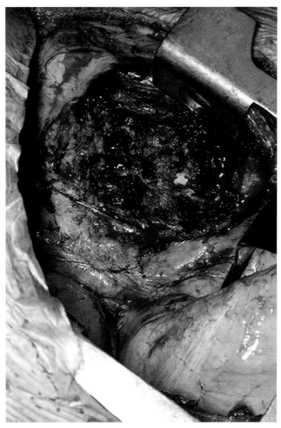

Figure 20-6

3. Reconstruction

◆ The primary methods for reconstruction of the chest wall include using a polytetrafluoroethylene (PTFE) patch (e.g., Gore-Tex) or polypropylene (Marlex) methylmethacrylate sandwich. The use of PTFE is somewhat easier because the patch can be used right out of the package.

◆ A 2-mm-thick piece is used and sutured in place with nonabsorbable monofilament sutures in an interrupted pattern. The patch should be taut. If a polypropylene sandwich is used, the shape of the chest wall defect is reproduced on a back table, and methylmethacrylate is placed on the Marlex with a centimeter free on the outer edges.

◆ Hardening of methylmethacrylate is an exothermic reaction; to avoid thermal injury, it should be allowed to harden on the back table. Once hard, it is sutured into place using the exposed edges of the Marlex mesh.

   ▲ CT scan demonstrates mass in the left chest wall. Needle biopsy proved this mass to be an isolated metastatic Hürthle cell carcinoma (Fig. 20-7).

   ▲ Defect in the chest wall measures 10 × 10 cm after resection of a metastatic Hürthle cell carcinoma (Fig. 20-8).

   ▲ Gore-Tex patch in place after chest wall resection; initial sutures have been placed (Fig. 20-9).

   ▲ Gore-Tex patch completed (Fig. 20-10).

◆ Coverage of the reconstruction is usually accomplished by muscle flaps. The latissimus dorsi is the most commonly used muscle. Almost any other chest wall muscle can and has been used.

   ▲ Example of a recurrence of breast cancer after chest wall irradiation. After excision the latissimus dorsi muscle will be used to cover the chest wall reconstruction. Vascularized muscle is necessary to cover resection and reconstruction after radiation therapy. This photograph shows the defect in the bed of the left mastectomy site after radiation therapy (Fig. 20-11).

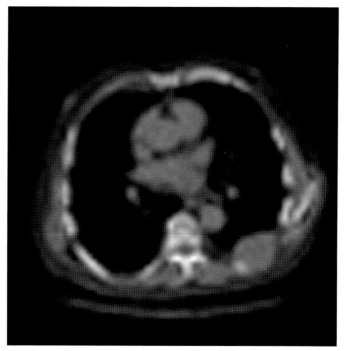

Figure 20-7

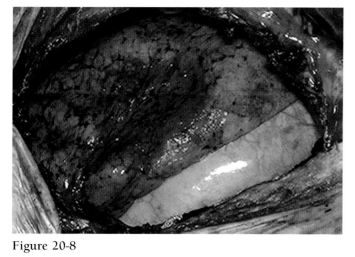

Figure 20-8

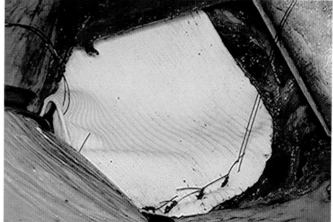

Figure 20-9

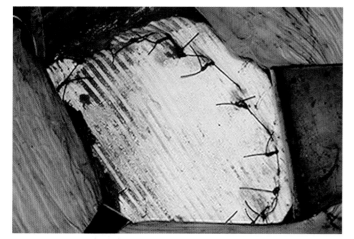

Figure 20-10

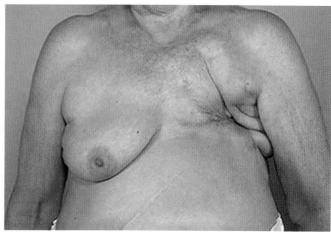

Figure 20-11

▲ The area of recurrence has been resected, and the left latissimus dorsi muscle has been elevated and detached from its insertion (Fig. 20-12).

▲ The muscle has now been passed under the skin bridge to cover the resected defect (Fig. 20-13).

▲ The muscle has been sutured into the bed of the reconstructed area to cover the reconstruction of the bony chest wall. A skin graft will be placed over the vascularized muscle (Fig. 20-14).

Step 4. Postoperative Care

◆ After the dressing is applied, an elastic wrap is placed around the chest, which is thought to decrease the chance of a seroma.

◆ Pain management is important and usually consists of epidural and patient-controlled analgesia.

Step 5. Pearls and Pitfalls

◆ Infected reconstructions usually present as increased pain, redness, or drainage from the incision. An infected foreign body such as a Gore-Tex patch or Marlex-methylmethacrylate sandwich usually needs to be removed. Fortunately, a thick membrane forms around the material, so removal does not result in an open pneumothorax. With proper antibiotics, removal of the artificial material, and careful wound care, the defect should heal. If there is significant flail of the chest or an unsightly cosmetic result, the defect can be repaired once the infection is healed.

◆ Follow-up should be a CT scan at least once a year to detect any recurrence. An advantage of PTFE reconstruction is that it is easy to see on follow-up CT scans.

Suggested Readings

Abbas AE, Deschamps C, Cassivi SD, et al. Chest wall desmoid tumors: Results of surgical intervention. Ann Thorac Surg 2004;78:1219-1223.
Fong Y, Pairolero PC, Sim FH, et al. Chondrosarcoma of the chest wall. Clin Orthop Relat Res 2004;427:184-189.

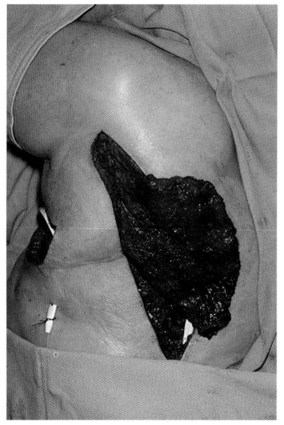

Figure 20-12

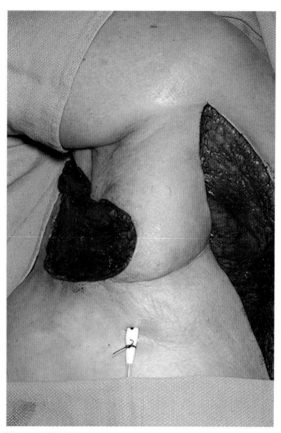

Figure 20-13

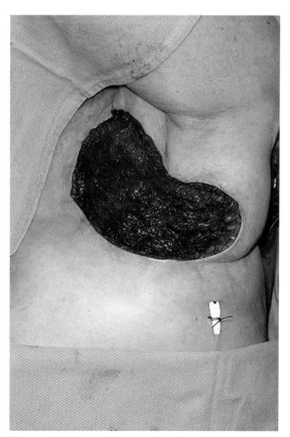

Figure 20-14

STERNAL-SPLITTING APPROACHES TO THYMECTOMY FOR MYASTHENIA GRAVIS AND RESECTION OF THYMOMA

Dawn E. Jaroszewski and Victor F. Trastek

Step 1. Surgical Anatomy

◆ The thymus is a lymphoid organ located in the anterior mediastinum overlying the pericardium and great vessels. It is a bi-lobed, H-shaped lymphoid organ, usually fused in the midline. The upper horns extend into the cervical outlet, and the lower horns often extend and attach to the pericardial fat pad. The phrenic nerve is the crucial lateral boundary of the thymus (Fig. 21-1). The arterial blood supply of the thymus superiorly is from the inferior thyroid arteries. Laterally branches from the internal mammary arteries and inferiorly pericardiophrenic arteries provide additional blood supply. Venous drainage is predominantly via branches to the innominate vein; these branches are of substantial size, requiring ties or clips.

1. History of Thymectomy and Myasthenia Gravis

◆ In 1939 Blalock and associates first reported remission of myasthenia gravis (MG) in a young woman after resection of the thymus. By 1944 more than 20 cases of MG treated by thymectomy had been reported. The relationship between MG and the thymus gland has been well established, although the mechanism for improvement of symptoms after thymectomy is less clear. Evidence supports surgery in severe disease refractory to medical treatment. Some

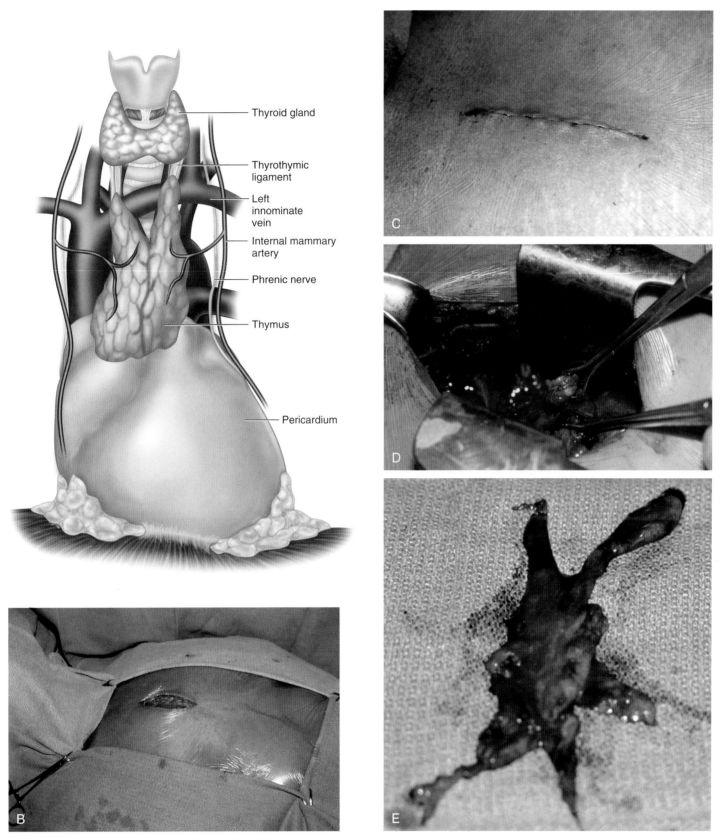

Thyroid gland

Thyrothymic
ligament

Left
innominate
vein

Internal mammary
artery

Phrenic nerve

Thymus

Pericardium

Figure 21-1

debate remains over the indications for thymectomy as a treatment of patients with milder symptoms and no evidence of a thymoma on chest imaging.

◆ Following thymectomy, up to 40% of patients with MG can be expected to have a complete response as measured by no requirement for medication. Continued resolution of symptoms can occur for up to 18 months after thymectomy. An additional 30% to 40% of patients will achieve a partial response, usually manifested by a significant reduction in the amount and type of medications required for controlling MG symptoms. In general, patients with non-thymomatous MG, of younger age, and with shorter disease duration have a better remission rate. No laboratory test or other diagnostic evaluation can predict a patient's response to thymectomy.

2. Patients with Thymoma

◆ Thymoma is the most common neoplasm of the adult anterior mediastinum, accounting for 20% to 25% of all mediastinal tumors. Thirty percent of patients who have a thymoma experience symptoms suggestive of MG, and 15% of patients with MG will have a thymoma. An additional 5% of patients with thymoma will have other systemic syndromes, including red cell aplasia, dermatomyositis, systemic lupus erythematosus, Cushing syndrome, and the syndrome of inappropriate antidiuretic hormone secretion.

◆ No clear histologic distinction between benign and malignant thymoma exists. The propensity of a thymoma to be malignant is determined by its invasiveness. Although considered to have an indolent growth pattern, thymoma has the ability for both local invasion and intrathoracic recurrence. Malignant thymomas can invade the vasculature, lymphatics, and adjacent structures within the mediastinum. Seemingly benign thymomas can also metastasize to the lungs and pleura. As a result, the evaluation and treatment of these tumors, particularly in locally advanced disease, require a multidisciplinary approach to improve long-term patient outcomes.

Step 2. Preoperative Considerations

1. A Multidisciplinary Approach

◆ Treatment and care of the MG patient undergoing thymectomy require multiple specialties. Neurology, anesthesia, critical care, and the entire surgical team should be involved both before and after surgery.

2. Preoperative Workup

◆ Computed tomography (CT) scanning of the chest to assess for the presence of a thymoma is helpful. In cases with thymoma, assessment of invasion is helpful for surgical planning. The diagnosis of thymoma is usually made based on radiologic findings. Chest CT scan is the imaging procedure of choice with intravenous contrast dye to show the relationship between thymoma and surrounding vascular structures. Magnetic resonance imaging can also be useful for evaluating the invasion of mediastinal structures.
◆ A measurement of pulmonary function should also be performed to ascertain whether any involvement of respiratory muscles exists. If severe disability of forced vital capacity is present, the possibility of postoperative mechanical ventilation should be discussed with the patient, anesthesia team, and critical care physicians.

3. Neurology

◆ Working closely with the neurologist is critical for medical optimization of the patient's condition before and after surgery. If the patient is unable to be medically optimized or respiratory dysfunction is present, preoperative plasmapheresis should be performed. This procedure significantly reduces the level of circulating anti–acetylcholine receptor antibodies and should be done the week before the planned surgery. Significant improvement in respiratory function and muscle strength has been shown postoperatively when plasmapheresis was performed preoperatively on MG patients.

4. Anesthesia

♦ Anesthesia administration by someone experienced in the care of patients with MG is necessary. Patients should take their MG medication the morning of the operative procedure. The use of succinylcholine or other nondepolarizing muscle relaxants should be avoided. A single-lumen tube is usually adequate, although a double-lumen tube may be helpful if a large thymoma is present or extends toward one side. A double-lumen tube is also used if pleural or lung metastases from thymoma are present and need to be simultaneously resected. Deep anesthesia is maintained by an inhalation agent and short-acting narcotics. Monitoring of neuromuscular transmission can be performed by peripheral nerve stimulation to aid in the titration of muscle relaxants and to ensure complete reversal of neuromuscular block following the surgical procedure.

Step 3. Operative Steps

1. Partial Sternal-Splitting Incision/Sternotomy

Discussion

♦ For open thymectomy in patients with MG, we most commonly perform a partial sternal-splitting incision. This incision provides adequate visualization of the entire intrathoracic and cervical portion of the thymus gland. If a thymoma is unexpectedly found or exposure is not adequate, the incision can easily be extended into a full sternal-splitting incision. It is critical for the MG patient that complete removal of all thymic tissue be performed. This procedure removes all thymic tissue as well as adipose tissue from the lower poles of the thyroid to the diaphragm and from phrenic nerve to phrenic nerve.

Steps

1. Positioning
♦ After induction of general endotracheal anesthesia, the patient is placed in the supine position and the neck, chest, and upper abdomen are sterilely prepped and draped.
2. Skin Incision
♦ A midline sternal incision is made down to the level of the fourth or fifth rib with a knife blade (see Fig 21-1A). The cosmetic appearance of this incision is very appealing (see Fig 21-1B).
3. Sternotomy
♦ With blunt finger dissection and electrocautery, the area below the sternal notch is freed. The sternum is then divided down the center to the fourth or fifth rib space. A single transverse incision is then made at the inferior aspect of the sternum at the lower interspace with an oscillating saw (Fig. 21-2). A retractor is then placed and the sternum spread open.

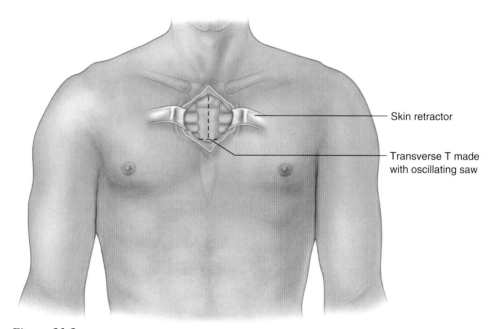

Skin retractor

Transverse T made
with oscillating saw

Figure 21-2

2. Full Median Sternotomy Incision

Discussion

+ For thymomas larger than 4 cm in diameter or with any evidence of invasion, patients should undergo exploration through a complete median sternotomy. Careful evaluation of invasion of surrounding structures must be made at the time of surgery. The mass and any associated structures should be resected en bloc and evaluation of margins performed by the pathologist as frozen specimens. One phrenic nerve should always be spared even if both are involved with the mass. Debulking as much of the mass as possible without injuring the remaining nerve is helpful. Areas surrounding the resection should be clipped for further radiation therapy. Any required vascular resections and reconstruction can also be easily performed through this sternotomy incision. If pleural or lung metastases are discovered, these should be resected.

Exploration

+ The overlying mediastinal pleurae are separated in the midline bringing the thymus and innominate vein into view. When a thymoma is present, a thorough exploration of the mediastinum, pleural spaces, and lungs is also performed.

Identification of Phrenic Nerves
+ The phrenic nerves are identified as the posterior-lateral margins of the thymic resection. Using a right-angled clamp, an incision approximately 1 cm superior to the phrenic nerve should be made along the mediastinal pleurae bilaterally (Fig. 21-3). This facilitates lateral dissection and prevents inadvertent injury to the phrenic nerve while dissecting out the thymus.

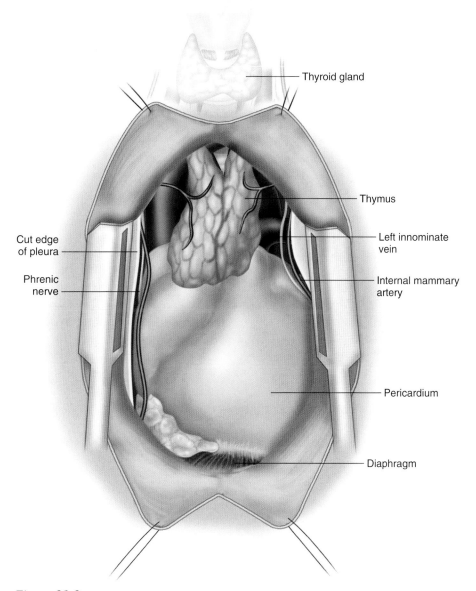

Thyroid gland

Thymus

Left innominate vein

Cut edge of pleura

Internal mammary artery

Phrenic nerve

Pericardium

Diaphragm

Figure 21-3

Dissection

Four Horns of the Thymus

▲ Thymectomy is often easily performed by first dissecting out the four horns of the gland. The right inferior horn is most easily identified and dissected off the pericardium (see Fig. 21-1C). Resection can then be continued in the dissection plane cephalad along the pericardium (Fig. 21-4). As the middle portion of the thymus is approached, the dissection plane becomes more fatty and difficult to visualize. All fatty tissue should be cleared from the pericardial surface and considered potential thymic tissue. As planes become more indiscrete, it is often easier to return to the left inferior horn and again dissect cephalad along the pericardium. On the left, the phrenic nerve is often much closer and a blunt dissection technique is necessary to separate the nerve from the fatty tissues and help prevent injury. It should require only blunt dissection to free the nerve because the mediastinal pleurae have been previously incised. Again, as the middle portion of the gland is approached and dissection becomes more difficult, return to freeing the remaining poles.

▲ The superior poles can be approached in the cervical area. The poles can be circumferentially freed from above the innominate vein until the thyrothymic ligaments are identified (Fig. 21-5). The horns are each disconnected from the thyroid gland and the ligaments ligated with 2-0 silk suture.

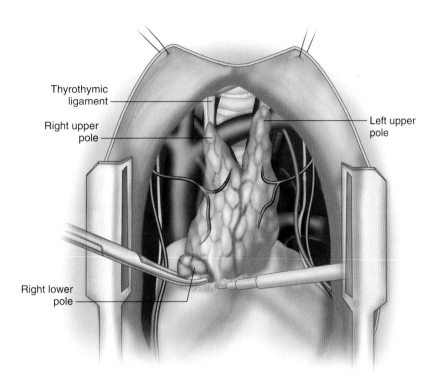

Figure 21-4

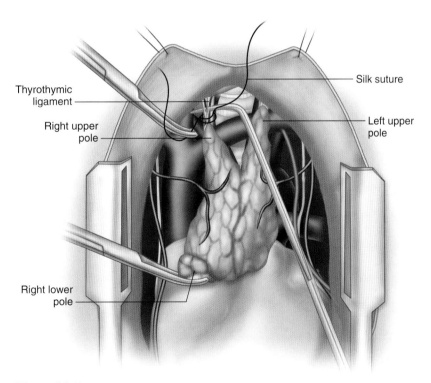

Figure 21-5

Middle Thymus and Ligation of Vessels

◆ Returning to the middle portion of the thymus, the associated fatty tissue is pulled back from the area above the phrenic nerve up to the junction of the innominate vein and superior vena cava (Fig. 21-6).
◆ Lateral vessels from the internal mammary are carefully divided and ligated with 3-0 silk ties. The thymus gland is then reflected further along the left innominate vein until the midline venous draining vessels are identified, divided, and tied (Fig. 21-7).

The Specimen

◆ The gland should be completely freed and the specimen removed intact with all four poles (see Fig 21-1D). It should be sent to pathology for gross evaluation and, if thymoma is present, for frozen evaluation of margins.

Closure

◆ After the thymus is removed, meticulous hemostasis should be obtained. Postoperative bleeding secondary to coagulopathy can be increased in patients who have undergone preoperative plasmapheresis.
◆ A chest tube should be place through the chest wall across the mediastinum. The sternum is approximated with interrupted stainless steel wires. At least two wires should be placed in the manubrium and the remainder around the interspaces of the sternum.
◆ A figure-of-eight wiring to incorporate and reapproximate the inferior T-division is recommended.
◆ The remainder of the soft tissue closure is completed with multiple layers of absorbable suture, including subcuticular closure of the skin.

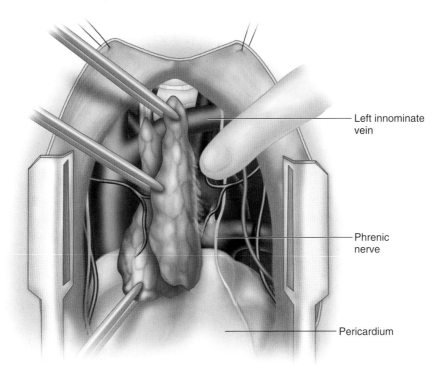

Figure 21-6

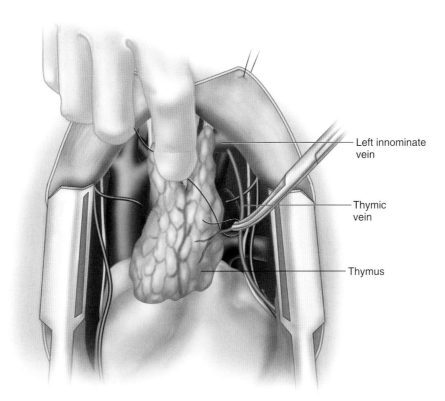

Figure 21-7

Step 4. Postoperative Care

- ◆ After the operation is completed, the patient is taken to the recovery room, awakened, and evaluated by the anesthesiologists.
- ◆ Immediate extubation is preferred, provided respiratory effort and blood gas values are acceptable. Most patients can be extubated and closely observed in intermediate or intensive care.
- ◆ Aggressive pulmonary toilet and early ambulation are important. Postoperative management by both neurology and surgery is critical. Once the patient achieves stable respiratory status, routine surgical floor care is appropriate.

Step 5. Pearls and Pitfalls

1. Preoperative

- ◆ Evaluate thoroughly and know what you are dealing with.
  - ▲ If thymoma is present, plan what surgical resection will entail.
  - ▲ If MG symptoms exacerbated or respiratory function poor, plan for preoperative plasmapheresis.
  - ▲ All team members should be on board.
  - ▲ Neurology to maximize patient
  - ▲ Anesthesia with experience
  - ▲ Critical care and recovery prepared if mechanical ventilation expected to be prolonged

2. Intraoperative

- ◆ All thymic tissue needs to be taken.
- ◆ Protecting the phrenic nerve should be a priority.
- ◆ Hemostasis is critical.

3. Postoperative

- Extubate early
- Team approach to care and medication management
- Close observation
- Aggressive pulmonary toilet
- Early ambulation
- Drains out early

Suggested Readings

Blalock A. Thymectomy in the treatment of myasthenia gravis: Report of twenty cases. J Thorac Surg 1944;13:316.

Blalock A, Mason MF, Morgan HJ, et al. Myasthenia gravis and tumors of the thymic region: Report of a case in which the tumor was removed. Ann Surg 1939;110:544.

D'Empaire G, Hoaglin DC, Perlo VP, Pontoppidan H. Effect of prethymectomy plasma exchange on postoperative respiratory function in myasthenia gravis. J Thorac Cardiovasc Surg 1985;89:592-596.

Eisenkraft JB, Papatestas AE, Kahn CH, et al. Predicting the need for postoperative mechanical ventilation in myasthenia gravis. Anesthesiology 1986;65:79-82.

Frist WH, Thirumalai S, Doehring CB, et al. Thymectomy for the myasthenia gravis patient: Factors influencing outcome. Ann Thorac Surg 1994;57:334-338.

Jaretzki A. Thymectomy for myasthenia gravis: Analysis of controversies regarding techniques and results. Neurology 1997;48(suppl 5):S52.

Masaoka A, Yamakawa Y, Niwa H, et al. Extended thymectomy for myasthenia gravis patients: A 20-year review. Ann of Thorac Surg 1996;62:853-859.

Mulder DG, Graves M, Herrmann C. Thymectomy for myasthenia gravis: Recent observations and comparisons with past experience. Ann Thorac Surg 1989;48:551-555.

Okkumura M, Miyoshi S, Takeuchi Y, et al. Results of surgical treatment of thymoma with special reference to the involved organs. J Thorac Cardiovasc Surg 1999;117:605-613.

Riedel RF, Burfeind WR. Thymoma: Benign appearance, malignant potential. Oncologist 2006;11:887-894.

Seggia JC, Abreu P, Takatani M. Plasmapheresis as preparatory method for thymectomy in myasthenia gravis. Arq Neuropsiquiatr 1995;53:411-415.

Shimizu N, Moriyama S, Aoe M, et al. The surgical treatment of invasive thymoma: Resection with vascular reconstruction. J Thorac Cardiovasc Surg 1992;103:414-420.

PECTUS EXCAVATUM: MINIMALLY INVASIVE NUSS PROCEDURE

Jacob E. Perry, James Hoskins, and Joseph A. Iocono

Step 1. Surgical Anatomy

- Pectus excavatum, or funnel chest, is the most common of all congenital chest wall deformities. It is defined as the posterior depression of the inferior portion of the sternum with posterior curving of the attached ribs at the affected levels. The defect may or may not be symmetric, but most eccentric defects have more severe depression of the right side of the sternum.
- Pectus excavatum affects 1 in 400 children and is three to five times more prevalent in boys than in girls. Associations with connective tissue disorders, particularly Marfan syndrome, have been demonstrated. Combined pectus excavatum with pectus carinatum defects are also possible.
- As with all chest wall deformities, pectus excavatum can have many effects on the patient, both physiologic and psychosocial. Physiologic impairments resulting from pectus excavatum include decreased exercise tolerance, mitral valve prolapse, decreased stroke volume, and restrictive-type pulmonary dysfunction. The major psychosocial effects are due to poor self-image and low self-esteem in adolescence as a result of the noticeable deformity of the anterior chest wall.
- Understanding the abnormal relationship of the chest wall structures is vital to planning the repair. Pectus excavatum is a congenital malformation of the anterior thorax characterized by a prominent depression of the body of the sternum, usually involving the lower one half to two thirds. Usually ribs 1 to 3 are spared, as is the manubrium, with most deformities involving the fourth through seventh ribs and their respective costal cartilages. Usually the deepest point of depression is just above junction with the xiphoid. The Nuss procedure corrects the anomaly by realigning the sternum in situ without resection of the costal cartilage. A personalized titanium bar is fashioned in the operating room to hold the sternum in correction for 2 years so that remodeling can take place. When the bar is removed, the chest wall has remodeled and stays in its new alignment.

Step 2. Preoperative Considerations

1. Preoperative Workup

- Assess severity of defect
- Imaging
  - ▲ Chest radiograph: anteroposterior (AP), lateral
  - ▲ Computed tomography (CT) (Fig. 22-1) chest measurement of Haller index (should be >3.5) (Fig. 22-2)
  - ▲ Transverse diameter of chest wall, AP diameter

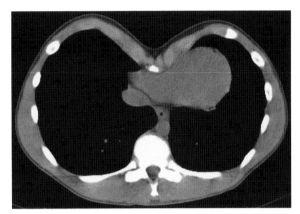

Figure 22-1

Haller index = A/C

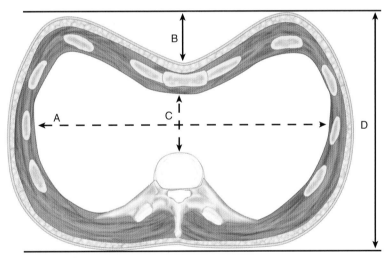

Figure 22-2

▲ Studies
▲ Echocardiogram
▲ Pulmonary function tests
▲ Exercise tolerance testing
◆ *Labs:* Complete blood cell count, bone morphogenetic protein, prothrombin time, partial thromboplastin time

Step 3. Operative Steps

1. Anesthesia

◆ Supplemental thoracic epidural for postoperative pain control
◆ Deep venous thrombosis prophylaxis for older patients
◆ Good intravenous (IV) access with two large-bore peripheral IVs
◆ Antibiotic prophylaxis

2. Positioning and Prepping

◆ The patient is placed supine on the operating room table with both arms abducted on arm boards so that the axillae are able to be prepped in the field.
◆ Foley catheter, nasogastric tube (NGT) remove at end of case
◆ Prep of choice should include bilateral chest to level of bed laterally to include both axillae, superiorly to chin and inferiorly to umbilicus (Fig. 22-3).

3. Landmarks and Measurements

◆ Mark the deepest portion of the deformity. If the deepest location is at the xiphoid, then use the base of the sternum as the level of incisions and bar placement.
◆ Mark the intercostal spaces laterally that correspond to this level, and draw planned transverse lateral incisions from anterior to midaxillary lines bilaterally (~2.5 cm long).
◆ Mark the location where the bar should enter the thoracic cavity bilaterally at the point of maximal excursion of the defect anteriorly (mark with X) (Fig. 22-4).
◆ Measure from midaxillary line to midaxillary line at the level of planned repair.
◆ Subtract 1 in. from the measurement for choosing the correct-size pectus bar template and pectus bar.
◆ Mold the pectus bar template to conform to desired correction of chest deformity. Place this on the back table to use to create customized pectus bar.

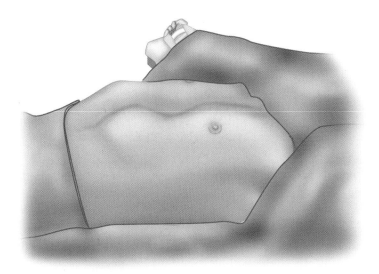

Figure 22-3

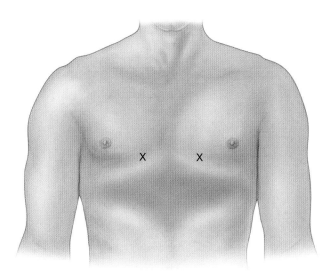

X's mark the point of maximal excursion of the
chest and are the locations where the bar transitions
from a subcutaneous level to an intrathoracic one.

Figure 22-4

4. Incision and Dissection

- Make two transverse lateral incisions from anterior to midaxillary line bilaterally at the level where the bar will be placed.
- Extend incisions to the level of muscle fascia and create subcutaneous pockets from incisions medially to the level of maximal excursion (marked previously with X).
- Create lateral pockets that are large enough to hold pectus bar stabilizers.
- On the right side, two intercostal spaces below the first incision, make a 5-mm incision in the midaxillary line for placement of trocar and port. We recommend a laparoscopic-type port with capability for CO_2 instillation.
- Use 8 to 10 mm Hg of pressure and create pneumothorax.
- Visualize chest, point of maximal excursion, and point of maximal depth inside the right thorax with 30-degree thoracoscope. You can perform the surgery with one port on the right side and visualize the bar going across from right to left or use two ports and watch from both sides of the chest.
- Under video guidance, place the pectus introducer, depending on the patient's size (three sizes are available) from the right-side incision into the pocket created, and then enter the thoracic cavity at the X while watching the monitor.
- Using upward traction, gently advance the introducer across the mediastinum in the plane immediately anterior to the pericardium and inferior to the point of deepest pectus defect.
- Watch for arrhythmias, and stop if any are seen.
- Assistant should be waiting on other side of the chest with a retractor (Army/Navy type), exposing the X spot on the left side.
- The pectus introducer should exit the chest at this exact location and then travel in the left-sided subcutaneous pocket and out the left-sided incision.
- Once in place, the introducer is firmly pulled "up" while pressing both sides above and below the defect down to remold the sternum with the introducer in place. Tie two lengths of heavy umbilical tape to the end of the introducer.
- Leave the introducer in place while molding patient's bar on the back table (Fig. 22-5).

5. Bar Measurement and Molding

- The size of the pectus bar itself is the length of the distance from midaxillary line to midaxillary line minus 1 in. It should be the same size as the pectus bar template.
- Mold the correct size pectus bar with a bar bender (there are hand-held and table-top choices), and fashion the bar to the exact shape of the template. Be careful about keeping the right and left sides of the bar correct. You may leave the most acute angle outermost bends to be done when the bar is in situ before flipping the bar.

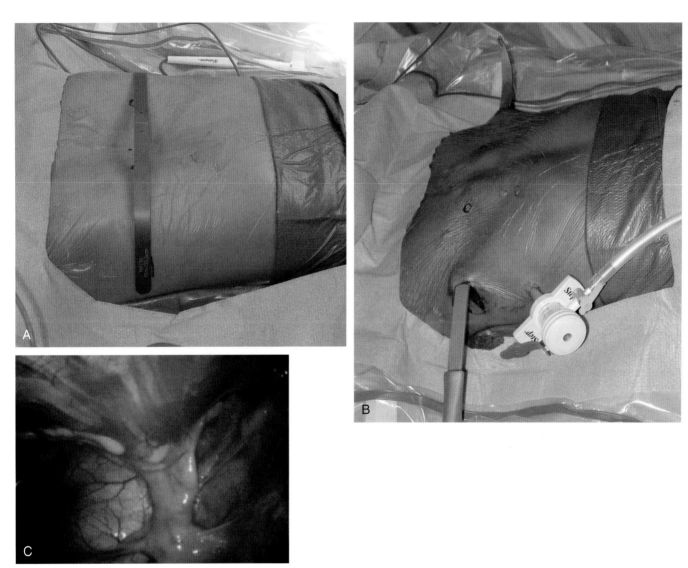

Figure 22-5

6. Passing the Pectus Bar

- Once the customized pectus bar is molded, remove the pectus introducer and leave the two strands of umbilical tape in the tract. Use one umbilical tape to tie to the customized pectus bar, and keep the other umbilical tape aside as a backup in case the first one breaks.
- Pass the customized pectus bar through the tract by advancing it across the mediastinal tract made by the pectus introducer. Gently pull on the umbilical tape (left-sided surgeon) while pushing the bar across (right-sided surgeon) while watching via the thoracoscope. Pass the bar with the ends facing up for easier passage and to allow for final hand bending of outer edges (Fig. 22-6).

7. Flipping and Securing the Bar

- Once the bar is in place with the tips facing up, flip the bar using two pectus flippers, which place the sternum and chest wall into the desired "chest-out" position.
- Check for precise bar placement and stability of the bar, which might need to be unflipped and hand modifications of the edges made while the bar is in situ. If the bar was molded correctly, these modifications will be minimal.
- Check for adequacy of the repair. If defect is still pronounced or the bar seems unstable, a second bar can be placed one or two intercostal spaces away from the first bar. Two new incisions, pockets, and tunnel will be necessary in most cases.

8. Pectus Bar Stabilizers

- Place one or two stabilizers in the lateral pockets made at the incision sites, and attach these to the pectus bar for improved security from bar dislodgement.
- There are two choices of shapes for stabilizers. Each type will slide over the bar in a "tongue-in-groove" fashion.
- Secure the bar and stabilizer in pockets with a figure-of-eight suture around the junction of the bar and stabilizer with either cardiac wire or large (0 or larger) absorbable suture.
- Secure muscle over the bar in the pocket with horizontal mattress sutures.
- Close the remainder of the wound with absorbable sutures.

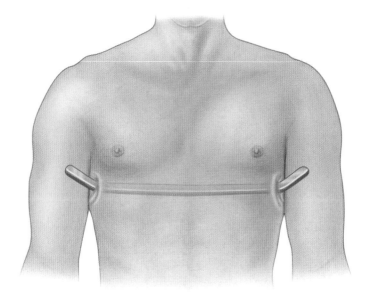

Figure 22-6

9. Removing Carbon Dioxide from the Chest

- ◆ Create a water seal by cutting the carbon dioxide tubing and inserting it in a container of sterile water or saline while the port is still in place.
- ◆ Have anesthetist give a series of large "handbag" breaths with peak inspiratory pressure of 40 and peak end-expiratory pressure of 10 to reexpand right lung and remove the pneumothorax. Place a horizontal mattress stitch around the port in the muscle layer during the evacuation breaths.
- ◆ Once carbon dioxide is evacuated, remove 5-mm port and tie the mattress stitch. Place a subcuticular stitch in the port site (Fig. 22-7).

Step 4. Postoperative Care

- ◆ Chest radiograph is taken either in operating room or in the recovery room to assess for pneumothorax and document placement of bar.
  - ▲ Floor bed with continuous pulse oximetry is usually sufficient.
  - ▲ Average hospital stay is 2 to 5 days
  - ▲ Activity is slowly increased.
    - Bed rest with head of bed elevated 30 to 45 degrees on the day of surgery
    - Out of bed to chair on postoperative day 1
    - Ambulate with assist (especially in and out of bed) on postoperative day 2
    - Transition to oral pain medication on postoperative day 3 or 4
    - Hospital stay dependent on pain control and activity
    - No bending of chest or waist, no twisting
    - Return to activities slowly: 2 weeks; begin noncontact exercise at 6 to 8 weeks

Step 5. Pearls and Pitfalls

- ◆ Complications
  - ▲ Pneumothorax approximately 10%
  - ▲ Hemothorax
  - ▲ Bar infection
  - ▲ Bar dislodgement
  - ▲ Much has been written about procedures for "extra" securing sutures around the bar and ribs; this may improve the stability of the bar and needs to be assessed on an individual basis.
- ◆ Improvement in symptoms
  - ▲ Subjective
  - ▲ Objective: difficult to measure

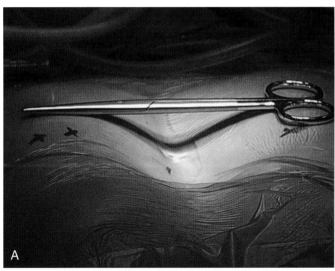

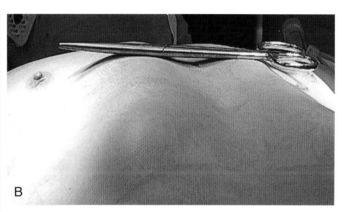

Figure 22-7

Suggested Readings

Brigato RR, Campos JR, Jatene FB, et al. Pectus excavatum: Evaluation of Nuss technique by objective methods. Interact Cardiovasc Thorac Surg 2008;7:1084-1088.

Croitoru DP, Kelly RE Jr, Goretsky MJ, et al. Experience and modification update for the minimally invasive Nuss technique for pectus excavatum repair in 303 patients. J Pediatr Surg 2002;37:437-445.

Croitoru DP, Kelly RE Jr, Goretsky MJ, et al. The minimally invasive Nuss technique for recurrent or failed pectus excavatum repair in 50 patients. J Pediatr Surg 2005;40:181-187.

Nuss D, Kelly RE Jr, Croitoru DP, et al. A 10-year review of a minimally invasive technique for the correction of pectus excavatum. J Pediatr Surg 1998;33:545-552.

Park HJ, Chung W-J, Lee IS, et al. Mechanism of bar displacement and corresponding bar fixation techniques in minimally invasive repair of pectus excavatum. J Pediatr Surg 2008;43:74-78.

Vegunta RK, Pacheco PE, Wallace LJ, et al. Complications associated with the Nuss procedure: Continued evolution of the learning curve. Am J Surg 2008;195:313-317.

CHAPTER 23

THORACOSCOPIC SYMPATHECTOMY

Mark J. Krasna and Lei Yu

Sympathectomy is a surgical procedure where portions of the sympathetic nerve trunk are destroyed to treat diseases such as hyperhidrosis (HH), facial blushing, and Raynaud disease. Sympathectomy itself is a relatively easy procedure to perform. It is difficult, however, to access the nerve tissue in the chest cavity by conventional surgical methods. Thoracoscopy has become a standard approach for performing sympathectomy and has led to a resurgence of this procedure for a variety of diseases.

Indications

There are several indications for the treatment of HH (palmar or axillary): craniofacial sweating, facial blushing, and social phobia. Other indications for sympathectomy include Raynaud disease, reflex sympathetic dystrophy (RSD), causalgia, long QT syndrome, and untreatable angina pectoris.

Nonsurgical Treatment

It is generally thought that patients undergoing thoracoscopic sympathectomy should have previously attempted a trial of nonoperative therapy. Patients with HH are generally offered topical agents such as Drysol (aluminum hydroxide). Occasionally a trial of iontophoresis is appropriate if the patient can tolerate the side effects of tingling and electrical shocks. Oral agents have been used with some success in patients with HH, including a trial of antidepressants or other psychotropic medications, which may allow the patient to "deal with" the psychological trauma caused by the socially debilitating symptoms of HH. Other medications, like β-blockers and cholinergics, do have a significant chance of resulting in some improvement in HH with, however, side effects such as fatigue, bradycardia, and dry mouth.

Surgical Techniques

Conventional approaches include the posterior approach and the supraclavicular approach, which is less painful than the posterior but is more prone to damaging important nerves and blood vessels. In recent years, minimally invasive surgical techniques have been developed that have made endoscopic thoracic sympathectomy (ETS) possible and popular.

Step 1. Surgical Anatomy

- Each sympathetic trunk consists of a long chain of nerve ganglia lying along either side of the spine and is broadly divided into three segments: cervical, thoracic, and lumbar. The autonomic nervous system controls involuntary body functions, such as breathing, sweating, and blood pressure. The most common area targeted in sympathectomy is the upper thoracic region, the part of the sympathetic chain lying between the first and fifth thoracic vertebrae (Fig. 23-1).
- The upper sympathetic thoracic ganglion (T1) is the ganglion most responsible for sweating and heat loss of the face, hands, and to a minor degree the axillae T1, in conjunction with the eighth cervical ganglion form the stellate ganglion, which is responsible for the eyelid and pupillary response. They should be preserved because an injury may cause Horner syndrome.
- The second thoracic ganglion (T2) controls the sweat response of the hands and face (except the interorbital portion), scalp, shoulders, and the anterior and posterior parts of the thorax above the breasts and contributes to facial blushing.
- The third ganglion (T3) affects the sweating of the hands, axillae, shoulders, and anterior and posterior parts of thorax above the breast and of the face to a minor degree.
- The fourth ganglion (T4) innervates the hands and the axillae. It should be noted that there is duplicate sympathetic innervation for the hands, face, and axillae.
- ETS cuts or destroys the sympathetic ganglia, the collections of nerve cell bodies in clusters along the thoracic or lumbar spinal cord.

Step 2. Preoperative Considerations

- Dermatologists, neurologists, endocrinologists, and cardiologists involved in diagnosing or treating HH should be consulted to evaluate the patient before referral to surgical treatment.
- Contraindications before surgery are rare but include severe cardiovascular insufficiency or pulmonary insufficiency; severe pleural diseases (tracheobronchitis, pleuritis, empyema); and uncontrolled diabetes. Prior thoracic surgery, although perhaps difficult, is not an absolute contraindication.[1]

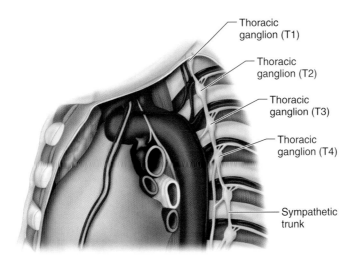

Thoracic
ganglion (T1)

Thoracic
ganglion (T2)

Thoracic
ganglion (T3)

Thoracic
ganglion (T4)

Sympathetic
trunk

figure 23-1

Level of Sympathectomy

♦ Currently, a T2 sympathectomy is performed for craniofacial hyperhidrosis and facial blushing and T3 and T4 for hyperhidrosis palmaris or axillary hyperhidrosis with palmar hyperhidrosis. For long QT syndrome, the sympathetic chain is sectioned from the level of the inferior third of the stellate ganglion (T1) to the sympathetic ganglia of T5, together with any branch that courses to the caudal region or in the lateral direction.

♦ We prefer cutting to clipping or coagulating the ganglia of the sympathetic trunk. The purported advantages of clipping are that the clips could be removed in case of severe side effects, such as compensatory HH and gustatory sweating and could also avoid lesions in the adjacent intercostal structures.

Step 3. Operative Steps

♦ ETS is performed with the patient under general anesthesia, generally using a double-lumen tube. After induction of general anesthesia and orotracheal intubation, patients are left in the supine sitting position (semi-Fowler) with the free arms abducted at right angles. Careful padding under both ulnar nerves and wrists should be employed.

♦ The operating thoracoscope is initially inserted via a single 10-mm trocar in the second to fourth intercostal space in the midaxillary line. Alternatively a second trocar can be introduced through a 5-mm incision at the third intercostal space.

♦ The lung is released of all adhesions with the use of cauterization, so it can be completely collapsed. We generally use a disposable 45-cm endoscopic scissors for this, taking care to cauterize and divide the often vascular adhesions to the apex of the thorax.

♦ The sympathetic chain is easily identified under the parietal pleura, running vertically over the head and neck of the ribs in the upper costovertebral region (Fig. 23-2). The second rib is the first to be seen easily inside the thorax, and it serves as a focal point. With a hook electrocautery, the parietal pleura is opened (Fig. 23-3). Dissection or coagulation of the ganglion is performed, isolating the communicating sympathetic rami anterior and posterior so that there is no transmission of heat or energy to the intercostal nerves (Fig. 23-4). Through these careful maneuvers, the sympathetic chain can be dissected from its bed (Fig. 23-5).

♦ The ganglia and their communicating branches must be carefully dissected, and attention must be given to avoid injuring the intercostal vessels, especially at the T4 level, where the vein enters the azygos arch.

♦ The resection bed of the sympathetic chain is inspected to ensure adequate hemostasis. At the end of the procedure, a chest tube or red rubber catheter is inserted through the lower port into the dissected area and removed after reinflation of the lung with positive pressure.

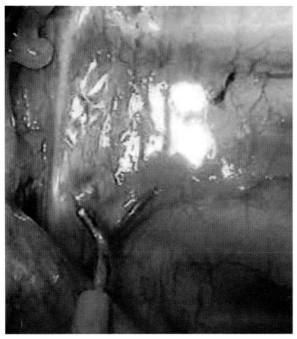

Figure 23-2

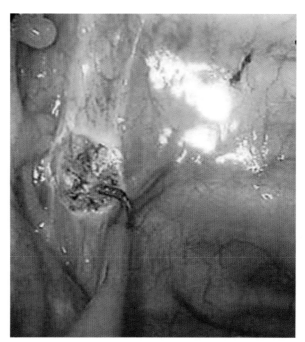

Figure 23-3

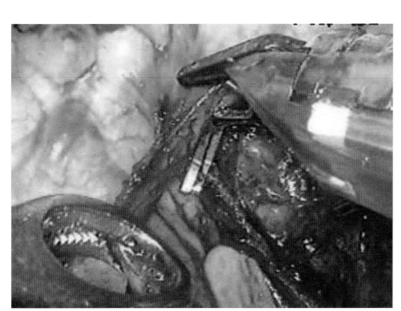

Figure 23-4

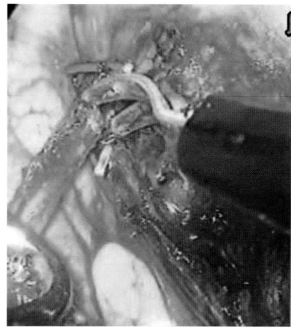

Figure 23-5

Step 4. Postoperative Care

- After complete recovery from anesthesia, patients are taken to the recovery room. According to their needs, analgesic medication will be administered. They generally are able to eat 2 to 4 hours after the surgery. Usually the patients are discharged later that day.
- We recommend 3 days of relative rest; patients may then increase regular physical activities gradually, avoiding intense physical activities for 15 days.
- All patients are examined before discharge for evidence of bradycardia or Horner syndrome, and a chest radiograph is done to rule out pneumothorax. Of approximately 10% of patients who get a small pneumothorax postoperatively, less than 10% require a catheter for drainage. This is generally kept in for several hours and the patient is discharged later that day.

Step 5. Pearls and Pitfalls

- Electrocautery, rather than mechanical resection, is preferred to divide the sympathetic chain because it is easier and quicker.
- Take great care to ensure that complete ablation of ganglia and severance of the sympathetic chain are achieved.
- Cauterize and divide the pleura for 5 cm laterally; in this way, if an aberrant nerve bundle of Kuntz is identified, it too is severed.
- Separate the transected ends of the sympathetic chain as far as possible to prevent regrowth of the nerve.
- Do not divide the sympathetic chain above the level of the second rib for the treatment of palmar and plantar HH; it increases the risk of Horner syndrome and contributes little benefit.

Results

Numerous international studies have shown that an incision on the sympathetic nerve gives a positive result when it comes to hand perspiration and also that the side effects are rare. Studies by ETS surgeons have claimed a satisfaction rate around 85% to 95%, with about 2% regretting the surgery,[2,3] generally because of compensatory sweating. The exact results of ETS, however, are impossible to predict because of considerable anatomic variations in sympathetic nerve function from one patient to the next and also because of variations in the surgical technique used.[4]

Permanent side effects, including compensatory sweating, gustatory sweating, Horner syndrome, and inability to raise the heart rate when working out physically, have left a negative impact on some patients.[5,6] The benefits of ETS to patients, however, far outweigh its disadvantages. A large majority of surgeons still believe that ETS should be performed on certain selected patients with severe palmar HH and RSD.

References

1. Lin C, Mo L, Lee L, et al. Thoracoscopic T2–sympathetic block by clipping—A better and reversible operation for treatment of hyperhidrosis palmaris: Experience with 326 cases. Eur J Surg Suppl 1998;13-16.
2. Herbst F, Plas E, Fugger GR, et al. Endoscopic thoracic sympathectomy for primary hyperhidrosis of the upper limbs: A critical analysis and long-term results of 480 operations. Ann Surg 1994;220:86-90.
3. Ponce González MA, Julià Serdà G, Santana Rodríguez N, et al. Long-term pulmonary function after thoracic sympathectomy. J Thorac Cardiovasc Surg 2005;129:1379-1382.
4. Reisfeld R. The importance of classification in sympathetic surgery and a proposed mechanism for compensatory hyperhidrosis: Experience with 464 cases. Surg Endosc 2007;21:1249-1250.
5. Reisfeld R. Video-assisted thoracic surgery sympathectomy for hyperhidrosis. Arch Surg 2005;140:99.
6. Schwartz PJ, Priori SG, Cerrone M, et al. Left cardiac sympathetic denervation in the management of high-risk patients affected by the long-QT syndrome. Circulation 2004;109:1826-1833.

CHAPTER 24

LUNG TRANSPLANTATION

Mark R. Bonnell

Step 1. Surgical Anatomy

- ◆ Solid working knowledge of the anatomy of the chest, in particular the hilar relationships of the left and right lung, is crucial. Other important structures whose anatomic relationships must be studied include the following:
  - ▲ Phrenic nerves
  - ▲ Pericardium and its reflections
  - ▲ Recurrent laryngeal nerve on the left side
- ◆ Because lung transplantation may require cardiopulmonary bypass (CPB) established either through the chest or the femoral vessels, it is key to understand anatomy relevant to CPB and to have a plan in mind if this is required, regardless of one's approach to the chest for the transplant (Fig. 24-1).

Step 2. Preoperative Considerations

- ◆ Lung transplantation is performed for end-stage lung disease. The decision for single or bilateral transplant is multifactorial but essentially depends on the disease and the patient's age. In general, suppurative lung disease (i.e., cystic fibrosis) requires bilateral transplant to prevent contamination of the other lung. Younger patients are generally considered for bilateral transplant because of modestly improved long-term survival.
- ◆ Candidacy for transplantation is decided by a multidisciplinary transplant committee after a protocol-driven evaluation. The full scope of this decision process is beyond the limits of this chapter; however, here follows a list of fairly standard inclusion criteria and contraindications. Realize that these are center specific.

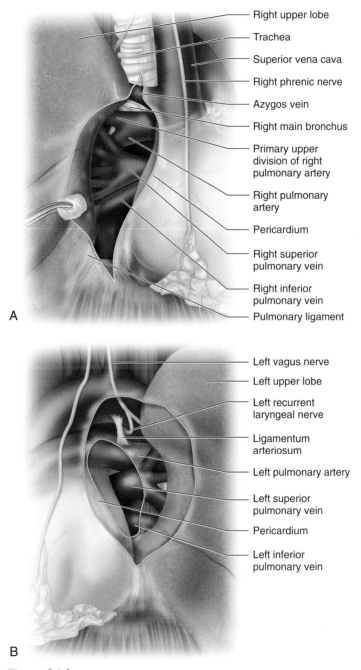

Right upper lobe

Trachea

Superior vena cava

Right phrenic nerve

Azygos vein

Right main bronchus

Primary upper division of right pulmonary artery

Right pulmonary artery

Pericardium

Right superior pulmonary vein

Right inferior pulmonary vein

Pulmonary ligament

A

Left vagus nerve

Left upper lobe

Left recurrent laryngeal nerve

Ligamentum arteriosum

Left pulmonary artery

Left superior pulmonary vein

Pericardium

Left inferior pulmonary vein

B

Figure 24-1

1. Inclusion Criteria

- High likelihood of death from lung disease within 2 to 3 years
- New York Heart Association functional class III or IV
- Acceptable psychosocial profile
- Normal metabolic profile
- Adequate nutritional status (body mass index [BMI] between 16 and 35)
- Ability to live within 4 to 6 hours of transplant center while awaiting transplant
- Ability to comply with a long-term disciplined medical regimen
- Normal heart assessment, including catheterization or appropriate stress monitoring
- No contraindication for immunosuppressive therapy
- Potential for rehabilitation
- Failure of maximum appropriate medical management
- Not amenable to other proven surgical treatment options

2. Absolute Contraindications

- Active malignancy
- Active extrapulmonary infection, including HIV and AIDS, hepatitis B, and hepatitis C
- Active pulmonary infection in patient considered for single-lung transplantation
- Significant acute or chronic cardiac insufficiency
- Significant hepatic or gastrointestinal disease
- Chronic renal disease (creatinine clearance <50 mL/min)
- Persistent colonization with *Burkholderia cepacia*
- Active fungal infection
- Known active substance abuse or history of substance abuse with failure to comply with rehabilitation
- Obesity (BMI >35)—refractory to weight-control programs
- Cachexia—not amenable to nutritional rehabilitation
- Acute illness that will adversely affect the outcome of transplantation
- Current use of mechanical ventilation for more than a very brief period
- Cigarette smoking within the past 6 months
- Insulin-dependent diabetes mellitus with evidence of end-organ damage, including the following:
  - ▲ Diabetic vasculopathy
  - ▲ Diabetic nephropathy

3. Relative Contraindications

◆ Older than 55 years for bilateral lung transplantation
◆ Steroid use greater than 10 mg/day; prednisone that cannot be weaned
◆ Previous cardiothoracic surgery or other bases for pleural adhesions
◆ Insulin-dependent diabetes mellitus with evidence of end-organ damage, including the following:
  ▲ Diabetic retinopathy
  ▲ Diabetic peripheral neuropathy
  ▲ History of noncompliance or psychiatric disorder likely to interfere significantly with a disciplined medical regimen
  ▲ Persistent colonization with pan-resistant *Pseudomonas aeruginosa*
  ▲ Ventilator dependency (if patient is already listed he or she will still be considered for lung transplant)
  ▲ Severe osteoporosis
  ▲ Systemic hypertension refractory to medical management

4. Donor Assessment

◆ By the time of operation, sidedness or bilaterality will already have been determined. You must determine the following:
  ▲ ABO compatibility
  ▲ Size matching (dimensions measured from apex to dome, across at the level of the aortic knob, and dome of diaphragm). Remember, with some diseases (e.g., chronic obstructive pulmonary disease) patients have hyperexpanded lungs, whereas patients with other diseases (e.g., idiopathic pulmonary fibrosis, pulmonary hypertension) tend to have normal to small lungs.
  ▲ Review donor history, arterial blood gases and trend, bronchoscopy, Gram stain, and chest radiograph.

5. Recipient-specific Considerations

▲ Location to hospital and transportation time
▲ Health at time of notification—any immediate new contraindications (i.e., fever)
▲ Previous thoracic operations or virgin chest
▲ Pulmonary artery (PA) pressures, hemodynamic stability, and risk of requiring CPB
▲ Patent foramen ovale
▲ Single or bilateral
▲ Drugs: induction protocol of the institution

Step 3. Operative Steps

1. Procurement

◆ View all radiographs and laboratory tests, confirm ABO blood type. Perform a bronchoscopy to ensure that anatomy is normal and all segments are clear of secretions. If mild to moderate amounts of purulent secretions are present, lavage with saline. If the secretions clear easily and do not reaccumulate, the lungs are generally still acceptable. This decision requires experience and is program specific.

◆ Exposure is made via median sternotomy in conjunction with abdominal teams. Widely open the pericardium in cruciform fashion and widely open each pleura, and take down the inferior pulmonary ligaments. Fully inspect both lungs for nodules, atelectasis, significant contusion or trauma, and other contraindications to transplant. Isolate superior vena cava (SVC) and encircle with umbilical tape, using care to avoid the azygos vein and right pulmonary artery (RPA). Isolate the aorta from the PA laterally and the RPA posteriorly and encircle with umbilical tape. Place pulmoplegia stitch in the main pulmonary artery (MPA) about 1 cm from bifurcation; we use a 4-0 Prolene U-stitch, a diamond purse string also works well. Systemically heparinize (coordinate with visceral team) (Fig. 24-2).

▲ Before cross-clamping, give 500 μg of prostaglandin E (PGE) into the MPA (Fig. 24-3) and wait for a systemic response drop in mean arterial pressure (MAP). Cross-clamp the aorta and amputate the left atrial appendage and divide 50% of the IVC for venting. Administer pulmoplegia (Perfadex at our institution) 3 L at 30 cm H_2O, and apply topical crushed ice. Use adequate suction so that the lungs are not bathed in the warm blood. Tie the SVC with the umbilical tape.

▲ Once plegia is complete, divide the IVC and then the SVC above the azygos. Next divide aorta above the innominate artery; include all head vessels if needed for reconstruction and the PA at the bifurcation (Fig. 24-4A). Incise the left atrium midway between the coronary sinus and left inferior pulmonary vein (Fig. 24-4B); continue cephalad and then toward the right side, ensuring an adequate atrial rim around right-sided veins. Be careful of the RPA when coming across the dome. This completes cardiectomy.

▲ Elevate the pericardium inferiorly, and incise the plane between the esophagus and the pericardium to the level of the carina (Fig. 24-5).

▲ Control the trachea and divide it between staple lines well above the carina with partial lung inflation to 20 cm H_2O (Fig. 24-6).

▲ Dissect the left pulmonary artery (LPA) free from the descending aorta by dividing the ligamentum arteriosum. Remove the entire lung block to separate left and right on back table.

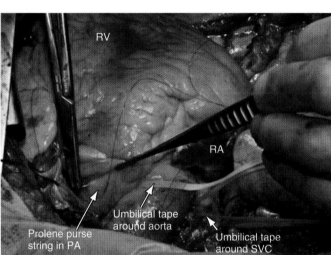

Figure 24-2

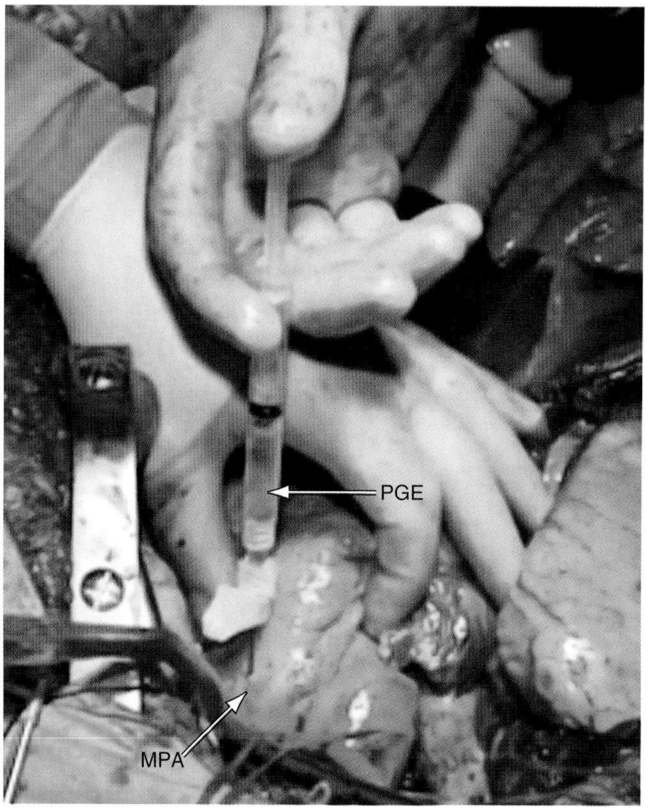

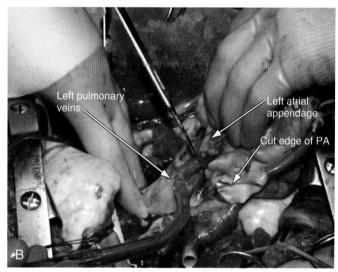

Figure 24-3

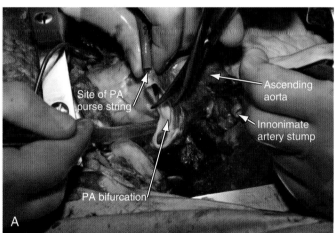

Figure 24-4

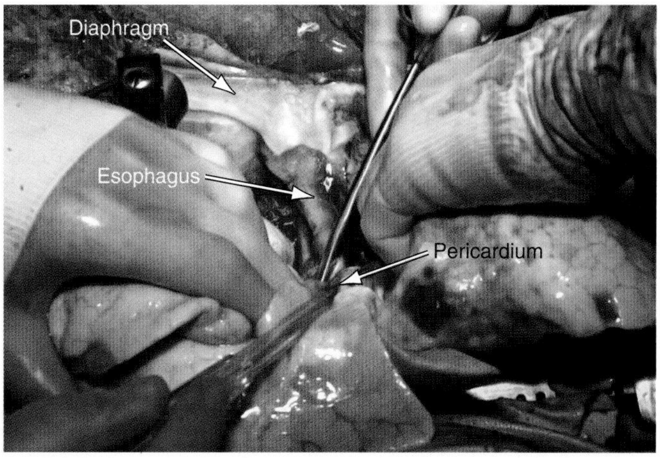

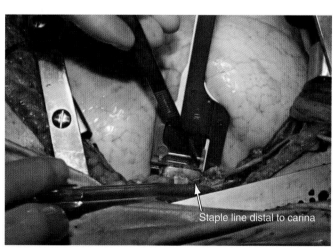

Figure 24-5

Figure 24-6

2. Back-Table Separation

- Flush retrograde plegia via each pulmonary vein and gently massage lungs to evacuate any remaining clot; this will be seen in effluent from the PA. Divide the pericardium from the inferior margin toward the carina. Divide the posterior wall of the left atrium similarly, leaving equal cuffs on the right and left.
- Free the PA from pericardial attachments back to the first branches to prevent distortion and divide at its bifurcation. Isolate but do not skeletonize the left mainstem bronchus, and divide between staple lines at its origin (Fig. 24-7).

3. Operative Steps Bilateral

- Incision: Our preferred approach for bilateral transplants is through a "clamshell" bilateral anterolateral thoracotomy. Some surgeons may prefer a staged bilateral posterolateral thoracotomy, which requires a "flip" of the patient between sides. The clamshell incision offers the advantage of saving modest amounts of ischemic time for the second organ and easy access for CPB if needed.
- Incision is made in the inframammary crease roughly following the fourth intercostal space and bisecting the sternum at this level (Fig. 24-8).
- Ligate both internal mammary arteries and veins.

4. Pneumonectomy

- Isolate the pulmonary veins and main PA by careful blunt dissection as you would for a pneumonectomy. Keep in mind that you need to reattach the new organ so save as much length as possible. The hilum of the recipient is usually quite stuck and crowded with large lymph nodes; take care. Obtain proximal control of each with umbilical tape.
- Before division of the vessels, we give about 100 units/kg of heparin. Typically we divide the PA first, but in some cases it is easier to divide one or both pulmonary veins first.
- Divide the pulmonary vasculature with an Endo-GIA with a vascular load. To gain length, you may divide it out at each major division if necessary.
- Divide the superior and inferior pulmonary veins separately using the same stapler.
- The bronchus is divided last and sharply with a No. 10 blade. Bulky nodes should be removed, but take great care not to skeletonize the bronchus, and keep in mind that the blood supply runs along the lateral aspects. This must be preserved. Trim it back until there are about three rings from the carina. The PA and left atrium should be released from their pericardial reflections.
- After pneumonectomy, irrigate well and make sure the hemithorax is hemostatic; many of these areas will be very difficult to visualize after the graft is in place.

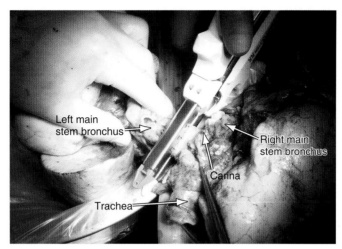

Figure 24-7

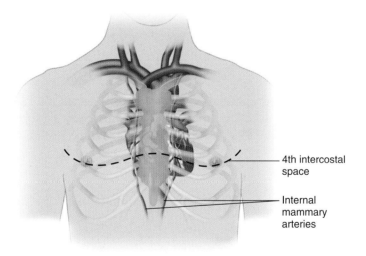

Figure 24-8

5. Implant

- Wrap the lung in an iced lap sponge.
- Open and trim the bronchus and send the remnant for culture.
- You may begin the anastomosis with the lung inside the chest or outside and then "parachute" it in after the first few stitches. We use 3-0 PDS and begin with a simple suture at each corner. Then proceed with a third stitch to run the posterior wall (membranous portion). The anterior wall is completed with interrupted figure-of-eight sutures. Intussusception of the donor bronchus inside the recipient should be done whenever possible. Taking deeper bites on the recipient side will facilitate this. Do not tie the sutures too tight because this may lead to necrosis.
- The PA is done second. Control the PA with a large vascular clamp, which may need to be placed within the pericardium. Be very mindful of the orientation; it is easy to twist this. We use 4-0 Prolene with an RB-1 needle.
- The left atrial cuff is last. Control with a large side-biting vascular clamp. Open each pulmonary vein separately at the staple line then "connect the dots" by opening the atrium between. Err on the side of leaving extra posteriorly. We use a 3-0 Prolene on an SH for this. Be careful not to purse-string this while your assistant follows the suture. Leave the last couple stitches lax for venting air and pulmoplegia (Fig. 24-9).
- If the donor atrial cuff is short or inadequate, we have utilized two different techniques using donor pericardium, as illustrated in Figure 24-10.

6. Venting

- Via the last two bites of the left atrial (LA) anastomosis, release the PA slowly first and allow the pulmoplegia and air to vent out, then the LA clamp slowly. Be sure to communicate with your anesthesiologist during this step because of the volume loss and potential for arrhythmias related to residual pulmoplegia or air.

7. Chest Closure

- Two 34 French chest tubes are left, one straight anteriorly to the apex and one angled in the sulcus. Be careful not to jam the apical tube all the way to the top. Pull it back a couple of centimeters to avoid injury to the stellate ganglia.
- Approximate the sternum with a single figure-of-eight wire. About four pericostal sutures are needed on each side using 1-0 PDS or Vicryl. Close the muscle layers with 2-0 and 3-0 Vicryl and the skin with staples. We do not routinely place drains.

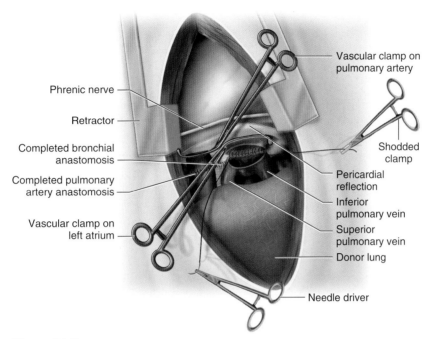

Vascular clamp on
pulmonary artery

Phrenic nerve

Retractor

Completed bronchial
anastomosis

Completed pulmonary
artery anastomosis

Vascular clamp on
left atrium

Shodded
clamp

Pericardial
reflection

Inferior
pulmonary vein

Superior
pulmonary vein

Donor lung

Needle driver

Figure 24-9

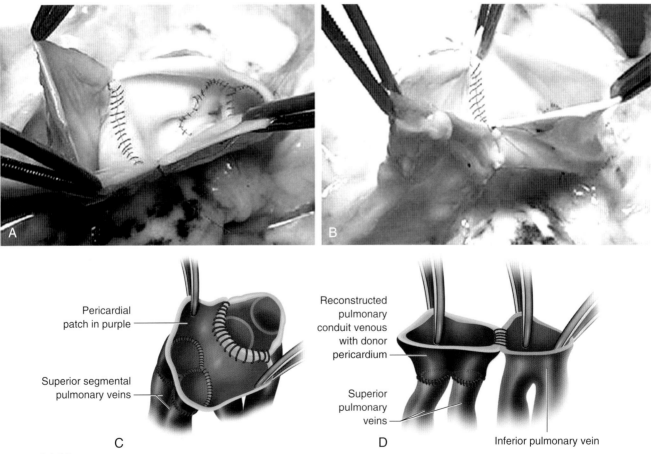

Pericardial
patch in purple

Superior segmental
pulmonary veins

C

Reconstructed
pulmonary
conduit venous
with donor
pericardium

Superior
pulmonary
veins

Inferior pulmonary vein

D

Figure 24-10

8. Alternative Approaches

◆ For a single-lung transplantation, we use a standard posterolateral thoracotomy through the fifth intercostal space (Fig. 24-11). An alternative for bilateral lung transplantation is to use staged posterolateral thoracotomies, turning the patient between sides. This approach provides somewhat better exposure to the hilum, the left atrium in particular, and may be preferred in some cases based on preoperative imaging. Care must be taken to prep and expose the groin for cannulation if bypass is needed during the operation.

Step 4. Postoperative Care

◆ Postoperative care begins in the operating room. The double-lumen endotracheal tube should be exchanged for a single lumen and fiberoptic bronchoscopy performed to confirm placement, check each anastomosis, and provide final bronchial suctioning before transport.

◆ In the intensive care unit (ICU), careful observation and monitoring, including continual assessment of blood pressure, oxygen saturation, urine output, and heart rate, are paramount. We routinely use PA catheters for the first 24 to 48 postoperative hours unless indicated to remain longer. Central filling pressures should be kept very low, and vasopressor or inotropic therapy continued or initiated as needed. The use of pulmonary vasodilating agents such as milrinone or nitric oxide may be very useful. Fluid resuscitation should be judicious. Early ventilator settings should use the minimum fraction of inspired oxygen necessary to maintain adequate oxygen delivery and minimize barotrauma. Usually a peak end-expiratory pressure of 5 cm H_2O is adequate. A feeding tube should be placed for early institution of nutrition. Use standard prophylaxis for deep venous thrombosis, holding heparin until there is no evidence of ongoing bleeding, especially if the patient required CPB.

◆ Extubate patients as soon as possible, and then mobilize them. Our practice is to do bronchoscopy just before extubation for anastomotic assessment and pulmonary toilet. Aspiration is a serious concern in these patients, and precautions as well as liberal evaluations for dysphagia are necessary. Pulmonary physiotherapy with vibropercussion and incentive spirometry is instituted after extubation.

◆ Immunosuppression begins preoperatively and continues throughout the perioperative period and lifelong. Each center has its own protocol, which in general consists of a calcineurin inhibitor (tacrolimus, cyclosporine), antiproliferative agent (CellCept, azathioprine, Myfortic), and steroids. Institutional bias, dogma, and regional environmental concerns affect the recipe that balances the fine line between infection and rejection with the long-term goals of minimizing bronchiolitis obliterans and lymphoproliferative disorders. Adherence to these protocols and "double-checking" is important to ensure that patients are being adequately immunosuppressed but not becoming overly neutropenic or have nephrotoxic doses of their calcineurin inhibitor, for instance. Check the intraoperative cultures, and guide the antibiotic prophylaxis accordingly.

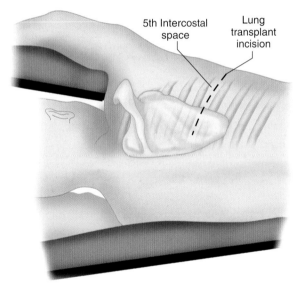

Figure 24-11

- On leaving the ICU area, the patient will be moved to a transplant unit that offers proper air filtration and isolation. Here physical therapy, pulmonary toilet, and education about their drug regimen and compliance are important. Surveillance for rejection will be done via biopsy. Noninvasive markers are being developed but have yet to be accepted as standard of care. More subtle clues, such as dropping O_2 saturation or decreasing forced expiratory volume in 1 second, may be early signs of rejection and should be noted. A spirometry device may be useful for daily testing of lung volume. Before release, the patient and family members should be educated on all aspects of caring for the patient, including information about medications, activity, follow-up, diet, and any other specific instructions, usually summarized in a patient handbook. Most of the discharge planning and education are provided by transplant coordinators.

Step 5. Pearls and Pitfalls

- It is better to undersize slightly than oversize.
- Avoid cell-saver when bronchus is open.
- Thoroughly lavage the donor lung with iced saline before bronchial anastomosis—best chance at pulmonary toilet.
- Opening pericardium allows for greater manipulation during dissection with less hemodynamic compromise.
- In some cases (especially on the left side), off-pump apical suction devices can be used to facilitate exposure, thereby avoiding need for CPB.
- If the recipient PA is much larger than the donor PA, superior or inferior division of the PA can be used.
- Be careful not to purse-string PA when tying.
- Clearly communicate the major steps (i.e., clamping and unclamping) with your anesthesia team.
- Limit volume resuscitation, even in the operating room.
- Have nitric oxide available because it may help to avoid the need for CPB.
- Check for the PA catheter before stapling the PA.
- Left-sided double-lumen tubes are preferred.

Suggested Readings

Christie JD, Edwards LB, Aurora P, et al. Registry of the International Society for Heart and Lung Transplantation: Twenty-fifth Official Adult Lung and Heart/Lung Transplantation Report—2008. J Heart Lung Transplant 2008;27:957-969.

Iribarne A, Russo MJ, Davies RR, et al. Despite decreased wait-list times for lung transplantation, lung allocation scores continue to increase. Chest 2009;135:928-935.

Mason DP, Batizy LH, Wu H, et al. Matching donor to recipient in lung transplantation: How much does size matter? J Thorac Cardiovasc Surg 2009;137:1241-1248.

Oto T, Rabinov M, Negri J, et al. Techniques of reconstruction for inadequate donor left atrial cuff in lung transplantation. Ann Thorac Surg 2006;81:1199-1204.

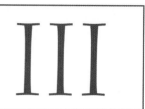

Esophageal Cancer

CHAPTER 25

TRANSTHORACIC ESOPHAGECTOMY

Daniel J. Boffa

Step 1. Surgical Anatomy

- The thoracic esophagus courses through the posterior aspect of the middle mediastinum. In most patients the esophagus lies in the midline; however, slight deviation to the right or left is not uncommon. Although the entire thoracic esophagus can be mobilized from either hemithorax, the ability to evaluate tissue planes at greatest risk for invasion dictates the approach. Tumors in the upper two thirds of the chest are most often approached from the right side of the chest (assess airway, azygos, pericardium), and tumors of the distal third are approached by several centers from the left side of the chest (assess aorta, pericardium, crus).

- The blood supply to the uppermost portion of the thoracic esophagus arises from the inferior thyroid arteries. The remainder of the thoracic esophagus is perfused by branches of the bronchial arteries and esophageal perforators directly from the aorta. Because of an extensive network of collaterals between the cervical, thoracic, and abdominal esophagus, the thoracic esophagus can be fully mobilized and left in situ if the operation is unable to be completed.

- An en bloc esophagectomy refers to the resection of all tissues from the hiatus to the arch of the azygos vein contained within the following borders: the left and right parietal pleura, the adventitia of the aorta, the vertebral bodies, the posterior pericardium, and the membranous airway at the carina. Included within this resection are the esophagus, the vagus nerves, periesophageal lymph nodes (levels 7 and 8), azygos vein (varies by surgeon), thoracic duct, bilateral parietal pleura, the base of bilateral inferior pulmonary ligament level 9 lymph nodes (bilaterally), and the posterior pericardium (Fig. 25-1).[1-3]

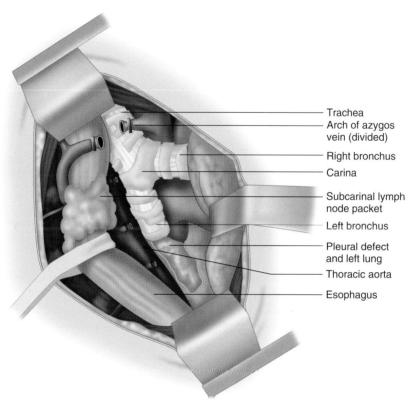

Trachea
Arch of azygos vein (divided)
Right bronchus
Carina
Subcarinal lymph node packet
Left bronchus
Pleural defect and left lung
Thoracic aorta
Esophagus

Figure 25-1

◆ A transthoracic lymph node dissection typically involves the periesophageal lymph nodes (level 8), bilateral inferior pulmonary ligament lymph nodes (level 9), subcarinal lymph nodes (level 7), and the right paratracheal lymph nodes (level 4) or the aortopulmonary (AP) window lymph nodes (level 5), depending on the approach. Typically, more than 15 lymph nodes can be expected with this type of resection.

Step 2. Preoperative Considerations

◆ Nutritional status should be evaluated by history (weight loss >20%) and chemistry (prealbumin <15). Nutritional supplements are typically administered orally, although percutaneous endoscopic gastrostomy tubes do not appear to affect subsequent reconstruction.[4] It should be noted that most patients receiving neoadjuvant therapy will experience sufficient improvement in dysphagia to maintain their weight.[5,6]

◆ The surgeon should perform an upper endoscopy (in the operating room or in the clinic) to plan the extent of resection. In addition to complete removal of the tumor, all Barrett mucosa should be removed. Both the gastric margin and esophageal margin should be grossly 5 cm from the tumor.[7]

◆ A bowel preparation is generally reserved for patients in whom the stomach is likely to be an inadequate conduit. A computed tomography angiogram can be helpful if there is a question of compromise of the right gastroepiploic arcade from previous gastric surgery.

◆ Surgical approach is dictated by the following:

   ▲ *Location of tumor:* Tumors in the upper and middle portions of the chest should be addressed from the right chest, in large part to be able to assess invasion into surrounding airway. Tumors of the lower thoracic esophagus could be approached through either side of the chest. The left-sided chest is particularly helpful if the tumor is growing into the left hemidiaphragm.

   ▲ *The ability to tolerate single-lung ventilation:* If a patient has an anatomic reason that limits single-lung ventilation to a particular side, this should be evaluated preoperatively and approach tailored accordingly (operate on the side of worse function).

   ▲ *Surgeon's preference and experience:* The oncologic differences between approaches appear to be subtle; safety should dominate this decision.

Step 3. Operative Steps

Tri-Incision Esophagectomy (Modified McKeown)

1. Thoracic Portion

- A right-sided posterolateral thoracotomy is performed in the sixth intercostal space. The lung is palpated to exclude occult pulmonary metastases. The early dissection should focus on regions at greatest risk for extramural invasion (T4).
- Incise the inferior pulmonary ligament up to the inferior pulmonary vein. Remove right level 9 lymph nodes. Continue the pleural incision along the posterior hilum, past the right main-stem bronchus up to the arch of the azygos vein. Caution should be used when cauterizing near the membranous airway. The arch of the azygos vein may or may not be divided (surgeon preference).

Anterior Dissection
- Begin by dissecting between the pericardium and the esophagus at a point just inferior to the inferior pulmonary vein (if a bulky tumor is present at this level, the posterior pericardium is incorporated into the en bloc specimen).
- Continue this dissection superiorly and laterally until the bulk of the posterior pericardium is free and the left pleura is reached (to avoid the *left*-sided inferior pulmonary ligament, wait to incise the left pleura until the posterior esophageal dissection).

- Elevating the subcarinal lymph node packet will expose the left mainstem at the carina, preventing injury to the left-sided airway as the esophagus is mobilized from below (often this will feel firm from the double-lumen endotracheal tube) (Fig. 25-2).

Posterior Dissection

- Incise the pleura along the posterior aspect of the esophagus, elevating the fatty streak off of the azygos vein towards the esophagus. Dissecting in the filmy plane just off the azygos vein will incorporate the thoracic duct in the en bloc specimen (as opposed to crease just posterior to the esophagus, which is a filmy plane that leaves the thoracic duct intact) (Fig. 25-3).
- Continue up the arch of the azygos superiorly and the hiatus inferiorly. The leftward extension of this dissection will reveal the anterior-lateral surface of the aorta. Careful dissection will expose esophageal perforators that can be ligated and divided.
- As the lateral dissection is carried further, the left pleura is reached and incised. The left lung will need to be adherent to the superior aspect of the incised pleura (the left inferior pulmonary ligament).
- The ligament is divided, allowing the left pleura to remain fixed to the en bloc specimen. This incision continues up the left inferior pulmonary vein.
- A left level 9 lymph dissection is performed. Passing a Penrose drain around the esophagus for retraction can facilitate exposure of the leftward aspect of the specimen.

Superior Dissection

- For tumors that arise in the mid to distal thoracic esophagus, all dissection cephalad to the arch of the azygos should be directly on the esophageal wall (to avoid injury to recurrent nerves).
- For tumors of the upper thoracic esophagus, the dissection should include as much peri-esophageal tissue as possible.
- Care should be taken as the dissection approaches the thoracic inlet because the right recurrent nerve can be injured at this level.
- The thoracic duct crosses over from right to left near the arch of the azygos vein. If the tumor mandates a wide dissection at this level, ligate the periesophageal tissue with ties to avoid a lymph leak.

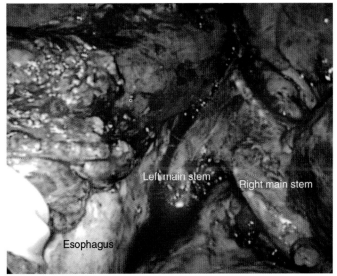

Figure 25-2

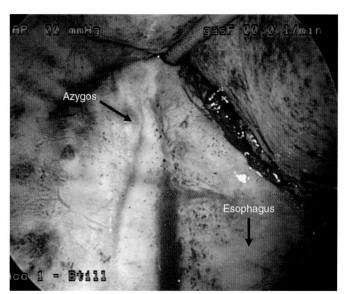

Figure 25-3

Inferior Dissection

- At the level of the hiatus the pleura is opened over the right crus.
- The phrenoesophageal ligament and peritoneum are incised to allow entry into the abdomen. This incision is carried circumferentially around the esophagus.
- The thoracic duct typically courses between the aorta and azygos vein. In this region the soft tissue must be suture ligated prior to division.
- If the tumor is locally invasive at this level, a rim of crus should be removed in continuity with the tumor. Care should be taken to avoid the phrenic nerve.

Closure

- The ribs are brought together with interrupted pericostal Vicryl sutures (No. 2 Vicryls).
- The soft tissue is reapproximated in multiple layers with absorbable suture.

Abdominal Dissection

- Through an upper midline laparotomy, the falciform ligament and the left triangular ligament are divided. This will allow the left lateral segments of the liver to be retracted into the right upper quadrant.
- Aggressive retraction of the xyphoid and costal arch superiorly and anteriorly will dramatically enhance the exposure of the epigastrium and hiatus.

Gastric Mobilization

- The pars flaccida, or clear membrane overlying the caudate lobe of the liver, is incised to expose the right crus.
- The periesophageal soft tissue is dissected off of the right crus, exposing the junction of the right and left crura posteriorly.
- The dissection continues anteriorly and the periesophageal tissue is dissected off of the left crus. With a little bit of blunt dissection, the esophagus should be easily mobilized circumferentially, allowing a Penrose drain to be passed around the esophagus.

Short Gastric

- The lesser sac can be entered at any point along the greater curvature; however, one must be aware of the transition from the right gastroepiploic to the short gastrics because the former must be preserved. It is often preferable to identify the right gastroepiploic arcade near the midportion of the greater curvature and start dividing the omentum 1 to 2 cm peripheral to the gastroepiploic arcade. This is continued up toward the fundus.
- Once the transition to the short gastrics is identified, the short gastrics are divided a centimeter off the stomach. Great care must be taken in the region of the splenic hilum because there are often adhesions to the splenic capsule. The dissection may be facilitated by dividing the adhesions in the lesser sac that tether the posterior wall of the stomach.

Left Gastric Artery

- As the stomach is elevated toward the hiatus, the left gastric artery can be identified in a band of fat between the retroperitoneum and lesser curvature (the vessels can also be approached from the right). The base of this pedicle should be thinned out to allow the left gastric lymph nodes to be contained within the specimen.
- The veins running alongside the artery are relatively fragile. Care should be taken to avoid the splenic artery because it courses laterally at the same level as the origin of the left gastric artery.

Gastric Conduit

- The shape of the conduit is dictated by the location of the tumor as well as by surgeon preference for whole stomach[8] or a narrow gastric tube.[9] In either case, the gastroesophageal junction must be resected, requiring division of at least the two highest vascular rami of the lesser omentum. The narrower the tube, the more rami that must be ligated toward the pylorus.

- A staple line is started on the lesser curve of the stomach and continued toward the fundus in a line that parallels the greater curvature (Fig. 25-4).
- Many surgeons think narrower tubes have better emptying, whereas wider tubes retain better perfusion. A tube should not be smaller than 4 cm because the stricture and leak rate increase substantially.

Kocher Maneuver

- The goal is to have the pylorus reach the caudate lobe when the conduit is pulled up.

Emptying Procedure

- A pyloroplasty or pyloromyotomy may be performed (either should be covered with a slip of omentum at the end of procedure).
- More recently we have been injecting the pylorus with 200 units of botulinum toxin A (BOTOX, Allergan, Irvine, CA) (divided into three injections at points along the muscle).

Jejunostomy

- A feeding jejunostomy (16 French or smaller, depending on the caliber of the bowel) is placed 30 cm distal to the ligament of Treitz. A short Weitzel tunnel should be used (<2 cm). The jejunum is secured to the abdominal wall, taking great care not to create an obstructive narrowing in the jejunum.

Anastomosis

Cervical

- The surgeon (standing on the patient's left) makes an oblique incision in the left neck along the anterior border of the sternocleidomastoid (SCM) muscle (originating 1 cm above the manubrium, extending half the distance to the mastoid process). The left neck is chosen because the course of the recurrent nerve is more predictable on the left side; however, a right neck dissection can be done as well.
- The dissected SCM muscle is retracted laterally to expose the omohyoid muscle, which is divided with cautery.
- The assistant retracts the trachea anteriorly and to the right (an index finger is the least traumatic). As the dissection extends more medially, the jugular vein is identified and retracted posteriorly. Change to Metzenbaum scissors.
- The assistant deepens his or her retraction into the tracheoesophageal groove (a nasogastric [NG] tube is helpful) (Fig. 25-5). The carotid artery is identified just medial to the jugular

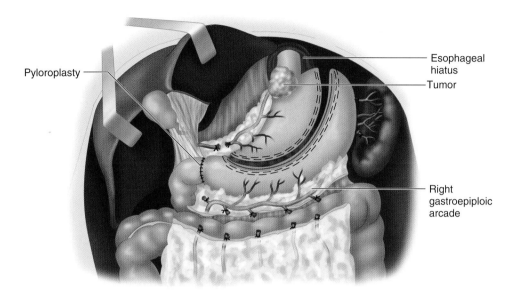

Pyloroplasty

Esophageal hiatus

Tumor

Right gastroepiploic arcade

Figure 25-4

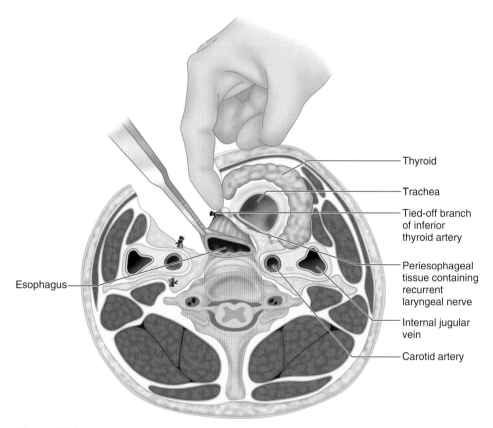

Thyroid

Trachea

Tied-off branch of inferior thyroid artery

Periesophageal tissue containing recurrent laryngeal nerve

Internal jugular vein

Carotid artery

Esophagus

Figure 25-5

vein. The prevertebral space is accessed between the carotid artery and the esophagus. An important arterial branch should be identified coursing under the carotid toward the tracheoesophageal groove (a branch of the inferior thyroid artery). This vessel is ligated and divided.

◆ The medial aspect (esophageal side) is a valuable landmark of the tracheoesophageal groove. The anterior dissection of the esophagus should begin just beneath this vessel. Blunt dissection with closed scissors is used to develop this plane between the esophagus and soft tissue anteriorly, which will elevate the left recurrent nerve off of the esophagus. This dissection continues bluntly around to the right lateral aspect of the esophagus to the prevertebral space. Breaking through the last layer of tissue to bring the anterior and posterior dissections into continuity can be difficult.

◆ In general, the mobilization is easier deeper into the thoracic inlet. A Penrose is placed around the esophagus and the soft tissue is dissected off of the esophagus bluntly into the thoracic inlet, connecting the thoracic and cervical mobilizations. A sign that the mobilization is complete is the ability to deliver several centimeters of esophagus through the cervical wound.

◆ The esophagus is divided with a stapler, leaving 4 cm of mobilized cervical esophagus. An umbilical tape is attached to the specimen side of the cervical esophagus, and the specimen is delivered into the abdomen (the umbilical tape maintains access through the closed chest). Proceed with anastomosis once the margins are negative.

◆ The umbilical tape is used to deliver a laparoscopic camera bag through the chest (open end in the abdomen, closed end in the neck). The conduit is placed in the bag and delivered into the neck by pulling the bag out of the cervical incision.

◆ A gastrostomy is made in the tip of the conduit. The esophagus is opened. The large end of an EndoGIA stapler (Ethicon Endo-Surgery Inc, Somerville, NJ) is inserted in the stomach side, the thin blade into the esophagus. The stapler is fired, leaving rows of staples as the back wall of anastomosis (Fig. 25-6A). The NG tube is advanced beyond the anastomosis.

◆ The anterior aspect is closed with a running 4-0 absorbable suture (see Fig. 25-6B). The redundant conduit is milked back into the abdomen by reaching up through the hiatus from the abdomen and pulling down gently as the anastomosis drops into the thoracic inlet. A Jackson-Pratt drain is placed in neck, spanning across the anastomosis and into the thoracic inlet.

Ivor Lewis Esophagectomy

Abdominal Portion

◆ An upper midline laparotomy is made and the gastric mobilization, conduit formation, jejunostomy tube, and gastric emptying procedure are performed as described for the tri-incision esophagectomy. Suture the tip of the conduit to the specimen in such a way that proper orientation can be maintained.

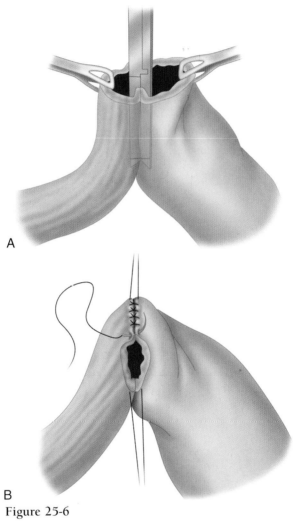

A

B

Figure 25-6

Thoracic Portion

- The incision and mobilization of the thoracic esophagus are as described in the section on tri-incisional esophagectomy (modified McKeown). At completion of the inferior portion of the dissection, bring the conduit up into the chest. Great care must be taken to maintain orientation (staple line of conduit should be facing rightward).

Anastomosis

- The thoracic esophagus is divided at least 3 cm above the arch of the azygos vein. The anastomosis is performed once the margins are negative.
- The appropriate end-to-end anastomosis (EEA) stapler is chosen (typically No. 28 or 25). The anvil is inserted into the cut end of the esophagus, and a purse string is placed to secure the esophagus around the stem of the anvil. Make sure that mucosa is included (if the purse string has a gap around the stem of anvil, place a second purse string).
- The conduit is brought into the right side of the chest without torsion and opened at the distal end along the side of the staple line (there will be extra length of conduit). The EEA stapler is inserted and the pin of the stapler is delivered through the wall of greater curvature of the conduit. The pin of the stapler and the stem of the anvil are engaged and the stapler fired (Fig. 25-7). The stapler is dialed out of the firing position, allowing the anvil to slip through the anastomosis. The stem of the anvil should have two complete rings of tissue on it (representing the gastric and esophageal wall).
- Attempt to keep the orientation set in the event the doughnuts are concerning and more sutures need to be placed. The redundant conduit containing the site of the gastrostomy is resected using an EndoGIA stapler. Care is taken not to pull the anastomosis into this stapling line.
- An NG tube is advanced into the conduit. A Jackson-Pratt drain is left in the posterior path of the conduit spanning the anastomosis.

Thoracic Esophagectomy Via Left Thoracoabdominal Approach

- The patient is positioned in the right lateral decubitus position. The left arm, left neck, chest, and abdomen are prepped into the field. An anterolateral thoracotomy is marked along the sixth interspace. The incision will extend through the costal arch and onto the abdomen obliquely for 5 to 8 cm (just enough to fit one hand in).
- Open the abdominal portion first, and assess for ascites, peritoneal implants, liver metastases, and local invasion that would preclude resection.

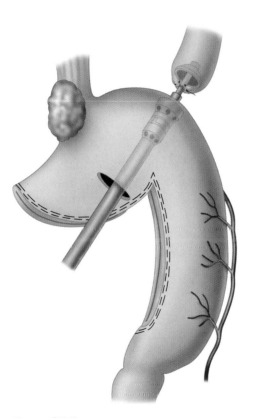

Figure 25-7

- Open the chest without dividing from the arch to feel for pulmonary metastases. The incision typically extends up to the anterior border of the latissimus dorsi muscle. If no metastases are identified, divide the arch with a scissors. A Finochietto retractor is placed to splay open the ribs. This is sutured to the chest wall to keep in place (Fig. 25-8).
- Incise the diaphragm radially approximately 2 to 3 cm from the insertion onto the chest wall. This will prevent significant denervation and maintain adequate tissue for closure. Typically the incision is continued until the dome of the spleen is visible (10 cm). Place two sutures on the rightward edge of the diaphragmatic incision to distract the diaphragm superiorly or inferiorly to expose the abdomen or chest, respectively.
- Begin the dissection in the area with the greatest concern for invasion to allow for rapid determination of resectability.

Thoracic Anterior Dissection

- Incise the inferior pulmonary ligament up to the inferior pulmonary vein. Resect the left level 9 lymph nodes. Continue by dissecting the esophagus off of the posterior pericardium. The exposure can often be facilitated by *carefully* placing a Kocher clamp on the pericardium to retract the pericardium anteriorly (avoid the phrenic nerve). Continue to advance until the right pleura is reached. The pleural incision can be made at this point; however, the right inferior pulmonary ligament is in this region. It is often better to enter the right side of the chest from the posterior dissection.

Thoracic Posterior Dissection

- Dissect the esophagus off of the aorta. Ligate any esophageal perforators. Just superior to the hiatus, enter the right pleural cavity. Divide the right inferior pulmonary ligament.
- Place a Penrose drain around the esophagus and dissect superiorly. Include the subcarinal lymph nodes in an en bloc specimen. Continue up under the arch of the aorta. At the level of the arch of the aorta, be careful to stay directly on the wall of the esophagus to avoid injury to the left recurrent nerve.
- Oversew the thoracic duct at the base of the right chest. Distract the aorta and mobilized esophagus anterolaterally, and place a mattress suture between the right lateral wall of the aorta and the azygos vein (may also include the azygos vein).
- Perform the gastric mobilization, gastric emptying procedure, and feeding jejunostomy as described above for the right chest approach (the sutures in the diaphragm can change the direction of the retraction to provide exposure to the abdomen or chest) (Fig. 25-9). When the abdominal portion is under way, ventilate the left lung.

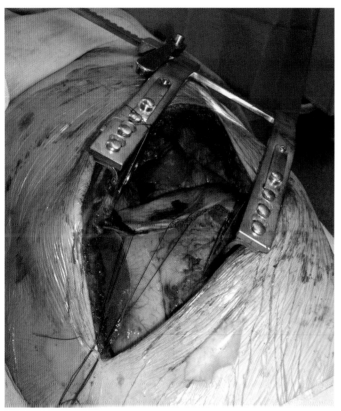

Figure 25-8

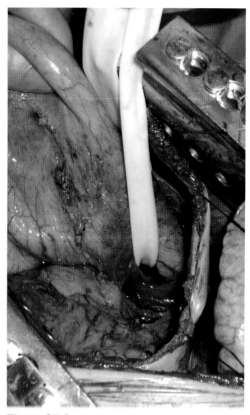

Figure 25-9

- Mobilize the cervical esophagus through an oblique left neck incision as described for tri-incisional, modified McKeown approach.
- A large Babcock clamp can be used through the neck incision to guide (not pull) as you push the conduit up to the neck from the left chest.
- Create a cervical anastomosis (once the margins are clear) as described for tri-incisional, modified McKeown approach.
- Milk the conduit down to remove any redundancy (typically the conduit has fallen into the right chest). Suture the conduit to the crus from the abdomen to prevent herniation around the conduit.
- Close the diaphragm with a running suture (No. 1 Vicryl or Prolene). The segment (roughly 5 cm) closest to the arch is particularly fragile. The suture should be run through this area but not pulled tight. Start a new suture on the internal oblique muscle just below the divided arch. Tie the pericostals, then cinch up on the diaphragmatic suture, and tie to the internal oblique suture. Close the arch with interrupted Vicryl mattresses. Close the abdominal portion in two layers.

Step 4. Postoperative Care

- Patients are typically extubated in the operating room and spend a single night in the intensive care unit.
- They should be out of bed the day of surgery and walking the first postoperative day.
- The tube feeding begins postoperative day 2 unless the abdomen is distended. On postoperative day 3, the tube feeds are advanced to goal unless there is evidence of a chyle leak. The chest tube is removed on day 2 or 3, as long as the drainage is less than 250 mL in 24 hours and does not suggest an anastomotic leak. The NG tube is removed on postoperative day 4 and the neck Jackson-Pratt on postoperative day 5.
- Clears liquids are given on postoperative day 5.
- Patients are typically discharged on postoperative day 8 to 10 on a clear liquid diet and tube feeding.

Step 5. Pearls and Pitfalls

- ◆ Nuisance bleeding from periesophageal tissues can be controlled by temporarily packing and working elsewhere in the thorax.
- ◆ The conduit should be handled as gently as possible, and care should be taken to avoid grasping the fundus in the region that will be used for anastomosis.

References

1. Rizzetto C, DeMeester SR, Hagen JA, et al. En bloc esophagectomy reduces local recurrence and improves survival compared with transhiatal resection after neoadjuvant therapy for esophageal adenocarcinoma. J Thorac Cardiovasc Surg 2008;135:1228-1236.
2. Mariette C, Castel B, Toursel H, et al. Surgical management of and long-term survival after adenocarcinoma of the cardia. Br J Surg 2002;89:1156-1163.
3. Altorki N, Kent M, Ferrara C, Port J. Three-field lymph node dissection for squamous cell and adenocarcinoma of the esophagus. Ann Surg 2002;236:177-183.
4. Margolis M, Alexander P, Trachiotis GD, et al. Percutaneous endoscopic gastrostomy before multimodality therapy in patients with esophageal cancer. Ann Thorac Surg 2003;76:1694-1697.
5. Steyn RS, Grenier I, Darnton SJ, et al. Weight gain as an indicator of response to chemotherapy for oesophageal carcinoma. Clin Oncol (R Coll Radiol) 1995;7:382-384.
6. Forshaw MJ, Gossage JA, Chrystal K, et al. Symptomatic responses to neoadjuvant chemotherapy for carcinoma of the oesophagus and oesophagogastric junction: Are they worth measuring? Clin Oncol (R Coll Radiol) 2006;18:345-350.
7. Barbour AP, Rizk NP, Gonen M, et al. Adenocarcinoma of the gastroesophageal junction: Influence of esophageal resection margin and operative approach on outcome. Ann Surg 2007;246:1-8.
8. Collard JM, Tinton N, Malaise J, et al. Esophageal replacement: Gastric tube or whole stomach? Ann Thorac Surg 1995;60:261-266.
9. De Giacomo T, Francioni F, Venuta F, et al. Complete mechanical cervical anastomosis using a narrow gastric tube after esophagectomy for cancer. Eur J Cardiothorac Surg 2004;26:881-884.

CHAPTER 26

TRANSHIATAL ESOPHAGECTOMY

James E. Lynch, Kiasha James, and Joseph B. Zwischenberger

History

Transhiatal esophagectomy (THE) has been gaining popularity for the past two and a half decades. In 1978 Orringer and Sloan renewed interest in this procedure, presenting it as an alternative approach to the more traditional transthoracic esophagectomy. THE is done without a thoracotomy and the physiologic impact on the body is minimized, resulting in decreased morbidity and mortality rates.

Indications

Patients under evaluation for an esophagectomy should be considered potential candidates for THE. The transhiatal approach to esophagectomy has been used for resection of tumors at any location; however, it is best for tumors in the lower esophagus distal to the membranous trachea and at the esophagogastric junction. This approach allows complete excision of the esophagus without the need for a thoracotomy. Patients post radiation treatment and those with peri-esophageal adhesions from various causes (caustic injuries, achalasia, previous surgeries) can still undergo THE; however, patients with local invasion of major structures or those with distant metastasis (stage IV disease) are considered unresectable because the risk from the surgery far outweighs the benefits derived from the procedure.

Step 1. Surgical Anatomy

- ◆ A comprehensive understanding of the anatomy of the esophagus is essential before any operation on the esophagus. Figure 26-1 outlines the key anatomic structures that must be identified before performing THE.

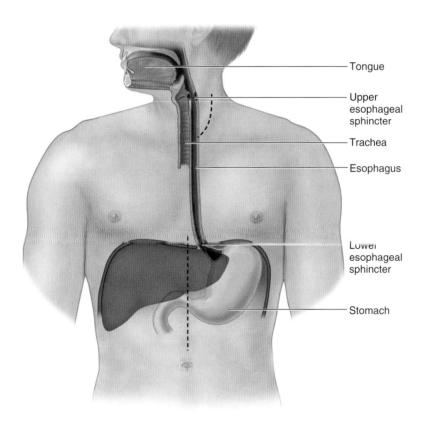

Tongue

Upper
esophageal
sphincter

Trachea

Esophagus

Lower
esophageal
sphincter

Stomach

Figure 26-1

Step 2. Preoperative Considerations

- Efficient preoperative evaluation should include a thorough assessment of the patient's cardiopulmonary reserve and their operative risk. Exercise stress testing, spirometry, and arterial blood gas should be considered.
- Before esophagectomy is performed, esophagoscopy with endoscopic ultrasound, contrast computed tomography (CT) of the chest and abdomen, and positron emission (PET) scan are required. A barium swallow, especially for initial diagnosis, may also be done.
- A barium swallow is useful for tumor location and assessment of whether there is extension into the proximal stomach. Esophagoscopy enables direct visualization and assessment of the mucosa and allows for procurement of samples for cytology and histology. Endoscopic ultrasound allows imaging and needle aspiration of periesophageal and celiac lymph nodes to complete preoperative staging. CT of the chest and abdomen is used to determine the extent of esophageal thickening and celiac or mediastinal adenopathy and to assess whether there is invasion into the tracheobronchial tree and aorta.
- PET is useful to identify the likelihood of distant metastases when positive, especially the lack thereof when negative. Smoking cessation at least 2 weeks before surgery is advised to minimize complications and facilitate early ambulation. Healthy dentition reduces risk of postoperative infection.
- Nasogastric feedings for nutritional supplementation should be instituted in patients with extensive weight loss and dehydration resulting from severe esophageal obstruction.
- Preoperative jejunostomy feeding tubes and percutaneous gastrostomy complicate gastric mobilization but are preferable to TPN.
- Discussing potential surgical complications with the patient (dysphagia, dumping, reflux, regurgitation, and early satiety) is extremely important to enable the patient to make informed decisions and to cultivate realistic expectations about the surgical outcome.

Anesthetic Management

- Continuous intra-arterial blood pressure monitoring with a radial artery catheter is performed to monitor hypotension caused by cardiac displacement by the surgeon's hand during intra-thoracic mobilization.
- Two large-bore intravenous (IV) catheters are placed in peripheral arm veins for rapid volume resuscitation during the operative procedure. Note that the average blood loss is less than 500 mL.
- An epidural catheter augments postoperative pain management to improve pulmonary function.
- A standard endotracheal tube is used. In the event of a posterior membranous tracheal tear during tumor dissection, the tube can be advanced into the distal trachea or left mainstem bronchus, allowing one-lung anesthesia while the repair is undertaken, thus avoiding a double lumen ET tube.

Step 3. Operative Procedure

- THE consists primarily of three phases: abdominal dissection, cervical dissection, and mediastinal dissection.

1. Abdominal Dissection

Incision

- This phase begins with a supraumbilical incision, which extends from the xiphoid to the umbilicus (see Fig. 26-1).

Dissection

- The triangular ligament is divided with retraction of the left lobe of the liver to the right (Fig. 26-2).
- Examine the stomach for tumor involvement and scarring or shortening from prior surgeries.
- Identify and protect the right gastroepiploic artery throughout this early procedure, particularly in patients with a history of prior abdominal surgeries.
- Begin separation of the greater omentum from the stomach along the greater curvature of the stomach where the right gastroepiploic terminates as it enters the stomach.
- The greater omentum is then separated from the right gastroepiploic artery with a 2-cm margin.
- The left gastroepiploic and short gastric arteries are ligated and divided, taking care to avoid injury to the gastric wall and the spleen.
- The peritoneum overlying the hiatus is incised, and the esophagogastric junction is mobilized and encircled with a rubber drain.
- The gastrohepatic omentum is mobilized and incised starting from the midpoint of the lesser curvature and moving toward the hiatus.
- After locating, ligating, and dividing the left gastric vein, the left gastric artery is ligated near its origin from the celiac axis.
- In patients with carcinoma, celiac lymph nodes are sent for pathologic staging. The presence of large celiac nodal metastasis is indicative of incurable disease and a biopsy is taken.
- The right gastric artery is protected throughout the mobilization of the stomach.
- A Kocher maneuver is performed to allow mobilization of the pylorus.
- A pyloromyotomy is then performed. Electrocautery and a fine-tipped mosquito clamp are used to dissect the gastric and duodenal muscle away from the underlying mucosa. Some prefer a Heineke-Mikulicz pyloroplasty, especially when adequate length is not a problem.
- Small metal clips are placed at the level of the pyloromyotomy to serve as markers for future radiographic studies.
- Via downward traction on the rubber drain encircling the esophagogastric junction, the distal 5 to 10 cm of esophagus is mobilized through the diaphragmatic hiatus.
- Mobility of the esophagus within the posterior mediastinum is assessed to ascertain that it is not fixed to the aorta, prevertebral fascia, or surrounding mediastinal structures. Three techniques for esophageal mobilization have evolved: (1) blunt dissection along the prevertebral fascia, (2) enlargement of the esophageal hiatus with direct visualization, and (3) thoracoscopic mobilization of the intrathoracic esophagus.
- If there are no contraindications to proceeding, a jejunostomy tube is placed.

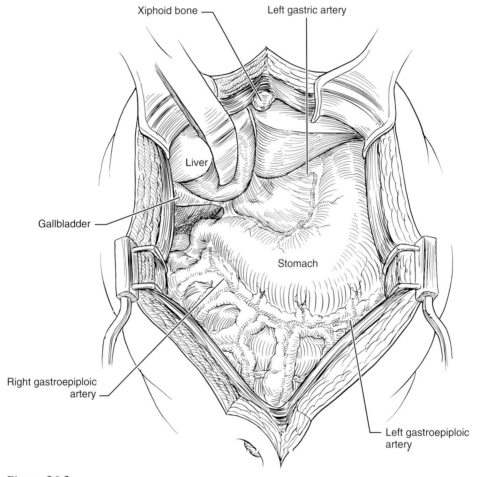

Figure 26-2
(From Townsend CM Jr, Evers MB. Atlas of General Surgical Techniques. Philadelphia: Saunders; 2010.)

2. Cervical Dissection

Incision

- A 5- to 6-cm hockey-stick incision along the anterior border of the left sternocleidomastoid (SCM) is made (Fig. 26-3).

Dissection

- The platysma is divided and the omohyoid is exposed.
- The SCM muscle and the carotid sheath are retracted laterally. Blunt dissection is used to reach the prevertebral fascia. If necessary, the middle thyroid vein and inferior thyroid artery may be ligated.
- The recurrent laryngeal nerve lies deep to these vessels; thus no retractor other than the surgeon's fingers should be placed against the tracheoesophageal groove to avoid injury to this vessel (Fig. 26-4).
- The tracheoesophageal groove is mobilized by dissecting close to the esophageal wall. Gentle finger traction can be used to elevate and move the thyroid cartilage to the right. Care must be taken to avoid injury to the recurrent laryngeal nerve.
- The cervical esophagus is then encircled with a rubber drain and retracted superiorly. Blunt dissection of the upper thoracic esophagus is then performed with the fingers kept against the esophagus
- Approximately a 10-cm length of esophagus is mobilized close to the level of the carina.

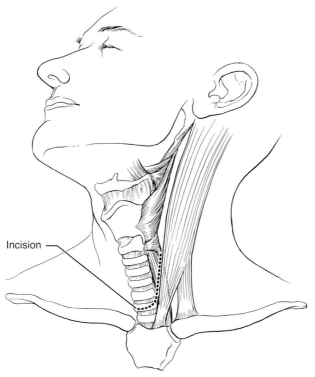

Figure 26-3
(From Townsend CM Jr, Evers MB. Atlas of General
Surgical Techniques. Philadelphia: Saunders; 2010.)

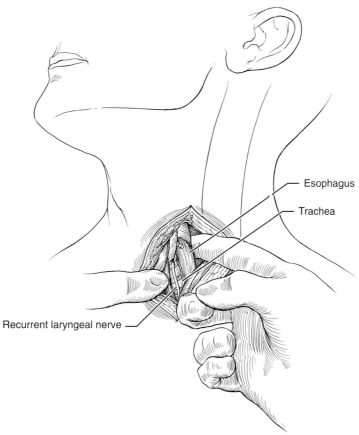

Figure 26-4
(From Townsend CM Jr, Evers MB. Atlas of General Surgical
Techniques. Philadelphia: Saunders; 2010.)

3. Mediastinal Dissection

- Three basic approaches to mediastinal dissection are available:
  - ▲ Thoracoscopy. The patient is positioned for a right-sided approach using video-assisted thoracoscopic surgery techniques. The esophagus is mobilized from the thoracic inlet to the hiatus. Visualization of the azygos vein, the aorta, and the membranous trachea allows each key structure to be mobilized and injury avoided. The azygos vein is divided with an EndoGIA (Ethicon Endo-Surgery Inc, Somerville, NJ). Lymph node localization and resection are also facilitated by this approach. Once the esophagus is mobilized, the cervical and abdominal portions are much easier. This technique is gaining popularity.
  - ▲ Transhiatal with direct visualization. On initial mobilization of the gastroesophageal junction at the hiatus, both the right and left crus are cut 1 to 2 cm at multiple sites to allow dilatation of the crus. The phrenic vein is directly above the crus and should be avoided or ligated. Once the crus is enlarged, the lower to mid mediastinum can be visualized to allow mobilization of the esophagus. Unfortunately, the azygos vein and membranous trachea are still difficult to visualize and must be mobilized at least partially using blunt technique.
  - ▲ Transhiatal blunt esophagectomy via the hiatus. One hand is inserted through the diaphragmatic hiatus posterior to the esophagus while the other hand or a half-sponge on a stick is inserted through the cervical incision, dissecting downwards along the prevertebral fascia (Fig. 26-5).

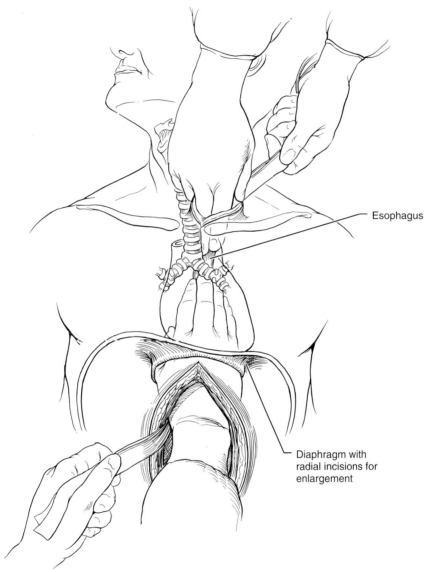

Esophagus

Diaphragm with
radial incisions for
enlargement

Figure 26-5
(From Townsend CM Jr, Evers MB. Atlas of General Surgical Techniques.
Philadelphia: Saunders; 2010.)

- The surgeon should keep his or her hands flattened posteriorly during the dissection to avoid anterior hand elevation, which would compress the left atrium and result in hypotension.
- From both the cervical and abdominal incisions, the esophagus is completely mobilized.
- The anterior esophageal dissection is undertaken first with gentle traction being applied to the rubber drains encircling the esophagus while dissection with the fingers against the anterior esophagus is performed.
- Care must be taken to avoid injury to the posterior membranous trachea as the esophagus is being mobilized.
- With the esophagus in the superior mediastinum, held between the index and middle fingers of the hand inserted through the hiatus, a downward motion is employed to lyse the remaining attachments (Figs. 26-6 and 26-7).
- A narrow retractor can now be placed into the diaphragmatic hiatus to facilitate the dissection of the lateral attachments of the esophagus.
- Upper traction is placed on the rubber drain encircling the esophagus, allowing dissection at the level of the thoracic inlet.
- Maintain dissection immediately adjacent to the esophagus to avoid injury to the azygos vein.
- After the esophagus is completely free, it is then allowed to retract back into the superior mediastinum.

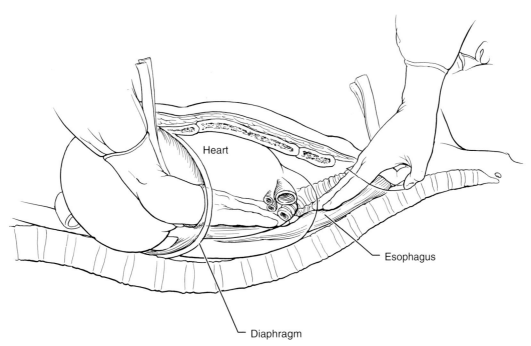

Figure 26-6
(From Townsend CM Jr, Evers MB. Atlas of General Surgical Techniques. Philadelphia: Saunders; 2010.)

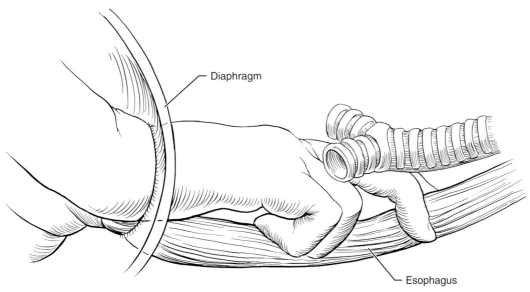

Figure 26-7
(From Townsend CM Jr, Evers MB. Atlas of General Surgical Techniques. Philadelphia: Saunders; 2010.)

- The esophagus is then gently pulled into the cervical wound and is divided obliquely in the neck 5 to 6 cm distal to the cricopharyngeus muscle using a GIA surgical stapler (Fig. 26-8).
- It is important to pay close attention to the blood pressure because compression of the mediastinum and transient impairment in cardiac venous return can induce hypotension.
- If hypotension occurs, the first steps would be to reposition the retractors or remove the dissecting hand. In most cases there would be prompt normalization of blood pressure.
- Deaver retractors are then placed into the diaphragmatic hiatus and the posterior mediastinum is assessed for bleeding. Check also for clear or cloudy fluid indicative of a lymph leak from a torn thoracic duct.
- To control minor bleeding, a large abdominal gauze pack can be inserted into the posterior mediastinum to tamponade any small bleeding vessels.
- The fully mobilized stomach and attached esophagus are positioned on the anterior chest, the gastric fundus is grasped, and gentle traction is applied along the length of the stomach.
- The distal resection margin must then be determined. Ideally the margin should be about 4 to 6 cm from the esophagogastric junction.
- The gastric fundus is retracted superiorly, and a 5-cm GIA stapler is used to transect the stomach proceeding from the lesser curvature toward the fundus.
- To maximize the length of the gastric tube, tension must be applied and the stomach must be progressively stretched in a cephalad direction with every application of the stapler.
- This technique in effect converts a J-shaped stomach into a straight tube.
- With tumors of the upper and middle esophagus and in cases of benign disease needing an esophagectomy, it is important to preserve as much stomach as possible to ensure continued collateral circulation to the gastric fundus.
- The esophageal specimen is then removed from the field, and an examination of the distal margins is done under frozen section.
- The completed gastric staple suture line is then oversewn with running Lembert suture of 4-0 polypropylene, or at least place a Z-stitch at the points of staple line juncture.
- Again, traction must be maintained along the stomach as the suture line is oversewn to prevent foreshortening or "purse stringing" of the lesser curvature, which would hinder the upward reach of the stomach.
- The large abdominal gauze pack placed in the posterior mediastinum earlier in the procedure is now removed.

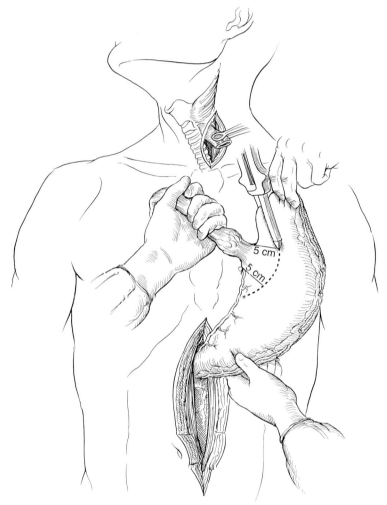

Figure 26-8
(From Townsend CM Jr, Evers MB. Atlas of General Surgical
Techniques. Philadelphia: Saunders; 2010.)

- The stomach is oriented such that the greater curvature is toward the patient's left side. Care must be taken to avoid torsion, which could complicate the surgical outcome (Fig. 26-9).
- The surgeon's hand is inserted through the posterior mediastinum with the palm faced down on the anterior surface of the stomach. The hand and forearm are advanced until three fingers emerge from the neck wound. This ensures that there is sufficient space in the posterior mediastinal tunnel to accommodate the gastric tube.
- The gastric fundus is grasped with finger tips of one hand and guided through the diaphragmatic hiatus, upward anterior to the spine, continuing beneath the aortic arch, and finally into the superior mediastinum.
- The fundus is then delivered into the neck using a Babcock clamp or ringed forceps inserted into the superior mediastinum and through the cervical incision (Fig. 26-10).

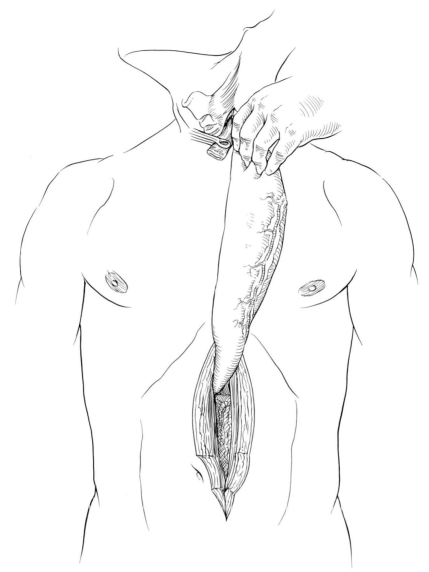

Figure 26-9
(From Townsend CM Jr, Evers MB. Atlas of General Surgical Techniques.
Philadelphia: Saunders; 2010.)

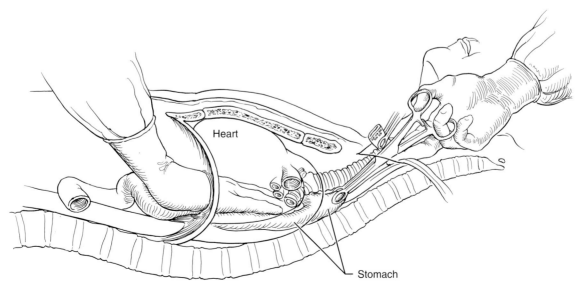

Figure 26-10
(From Townsend CM Jr, Evers MB. Atlas of General Surgical Techniques. Philadelphia: Saunders; 2010.)

- The fundus can be further advanced into the neck by gently pushing from below.
- Approximately 4 to 5 cm of stomach is drawn into the neck (Fig. 26-11).
- A moistened gauze pack can be inserted into the thoracic inlet posterior to the stomach or sutured to the skin to prevent the stomach from sliding back into the posterior mediastinum.
- The viability of the gastric tip, indicated by a healthy pink color, is then confirmed.
- 2-0 figure-of-eight silk sutures are used to narrow the diaphragmatic hiatus such that only two fingers of the surgeon's hand can be accommodated alongside the stomach. Interrupted stitches using 3-0 silk are then used to secure the anterior gastric wall to the diaphragmatic hiatus. This is done to prevent herniation of the abdominal contents alongside the intrathoracic stomach.
- The next step in the procedure is the construction of the esophagogastric anastomosis.
- The site of the anterior gastrostomy is selected at a point halfway between the oversewn lesser curvature of the stomach staple line and the greater curvature of the fundus. The ligated ends of the short gastric ends can be used as a marker to identify the greater curvature of the fundus.
- The cervical esophagus staple line is then sharply incised using a straight vascular clamp as a guide.
- Two 4-0 Vicryl sutures are then used to place two stitches: one at the midpoint of the anterior cut edge of the esophagus and one at a similar location on the posterior edge. The posterior stitch, however, is placed from inside the lumen, and the needle is not removed from the suture because it is reused at a later point in the procedure (Fig. 26-12).

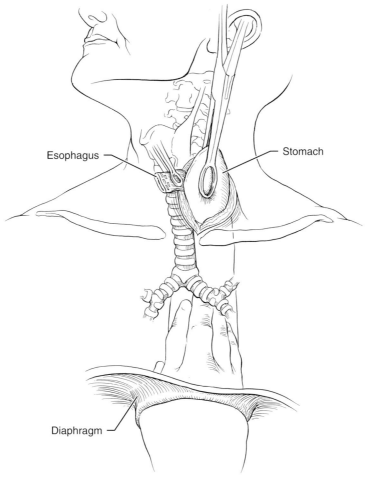

Esophagus

Stomach

Diaphragm

Figure 26-11
(From Townsend CM Jr, Evers MB. Atlas of General Surgical Techniques. Philadelphia: Saunders, 2010.)

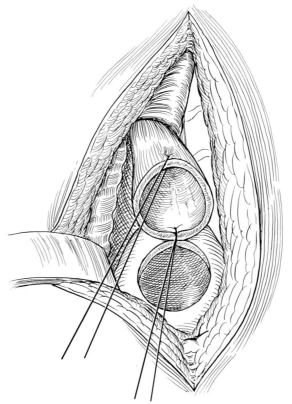

Figure 26-12
(From Townsend CM Jr, Evers MB. Atlas of General Surgical Techniques. Philadelphia: Saunders; 2010.)

- ◆ The next step involves the creation of a 2-cm gastrostomy using a needle-tipped electrocautery.
- ◆ This incision is oriented transversely, and the needle from the posterior esophageal suture is placed in the 6-o'clock position of the gastrostomy wall and then inserted through the full thickness of the cephalad aspect of the gastrostomy. By applying traction to this suture, the esophagus is brought toward the stomach.
- ◆ The posterior portion of the esophagogastric anastomosis is now performed using a 3-cm-long 3.5-mm EndoGIA stapler (Ethicon Endo-Surgery Inc, Somerville, NJ).
- ◆ The thicker portion of the stapler, known as the *cartridge*, is advanced into the stomach in a cephalad direction; the narrower portion, known as the *anvil*, is in the esophageal lumen (Fig. 26-13).
- ◆ With the tip of the stapler aimed toward the patient's right ear, tension is applied to the stay suture holding the esophagus and stomach together in an effort to bring them closer into the jaws of the device.
- ◆ It is important to keep this staple line away from the one earlier placed on the lesser curvature of the stomach as crossing of the two lines can create an area susceptible to ischemia.
- ◆ The stapler is now closed around the esophagus and stomach without being fired.
- ◆ The stapler is fired, completing the posterior anastomosis.

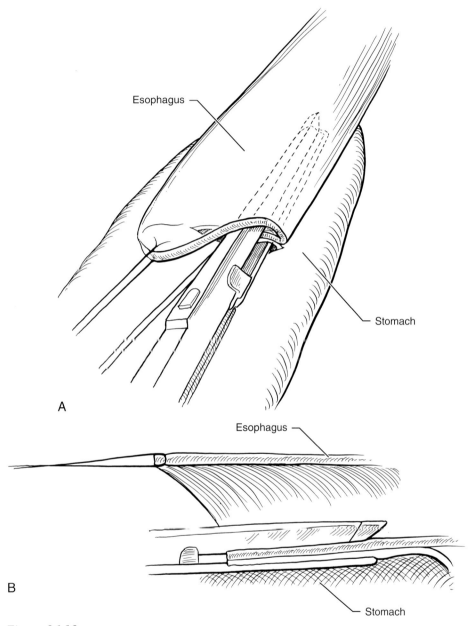

Esophagus

Stomach

A

Esophagus

Stomach

B

Figure 26-13
(From Townsend CM Jr, Evers MB. Atlas of General Surgical Techniques. Philadelphia: Saunders; 2010.)

- The anterior portion of the anastomosis is now completed with simple full-thickness inter-rupted sutures with 4-0 polydioxanone (PDS) suture (Fig. 26-14).
- A nasogastric is inserted before completion of the anastomosis so that the tip can be directed past the anastomosis. Special attention must be directed to lateral and medial corners where the handsewn portions meet the staple line because excessive traction can result in dehiscence along the staple line, complicating the outcome and requiring reentry to close.
- The nasogastric tube is positioned 4 to 6 cm above the pylormyotomy.

Drainage and Closure

- A Jackson-Pratt drain is placed in the thoracic inlet below the level of the anastomosis and is brought out through the inferior end of the neck incision.
- Two interrupted 4-0 Vicryl sutures are used to attach the strap muscles loosely to the under-side of the SCM muscle.
- The platysma is then returned to its native position using interrupted 4-0 Vicryl sutures and the skin closed.

Step 4. Postoperative Care

- An immediate postoperative chest radiograph should be performed to verify position of the drains and to assess whether there is hemothorax, pneumothorax, or mediastinal widening suggestive of postoperative hemorrhage.
- In most cases patients with a thoracic epidural can be extubated immediately post surgery.
- Incentive spirometry is strongly encouraged to improve and maintain airway patency and prevent atelectasis.
- Ambulation (three or four times per day) should begin on postoperative day 1.
- Jejunostomy tube feedings should begin on postoperative day 2. Feedings should consist of 5% dextrose and run at 30 mL per hour. If well tolerated by the patient, the rate may be increased to 60 mL per hour after 12 hours.
- On postoperative day 4, half-strength feedings can begin and the transition to full strength can begin the day after.
- The nasogastric tube, Foley catheter, and epidural and arterial catheters are removed at some point between postoperative day 3 and day 5.
- Approximately 24 hours after the nasogastric tube is removed, tube feedings are decreased and an oral liquid diet is begun. If patient is not tolerating oral feedings, nocturnal supple-mentation via the jejunostomy tube is instituted.
- Assessment of the anastomotic site is confirmed with a barium swallow on postoperative day 7. The barium swallow is also useful in confirming adequate gastric emptying.
- Most patients are discharged on postoperative day 7.
- Removal of the jejunostomy tube is done 4 weeks postoperatively.

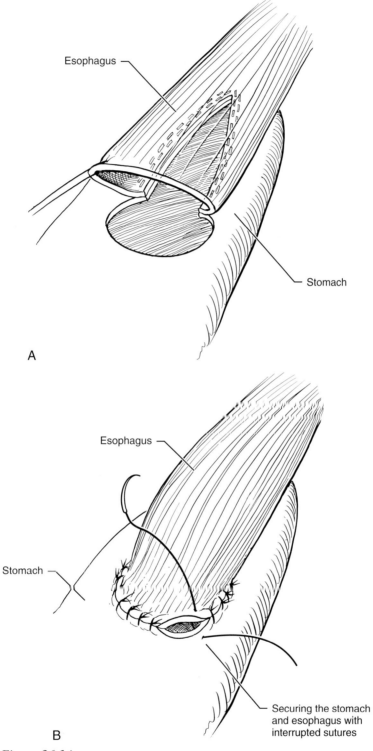

Esophagus

Stomach

A

Esophagus

Stomach

Securing the stomach
and esophagus with
interrupted sutures

B

Figure 26-14
(From Townsend CM Jr, Evers MB. Atlas of General Surgical
Techniques. Philadelphia: Saunders; 2010.)

Possible Postsurgical Complications

◆ Most postsurgical complications occur within the first 10 days of surgery. These include hoarseness and cervical dysphagia (due to recurrent laryngeal nerve injury), arrhythmias, chylothorax, anastomotic site disruption, and pleural effusion. Very early complications occurring in less than 1% of patients include epidural abscess, vertebral osteomyelitis, tracheogastric anastomotic fistula, pulmonary microabscess, and gastric tip necrosis.

Step 5. Pearls and Pitfalls

◆ THE spares the patient a thoracotomy and is therefore much better tolerated with reduced risk of pulmonary complications encountered compared with when the chest is entered.
◆ Anastomosis is placed in the neck, thus avoiding the fatal complication of mediastinitis, if a leak occurs.
◆ THE may not, however, offer adequate exposure of the mediastinum. Many have adopted VATS for transthoracic esophageal mobilization.
◆ Patients may have trouble with regular diet following the procedure, and frequent small feedings may be required.
◆ Dysphagia is common and patients may need to stay upright for 1 to 3 hours following eating; reflux-type symptoms may be encountered.

Suggested Readings

Goh A, Park K. Transhiatal oesophagectomy: A simple technique to carry out gastric or colonic conduit pull-up. Surgeon 2007;5:51-53.

Lin J, Iannettoni M. Transhiatal esophagectomy. Surg Clin North Am 2005;85:593-610.

Low D, Kunz S, Schembre D, et al. Esophagectomy—it's not just about mortality anymore: Standardized perioperative clinical pathways improve outcomes in patients with esophageal cancer. J Gastrointes Surg 2007;11:1395-1402.

Orringer MB. Transhiatal esophagectomy without thoracotomy. In Shields TW, LoCicero J, Ponn RB, Rusch V, eds. General Thoracic Surgery, 6th ed. Philadelphia: Lippincott Williams & Wilkins; 2005:2004-2022.

Vita M, Piraino A, Tessitore A, et al. Transhiatal esophagectomy (THE). Rays 2006;31:63-66.

Yee J, Finley RJ. Open esophageal procedures. In Souba WW, Fink MP, Jurkovich GJ, eds. ACS Surgical Principles and Practice. New York: WebMD; 2005:446-461.

CHAPTER 27

MINIMALLY INVASIVE ESOPHAGECTOMY

Joseph J. Wizorek, Omar Awais, and James D. Luketich

Step 1. Surgical Anatomy

- The esophagus includes cervical, thoracic, and abdominal segments and travels through the posterior mediastinum to join the stomach via the esophageal hiatus of the diaphragm. It is accompanied along its course by the anterior and posterior vagal trunks.
- The esophagus is a muscular tube, approximately 25 cm long and lacks a serosal layer. It is lined with squamous epithelium and transitions from striated muscle to smooth muscle as it courses through the thoracic cavity. The blood supply of the esophagus is segmental with limited overlap. The lymphatic anatomy is rich in intramural, extramural, and transmural channels, thus allowing for the rapid spread of an early localized tumor to metastatic disease.
- Surgical resection remains the primary treatment modality for resectable esophageal cancer, and transhiatal esophagectomy and Ivor Lewis esophagogastrectomy are the two most commonly performed operations.
  - ▲ A transhiatal esophagectomy is performed through a midline abdominal incision with blunt dissection of the thoracic esophagus through the esophageal hiatus, a gastric pull-up, and a cervical esophagogastric anastomosis.
  - ▲ An Ivor Lewis esophagectomy is performed through an upper midline abdominal incision with mobilization and creation of the gastric conduit followed by a right thoracotomy with dissection and removal of the thoracic esophagus and construction of an intrathoracic esophagogastric anastomosis.
  - ▲ Both transhiatal and Ivor Lewis esophagectomy are complex operations that have considerable morbidity and mortality in the range of 6% to 7% in experienced centers. However, in a national review, the mortality rate from esophagectomy ranges from 8% in high-volume centers to as high as 23% in low-volume centers.
- Laparoscopy has become the standard approach in the treatment of a variety of benign esophageal diseases, such as reflux and achalasia. This shift has been driven by a consistent observation that minimally invasive surgery is associated with equal efficacy, less pain, and an earlier return to work compared with open surgery. However, an open approach is still the standard of care for patients with esophageal cancer because of concerns that (1) minimally invasive surgery may not be equivalent in terms of nodal clearance and completeness of resection, (2) a minimally invasive approach may not have a measurable impact on morbidity, and (3) most esophageal surgeons have not been trained to perform the procedure minimally invasively.

◆ Data to support the claim that minimally invasive esophagectomy (MIE) is associated with less morbidity and mortality than the open approach exist and continue to accumulate. Two of the more frequent complications following esophagectomy are pneumonia (which carries a 20% mortality risk) and pulmonary failure. The avoidance of synchronous laparotomy and thoracotomy incisions may reduce the incidence of these complications. Although no randomized studies have been performed, our experience and that of others has suggested that MIE is associated with a lower rate of complications and mortality than that following open esophagectomy.

Step 2. Preoperative Considerations

◆ The preoperative evaluation for a patient undergoing an MIE is no different from that for a patient undergoing an open procedure.
◆ The two primary issues are whether the esophageal tumor is resectable and whether the patient has sufficient cardiopulmonary reserve.
◆ Staging of esophageal cancer includes an upper endoscopy, endoscopic ultrasound (EUS), computed tomography (CT) scanning, and positron emission tomography (PET) scanning. Upper endoscopy is performed to identify the proximal and distal extent of the tumor, which may impact the type of procedure performed; this is often done in the operating room at the time of the operation.
◆ The primary benefit of EUS is to determine the degree of invasion of the esophageal wall. Patients with T3 or N1 disease are usually treated with induction chemotherapy before esophagectomy. CT imaging is useful to determine the presence of bulky nodal disease within the abdomen. Bulky disease limited to the celiac nodal basin does not preclude esophagectomy, provided there is significant response to induction therapy. Finally, PET scanning, along with CT imaging, is primarily used to assess distant metastatic disease, which would preclude esophagectomy. We have not found PET particularly helpful in identifying periesophageal nodal disease because activity within these nodes is often obscured by the primary tumor.

- ◆ A final staging modality is laparoscopy. Typically patients undergo laparoscopy at the time of placement of an infusaport for induction chemotherapy. We have found laparoscopy to be a simple and safe method to identify abdominal metastases (liver or peritoneal) that might not be seen on CT imaging. In addition, the presence of bulky nodal disease can be assessed by laparoscopy and confirmed by biopsy. For these patients, additional radiation therapy may be included to the neoadjuvant treatment plan. Laparoscopy usually can be completed within 30 minutes, and patients can be discharged home on the same day.
- ◆ Patients should undergo a thorough evaluation to determine medical suitability for operation. This includes a cardiac stress test and, if indicated, coronary angiography. Patients with a significant tobacco history also should undergo pulmonary function testing. In addition, most patients with locally advanced cancer will have some degree of dysphagia and weight loss before diagnosis. Dysphagia often improves with induction therapy. If the patient has severe dysphagia, we place a jejunostomy tube during laparoscopic staging, although this has not been common for us. We strongly discourage the placement of either an esophageal stent or percutaneous gastrostomy tube for any patient who might be an operative candidate. Although esophagectomy is still possible in these situations, it is technically more challenging.

Step 3. Operative Steps

- ◆ Our early technique consisted of thoracoscopic esophageal mobilization followed by laparoscopic construction of the gastric conduit, gastric pull-up, and a neck anastomosis. A minimally invasive Ivor Lewis technique was reported by Watson and colleagues in 1999, who described the laparoscopic construction of a gastric conduit followed by thoracoscopic esophagectomy with construction of an intrathoracic esophagogastric anastomosis.
- ◆ The benefit of the minimally invasive Ivor Lewis approach is that it avoids a neck incision, therefore lowering the likelihood of a recurrent laryngeal nerve injury. There is also an absence of anastomotic tension, improved conduit perfusion, and a subsequent decrease in dehiscence rate. Initially, the operation was a hybrid, encompassing laparoscopy with a right mini thoracotomy. As our experience grew, we began to perform the operation completely minimally invasively. We have performed close to 250 minimally invasive Ivor Lewis esophagectomies. The operative details are similar to the three-hole approach, but we start the operation with laparoscopic construction of the gastric conduit followed by right video-assisted thoracoscopic surgery.

1. Abdominal Dissection

- The patient is positioned supine and intubated with a double-lumen endotracheal tube. On-table endoscopy is performed to assess tumor location and extension. The suitability of the stomach as a gastric conduit is also evaluated. Care must be taken to avoid undue insufflation during endoscopy.
- Proceeding with laparoscopy, the surgeon remains on the right while the assistant is positioned to the patient's left side.
- Six abdominal ports are used for the gastric mobilization (Fig. 27-1). The initial port is placed via an open technique while the remaining ports are placed under direct visualization. After an initial inspection of the peritoneal surfaces and the liver to rule out metastatic disease, the gastrohepatic omentum is opened.
- The left gastric pedicle is identified, and the celiac nodes are examined. If there are any enlarged nodes suspicious for metastatic implants, they are dissected and sent for frozen section analysis. If the nodes are not worrisome or return negative, the right crus is dissected free, mobilizing the lateral aspect of the esophagus.
- The dissection is then carried anteriorly and superiorly, mobilizing the anterior hiatus. Continuing this dissection toward the left crus, the fundus of the stomach begins to be mobilized. Avoid complete division of the phrenoesophageal ligament until conclusion of laparoscopy to maintain optimal pneumoperitoneum.
- After creating a retroesophageal window by completing the dissection of the inferior aspect of the right crus, attention is turned to the gastrocolic omentum. By carefully retracting the antrum of the stomach, a window is created in the greater omentum, allowing access to the lesser sac. This is done while carefully preserving the right gastroepiploic vessels.
- The dissection is carried along the greater curve of the stomach until the end of the gastroepiploic arcade is reached. The short gastric vessels are taken with a combination of the ultrasonic shears (Harmonic Scalpel, Ethicon Endo-Surgery Inc, Somerville, NJ) or the LigaSure device (Covidien, Mansfield, MA). Occasionally, clips are used to control large-diameter, short gastric vessels. With the greater curve mobilized, the fundus of the stomach is rotated toward the liver, exposing the retrogastric attachments. These are dissected free until the left gastric artery and vein are encountered. The retrogastric attachments are also divided toward the hiatus, completely mobilizing the fundus and the distal esophagus. The mobilization of the stomach is then carried back towards the pyloroantral region, where the dissection must be meticulous.
- An injury to the gastroepiploic arcade or the gastroduodenal artery renders the gastric conduit unusable. There are significant retroantral and periduodenal adhesions that must be divided to allow for adequate mobilization of the stomach. Since we have transitioned to an intrathoracic anastomosis, we have noted that an extensive Kocher maneuver is not necessary. The pylorus is considered adequately mobilized when it can reach the right crus under no tension.
- Once the stomach is completely mobilized, the left gastric artery and vein are divided with a vascular load on the EndoGIA stapler (Ethicon Endo-Surgery Inc, Somerville, NJ). This is done by approaching the pedicle from the lesser curve. It is important that the pedicle be dissected completely, with all celiac nodes swept up onto the specimen (Fig. 27-2). Once the pedicle is divided, the distal esophagus and the gastric fundus and antrum are completely mobilized.

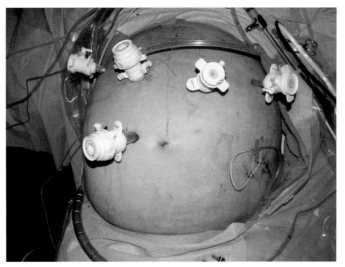

Figure 27-1

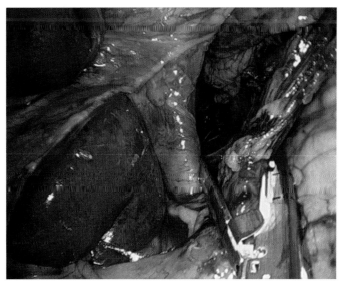

Figure 27-2

- The gastric tube is created before completion of the pyloroplasty and placement of the jejunostomy tube because this provides time to assess the conduit before bringing it into the chest.
- The initial staple line in creating the gastric conduit is a vascular (white) load across the vessels on the lesser curve (but not onto the gastric antrum). The initial 5- to 12-mm blunt right midclavicular port is changed to a 15-mm port to allow for the placement of a 4.8-mm (green load) EndoGIA stapler.
- An additional 12-mm port is placed in the right lower quadrant to assist with the creation of the gastric tube. During this step, it is important to have the first assistant grasp the proximal fundus along the greater curve and gently stretch it toward the spleen, while a second grasper is placed on the antral area with slight downward retraction applied. This places the stomach on a slight stretch and assists in creating a straight staple line.
- The staple line should parallel the gastroepiploic arcade–greater curve of the stomach. Initially, using 4.8-mm staple loads, the stomach is divided across the antrum with the goal to create a 5- to 6-cm-wide conduit (Fig. 27-3). Early in our experience, we discovered a significant increase in gastric tip necrosis and anastomotic leaks with a 3- to 4-cm-wide conduit. Once the antrum is divided, the right midclavicular port is changed back to a 5- to 12-mm port and the fundus is divided using a 3.5-mm (blue load) stapler. The graspers are readjusted as the fundus is divided, again to keep the stomach on stretch. If there is any concern about extension of tumor onto the gastric cardia, a wider margin is left in this region. It has not been our routine practice to oversew the staple line. The right gastric vessels are preserved.
- Next, a pyloroplasty is performed. Stay sutures are placed on the superior and inferior aspect of the pylorus. Once the pylorus has been placed on stretch, it is opened with ultrasonic shears. The pyloroplasty is then closed in a Heineke-Mikulicz fashion using the Endostitch device (Covidien, Mansfield, MA). This usually takes three to four stitches (Figs. 27-4 and 27-5). At the conclusion of the abdominal portion of the operation, the pyloroplasty is covered with omentum. In our experience, a laparoscopic pyloromyotomy is difficult to perform and more time consuming.
- Using a needle catheter kit, a 7 French feeding jejunostomy tube is placed via Seldinger technique in the left lower quadrant. Reflection of the transverse colon anterior and cephalad reveals the ligament of Treitz. A loop of small bowel 30 to 40 cm distal to this is tacked to the abdominal wall using the Endostitch device. Facilitating this step is the additional 10-mm port placed in the lower right quadrant. A needle and then a guidewire are passed into the jejunum under laparoscopic vision. Proper placement of the catheter is confirmed by observing distention of the jejunum as air is insufflated into the needle catheter. The jejunum surrounding the feeding tube is then tacked to the abdominal wall using several additional Endostitches. An additional segment of jejunum, 5 cm distal to the tube insertion site, is also tacked to the anterior abdominal wall as an anti-torsion stitch (Fig. 27-6).

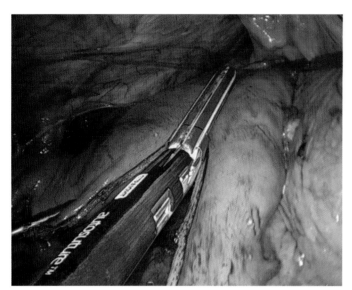

Figure 27-3

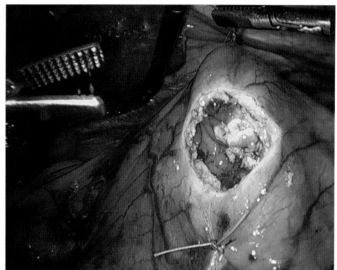

Figure 27-4

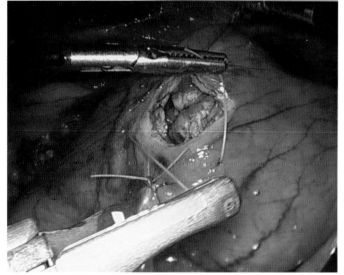

Figure 27-5

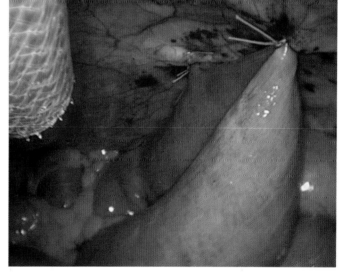

Figure 27-6

◆ Finally, using an Endostitch, the most superior portion of the gastric tube is anchored to the specimen (Fig. 27-7). The stitch maintains correct orientation of the gastric conduit as it is delivered into the chest (Fig. 27-8). The laparoscopic portion of the procedure is completed by dividing the phrenoesophageal membrane. The crura are also assessed to determine if a reapproximation/hiatal closure should be performed to prevent delayed herniation of the conduit into the chest.

2. Chest Dissection and Anastomosis

◆ The patient is then turned to the left lateral decubitus position for the thoracoscopic mobilization of the esophagus and creation of the intrathoracic anastomosis. The operating surgeon stands on the right side of the table (facing the patient's back) and the assistant on the left side of the table. A total of five thoracoscopic ports are used (Fig. 27-9). A 10-mm camera port is placed in the seventh or eighth intercostal space, just anterior to the midaxillary line. A 10-mm port is placed at the eighth or ninth intercostal space, posterior to the posterior axillary line, for the surgeon's right hand. A 10-mm port is placed in the anterior axillary line at the fourth intercostal space, through which a fan-shaped retractor retracts the lung anteriorly to expose the esophagus. A 5-mm port is placed just anterior to the tip of the scapula and is used for retraction by the surgeon. A final port is placed in the sixth intercostal space at the anterior axillary line for suction and is also important in the creation of the anastomosis. The initial step is the placement of a retracting suture through the central tendon of the diaphragm, brought out through a 1-mm incision on the anterior chest wall at the level of the insertion of the diaphragm. This suture retracts the diaphragm inferiorly, allowing visualization of the hiatus and gastroesophageal junction (GEJ).

◆ Dissection in the chest begins by dividing the inferior pulmonary ligament to the level of the inferior pulmonary vein. The inferior pulmonary vein is retracted anteriorly, and the dissection is carried cephalad along the pericardium, mobilizing the subcarinal lymph nodes in the process. At risk during the mobilization of the subcarinal nodal packet is the membranous wall of the right mainstem bronchus, which should be clearly identified. With complete dissection of the subcarinal space, the left mainstem bronchus is exposed. The subcarinal nodal package is removed with the specimen. The pleura is then opened along the hilum to the level of the azygos vein. The parietal pleura is then opened cephalad to the azygos vein and toward the thoracic inlet. The vein is then mobilized off of the chest wall and then divided with a vascular load of the EndoGIA stapler. The esophagus can be encircled with a Penrose drain to facilitate traction and exposure (Fig. 27-10).

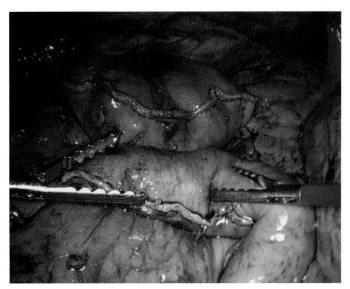

Figure 27-7

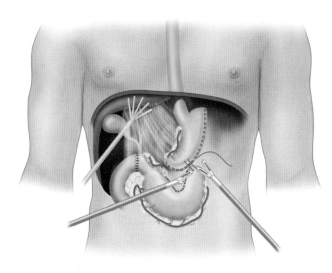

Figure 27-8

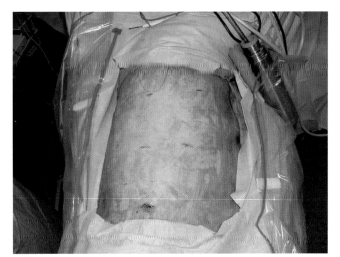

Figure 27-9

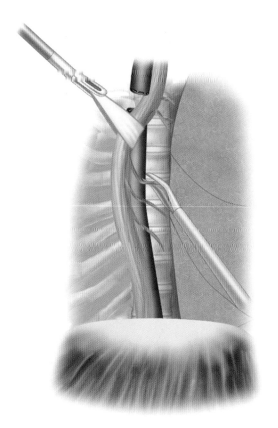

Figure 27-10

- Attention is then turned to mobilizing the posterolateral aspect of the esophagus. Generally a discrete identifiable groove in the parietal pleura delineates the plane between the esophagus and aorta. The pleura is opened along this groove to avoid injury to the thoracic duct and underlying aorta. It is often helpful at this point of the operation for the assistant to exchange the right-handed instrument from the fan lung retractor to a grasper. The grasper is then used to retract the esophagus anteromedially, allowing better visualization of the groove. Any tissue suspicious for branches of the thoracic duct or aortoesophageal vessels are clipped before being divided with the ultrasonic shears. The lateral dissection is carried from the azygos vein to the GEJ and the deep margin of the dissection is the contralateral pleura, which is occasionally entered in the setting of a bulky tumor.
- The esophagus is then nearly circumferentially mobilized throughout its course. The specimen is pulled into the chest with the attached gastric conduit. It is extremely important that the gastric tube remain properly oriented with the staple line continuing to face the lateral chest wall. The stitch is cut between the specimen and the conduit, and the specimen is retracted anteriorly and superiorly, thus exposing any remaining attachments between the esophagus and mediastinum. Above the level of the azygos vein, the dissection plane must be directly on the wall of the esophagus. This prevents injury to the recurrent laryngeal nerve.
- With the esophagus completely mobilized, the inferior posterior port is enlarged to approximately 3 cm and a wound protector is placed. The esophagus is divided using EndoShears at a level appropriate for the tumor. The specimen is removed through the wound protector, opened on the back table, and then sent for pathologic analysis of the margins. The anvil of a 28-mm end-to-end anastomosis (EEA) stapler is inserted into the cut end of the proximal esophagus (Fig. 27-11), and a purse-string suture is sewn and tied to secure the anvil in position. A second purse-string suture to secure the anvil further is also placed. The gastric conduit is then pulled up to the apex of the chest, and the ultrasonic shears are used to open the tip along the staple line. The EEA stapler is introduced through the posterior inferior port and passed through the gastrotomy and into the conduit. The stapler tip is brought out along the greater curve of the gastric conduit and docked to the anvil (Fig. 27-12).
- Before creating the anastomosis, we carefully ascertain the amount of conduit that will lie in the chest. It is a common mistake to bring an excess amount of stomach into the chest in an effort to minimize tension on the anastomosis. This excess conduit will often assume a sigmoid curve above the diaphragm and may lead to significant problems with gastric emptying.

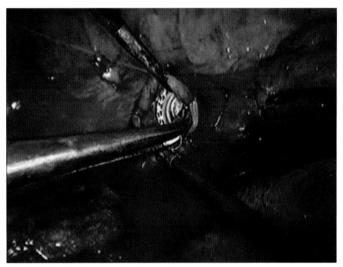

Figure 27-11

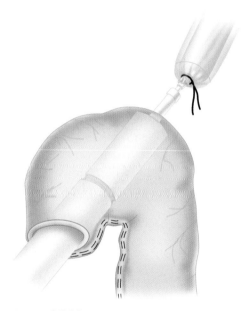

Figure 27-12

◆ In addition, ensuring proper orientation of the stomach is critical (Fig. 27-13). The stapler is fired, creating a circular esophagogastric anastomosis (side of gastric conduit to end of esophagus). The gastrostomy and conduit tip are then resected using two or three loads of an articulating linear EndoGIA stapler (Fig. 27-14). A 28 French chest tube is left in the right hemithorax and a Jackson-Pratt (JP) drain is placed along the conduit and across the anastomosis (Fig. 27-15). The potential space between the conduit and the right crus of the diaphragm is then closed with a single interrupted stitch to prevent delayed herniation. Intercostal nerve block with a long-acting analgesic is injected, and a nasogastric tube is advanced across the anastomosis under direct thoracoscopic vision. Most patients are extubated in the operating room after bronchoscopy.

Step 4. Postoperative Care

◆ Postoperatively the patients routinely spend 12 to 24 hours in an intensive care setting and are then transferred to the regular ward. Tube feedings are started on postoperative day 2 and advanced to target cycle feeds by postoperative day 3. A barium swallow is obtained and, if satisfactory, the chest tube is removed, and clear liquids of 1 to 2 oz. per hour are started on postoperative day 3 or 4. The patients are routinely discharged to home on postoperative day 5 or 6. Before discharge the JP drain is pulled back. Initial follow-up in the clinic is in approximately 2 weeks after discharge.

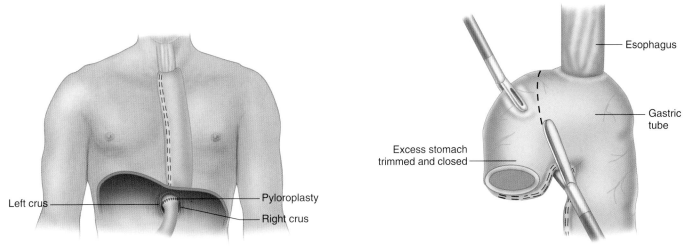

Left crus — Pyloroplasty — Right crus

Figure 27-13

Esophagus

Gastric tube

Excess stomach trimmed and closed

Figure 27-14

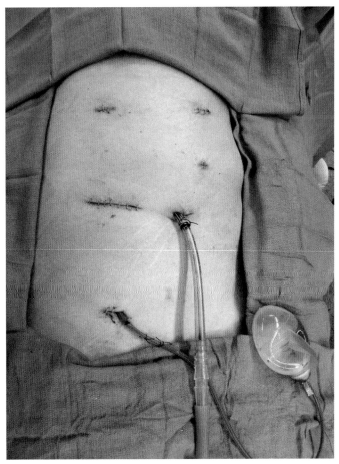

Figure 27-15

Step 5. Pearls and Pitfalls

- Preoperative evaluation requires CT imaging, EUS, and PET imaging. On-table endoscopy is also performed to evaluate tumor extension.
- Careful preservation of the gastroepiploic artery is essential in the creation of the gastric conduit, and the arcade must not be injured during the gastric mobilization.
- Adequate mobilization of the stomach and pylorus is essential. The pylorus should reach the right crus once mobilized.
- All celiac nodes should be dissected and kept with the specimen before dividing the left gastric artery and vein.
- Proper orientation of the conduit when it is tacked to the specimen is important because the conduit must not come into the chest twisted.
- The margins of dissection in the chest include the pericardium, the contralateral pleura, and the aorta–thoracic duct. We do not routinely take the thoracic duct as part of the specimen.
- Above the azygos vein, it is important for the dissection to stay on the wall of the esophagus to avoid injury to the recurrent laryngeal nerve.
- Avoid pulling excess gastric conduit into the chest for the esophagogastric anastomosis.
- An epidural catheter is not routinely used. Instead, intercostal rib blocks are placed at the conclusion of the chest portion of the procedure.
- Tube feedings are started on postoperative day 2, and a barium swallow is obtained on postoperative day 4 or 5, before starting oral intake.

Suggested Readings

Birkmeyer JD, Siewers AE, Finlayson EV, et al. Hospital volume and surgical mortality in the United States. N Engl J Med 2002;346(15):1128-1137.

Bonavina L, Bona D, Binyom PR, Peracchia A. A laparoscopy-assisted surgical approach to esophageal carcinoma. J Surg Res 2004;117(1):52-57.

Collard JM, Lengele B, Otte JB, Kestens PJ. En bloc and standard esophagectomies by thoracoscopy. Ann Thorac Surg 1993;56(3):675-679.

Cuschieri A, Shimi S, Banting S. Endoscopic oesophagectomy through a right thoracoscopic approach. J R Coll Surg Edinb 1992;37(1):7-11.

Daly JM, Karnell LH, Menck HR. National Cancer Data Base report on esophageal carcinoma. Cancer 1996;78(8):1820-1828.

de Paula AL, Hashiba K, Ferreira EA, et al. Laparoscopic transhiatal esophagectomy with esophagogastroplasty. Surg Laparosc Endosc 1995;5(1):1-5.

Enzinger PC, Mayer RJ. Esophageal cancer. N Engl J Med 2003;349(23):2241-2252.

Jagot P, Sauvanet A, Berthoux L, Belghiti J. Laparoscopic mobilization of the stomach for oesophageal replacement. Br J Surg 1996;83(4):540-542.

Kelsen DP, Ginsberg R, Pajak TF, et al. Chemotherapy followed by surgery compared with surgery alone for localized esophageal cancer. N Engl J Med 1998;339(27):1979-1984.

Luketich JD, Nguyen NT, Weigel T, et al. Minimally invasive approach to esophagectomy. JSLS 1998;2(3):243-247.

Luketich JD, Alvelo-Rivera MA, Buenaventura PO, et al. Minimally invasive esophagectomy: Outcomes in 222 patients. Ann Surg 2003;238:486-495.

Swanstrom LL, Hansen P. Laparoscopic total esophagectomy. Arch Surg 1997;132(9):943-947; discussion 947-949.

Watson DI, Davies N, Jamieson GG. Totally endoscopic Ivor Lewis esophagectomy. Surg Endosc 1999;13(3):293-297.

CHAPTER 28

ROBOTIC ESOPHAGECTOMY

Raymond J. Gagliardi and Almudena Moreno Elola-Olaso

- ◆ Esophagectomy is associated with high morbidity and mortality rates, not only because it involves the manipulation of both abdominal and thoracic-mediastinal structures but also because the patients are often malnourished or suffer from a variety of co-morbidities.
- ◆ During the early 1990s, minimally invasive approaches, either transthoracic or laparoscopic-transhiatal, were proposed as a way to reduce morbidity and mortality associated with this operation. Still, the difficult manipulation of the rigid instruments in the upper mediastinum and the two-dimensional vision limited the application of these approaches. Moreover, they are not advisable for all surgeons because advanced skills in both open and minimally invasive techniques are mandatory.
- ◆ The application of robotic techniques overcomes the deficiencies of laparoscopy and thoracoscopy. It offers high-definition three-dimensional vision and full range of motion of the articulated instruments, allowing precise dissection in a confined operating space.
- ◆ A mobile cart with four arms holds the robotic instruments that are inserted through specific trocars. The surgeon is located at a remote console that transmits the surgeon's finger and hand movements to the instruments of the da Vinci robot. Finally, standard laparoscopic equipment allows the assistant surgeon to follow the operation through a laparoscopic camera (Fig. 28-1).

Step 1. Surgical Anatomy

- ◆ Knowledge of the anatomy of the esophagus and its relationships is critical for minimally invasive and robotic-assisted esophagectomy. Each anatomic portion of the esophagus is best dissected through a different approach, so this is extremely important in order to plan the operation.
- ◆ The cervical esophagus and the proximal 3 to 4 cm of the thoracic esophagus are best approached through the cervical incision. Anteriorly the cervical esophagus is closely related to the trachea. At this point, blunt dissection is recommended to avoid the injury of the left recurrent nerve, which lies in the groove between the trachea and the esophagus.
- ◆ The abdominal esophagus and distal thoracic esophagus are best manipulated from the abdominal approach; thus laparoscopic dissection is usually preferred. Dissection of the esophageal hiatus is performed easily, and the length of laparoscopic instruments allows approach of the distal esophagus up to the level of the carina.

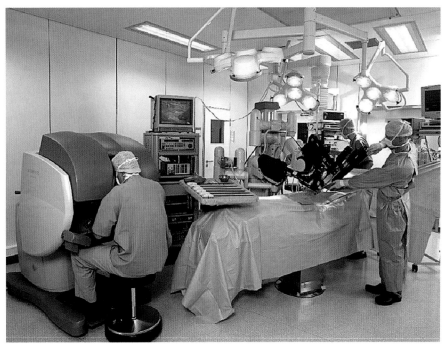

Figure 28-1
(From Intuitive Surgical Inc, Sunnyvale, CA.)

- Proximal thoracic esophagus is the most difficult portion to dissect with minimally invasive techniques. Anteriorly it is closely related to the trachea and main left bronchus, and posteriorly it must be separated from the thoracic aorta. The thoracic duct ascends posteriorly and to the right of the thoracic esophagus up to the level of T5, where it ascends on the left side of the esophagus. Video-assisted thoracoscopic techniques allow an easier dissection through direct visualization of the esophagus, but they involve a more invasive technique, requiring a small thoracotomy and insertion of two chest tubes. A laparoscopic approach is more difficult because vision is limited; the upper mediastinum is a narrow space that makes dissection from adjacent structures difficult. Robotic-assisted minimally invasive techniques allow better visualization of the operative field, and a fuller range of motion of its articulated instruments makes dissection easier.

Step 2. Preoperative Considerations

- Preoperative evaluation at the anesthesia clinic is advisable for all patients to define the patient's functional status and operative risk. Smoking cessation is advised in all patients.
- Deep vein thrombosis prophylaxis is accomplished with intraoperative and postoperative pneumatic compression stockings and subcutaneous heparin.

Step 3. Operative Steps

1. Transhiatal Approach

- Patient positioning: The patient is placed in a modified dorsal lithotomy, reverse Trendelenburg position, with the patient's head turned slightly to the right during the surgical procedure.
- Robot positioning: The da Vinci robot is docked over the left shoulder of the patient. Operating room setup is shown in Figure 28-2.
- Port placement (Fig. 28-3)
  - ▲ *Laparoscopic camera:* A 12-mm optically guided trocar is placed in the midportion of the abdomen, approximately one third of the distance between the umbilicus and the xiphoid.
  - ▲ *Working ports:* An additional right-sided, subcostal, reusable robotic 8-mm trocar is placed. Similarly, a left-sided, subcostal, reusable 8-mm trocar is placed. These serve as working ports. These ports will hold the robot trocars during the robotic dissection of the upper mediastinum.
  - ▲ *Additional ports:* One right-sided 5-mm trocar is placed for an articulated liver retractor, and a left-sided 5-mm trocar is placed on the left-hand side of the patient for an auxiliary retraction port, which will be performed by the first assistant.

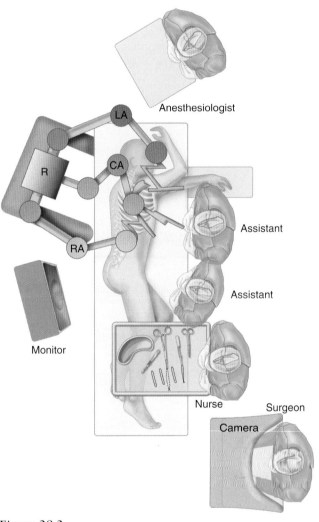

Figure 28-2

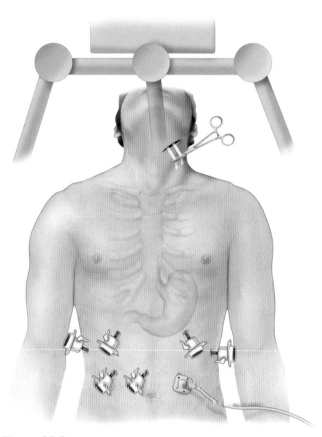

Figure 28-3

Laparoscopic Dissection

- The esophageal hiatus is exposed by retracting the left lobe of the liver upward, using a Nathanson Liver Retractor (Mediflex Surgical Products, Islandia, NY). The dissection is started at the lesser omentum, and progressed towards the gastroesophageal junction (GEJ). The phrenoesophageal ligament is taken down beginning at the right crus of the diaphragm. We continue our dissection around the hiatus until the right crus is completely exposed. Next we move our dissection to the left-hand side of the hiatus. A retroesophageal window is created, and a band is passed and placed circumferentially around the distal esophagus and clipped anteriorly for downward traction of the GEJ (Fig. 28-4).
- The dissection continues toward the junction of the gastroepiploic and the most inferior short gastric vessels, which are completely ligated, preserving the right gastroepiploic vessels to ensure vascular supply to the gastric conduit.
- The left crus is completely exposed and freed up from the esophageal tissues, and the stomach is lifted upward such that the tissue near the celiac axis is taken down and the lymphadenectomy is extended to the celiac trunk. The left gastric vessels are clipped using a vascular stapler. Once this is accomplished, the stomach is completely mobilized.
- A laparoscopic Kocher maneuver is performed, but a pyloroplasty is not usually required.
- We continue our dissection toward the thoracic esophagus laparoscopically, carefully avoiding the pleura on either the right or left sides while using the Penrose drain for downward traction on the stomach at the GEJ (Fig. 28-5). At this point, we remove the laparoscopic instrumentation and replace our left-handed and right-handed ports with 8-mm da Vinci trocars.

Robotic Mediastinal Dissection

- The da Vinci robot (Intuitive Surgical Inc, Sunnyvale, CA) is brought into position cephalad to the patient. We place a hook cautery on the right-hand arm of the da Vinci and a ProGrasp grasping device (Intuitive Surgical Inc, Sunnyvale, CA) on the left-hand side of its arm, and these are placed in the patient. The laparoscope is replaced with a straight da Vinci camera. Our auxiliary left-handed abdominal laparoscopic port is used to retract the stomach in a downward fashion at the GEJ, allowing us to continue our dissection up the hiatus into the mediastinum.
- The periesophageal tissues are dissected circumferentially around the esophagus up to the level of approximately the thoracic inlet, keeping all periesophageal and mediastinal lymph nodes intact with the specimen. At the conclusion of the robotic dissection, the da Vinci robot devices are removed from the patient and the robot is backed away from the operative table (Fig. 28-6).

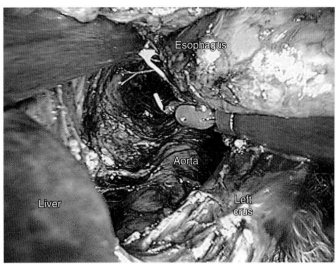

Figure 28-4
(With kind permission from Springer Science+Business Media:
Galvani, CA. Robotically assisted laparoscopic transhiatal
esophagectomy. Sur Endosc 2008;22:188-195, Figure 4.)

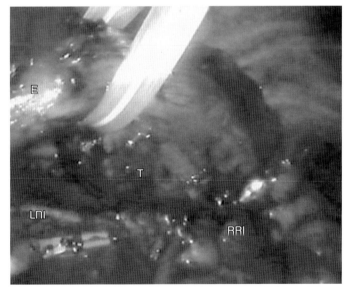

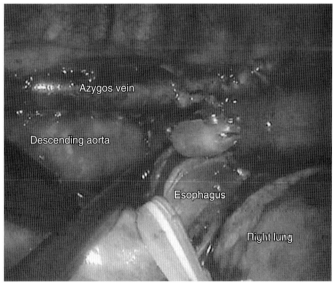

Figure 28-5
E, esophagus; LRI, left robotic instrument; RRI, right robotic
instrument; T, tumor.
(From Boone J, Draaisma WA, Schipper ME, et al. Robot-
assisted thoracosecopic esophagectomy for a giant upper
esophageal leiomyoma. Dis Esophagus 2008;21:90-103,
Figure 4.)

Figure 28-6
(With kind permission from Springer Science+Business Media:
Van Hillegersberg R. First experience with robot-assisted
thoracoscopic esophagolymphadenectomy for esophageal
cancer. Surg Encosc 2006;20:1435-1439, Figure 3.)

Laparoscopic Creation of the Gastric Conduit

- The stomach is tubularized, using multiple EndoGIA (Covidien, Mansfield, MA) firings perpendicular to the lesser curvature, and then continued along the greater curvature, creating a curvilinear gastric conduit that is approximately 30 to 40 mm in diameter, based on the gastroepiploic artery.
- A narrow attachment is left between the tube and the gastric fundus, and the gastric conduit is pulled up through the chest by bringing this up in a transhiatal fashion; the specimen is extracted through the cervical incision.
- A feeding jejunostomy tube is created laparoscopically, approximately 30 to 40 cm distal to the ligament of Treitz.

Cervical Dissection

- A linear incision is made on the left side of the neck along the anterior border of the sternocleidomastoid, down through the subcutaneous platysmal tissue, and the sternocleidomastoid muscle is retracted laterally.
- The omohyoid muscle is either ligated or retracted laterally, and the esophagus is mobilized with blunt dissection in the tracheoesophageal groove down to the level of the anterior cervical spine. A Penrose drain is placed around the cervical esophagus at the level of the thoracic inlet.
- Following completion of the gastric conduit, the thoracic esophagus and the stomach are brought up through the thoracic inlet with gentle upward traction, under direct laparoscopic vision to avoid twisting of the conduit and therefore monitoring its proper positioning.
- Using an EndoGIA heavy tissue stapler, the cardia of the stomach is then divided (Fig. 28-7).
- The cervical esophagus is also divided with removal of the surgical specimen through the cervical incision. The esophagogastric anastomosis is created proximal to the thoracic outlet, either hand sewn or stapled. A nasogastric tube is placed through the esophagogastrostomy under palpation before closure.

2. Transthoracic Approach

Robotic-Assisted Thoracoscopic Dissection

- Patient positioning: Patient is intubated with a left-side double-lumen endotracheal tube and positioned in the left lateral decubitus position.
- Robot positioning: Robot is placed at the right upper side of the patient.

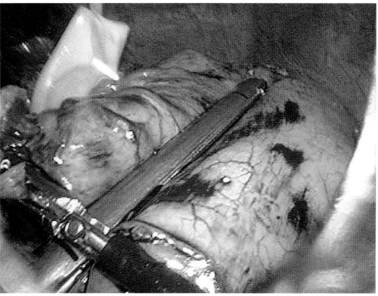

Figure 28-7
(With kind permission from Springer Science+Business Media: Galvani
CA. Robotically assisted laparoscopic transhiatal esophagectomy. Sur
Endosc 2008;22:188-195, Figure 5.)

- ◆ Port positioning
  - ▲ Robotic camera port: 10-mm camera port at the sixth intercostal space in the posterior axillary line
  - ▲ Robotic instrument ports: Two 8-mm trocars—one anterior to the scapular rim in the fourth intercostal space, another more posteriorly placed in the eighth intercostal space
  - ▲ Two thoracoscopic trocars for additional assistance in the fifth and seventh intercostal spaces, both posterior to the posterior axillary line

Surgical Technique

- ◆ The right lung is retracted laterally, facilitating the exposure of the esophagus.
- ◆ The right parietal pleura is divided at the anterior side, up to the level of the azygos vein, which is ligated using a vascular stapler, and the thoracic duct is clipped to prevent leaks.
- ◆ The esophagus is dissected circumferentially, and a Penrose drain is placed around it to perform traction and facilitate the dissection, which involves the esophagus and the periesophageal tissue from the hiatus to the thoracic inlet. During the dissection, all aortoesophageal vessels are clipped. All periesophageal lymph nodes are resected en bloc with the specimen.
- ◆ Two thoracostomy chest drains are left in the right thorax.

Cervical Dissection

- ◆ Patient position: The patient is repositioned in a dorsal lithotomy, reverse Trendelenburg position with the patient's head turned to the right side. The patient is also reintubated with a single-lumen endotracheal tube to allow right-sided lung reinsufflation.
- ◆ Surgical technique is resumed the same as with the transhiatal approach.
  - ▲ An incision along the anterior border of the sternocleidomastoid muscle is performed, and the omohyoid muscle is transected. Identification of the cleavage planes is facilitated by the pneumomediastinum.
  - ▲ The esophageal dissection is completed circumferentially and distally into the cervicomediastinal space.

Laparoscopic Dissection

- Port positioning
  - ▲ Camera port: An 11-mm trocar is located at the midline, approximately one third of the distance from the umbilicus to the xiphoid process.
  - ▲ Working ports: An additional 5-mm trocar is placed in the subxiphoid region on the right-hand side. Another 11-mm trocar is placed on the left-hand side of the subxiphoid region. Lateral to this, a 5-mm trocar is placed for retraction, and on the extreme right-hand side, a 5-mm trocar is placed for liver retraction.
- Surgical technique is similar to the minimally invasive esophagectomy.

Step 4. Postoperative Care

- After the operation, the patient is transferred to the intensive care unit for close observation.
- The nasogastric tube is usually not removed until postoperative day 6 or 7 at least. Jejunal feeding is started on postoperative day 1.
- Deep venous thrombosis prophylaxis is recommended in all patients, using both heparin and sequential compression devices (SCDs), and early ambulation is encouraged
- A barium swallow study is performed at postoperative day 6 or 7; if a leak is ruled out, clear liquids are started.

Step 5. Pearls and Pitfalls

- Robotic technology provides high definition three-dimensional vision and allows precise dissection in a confined operating space such as the upper mediastinum. Visualization of the operative field is also improved by optic motion scaling.
- It allows enhanced dexterity because of the full range of motion of the articulated instruments, and the robotic technology reduces surgeon tremor, providing a more precise dissection.
- Robotic techniques involve the loss of tactile sense that is provided in conventional operations, and the availability of instrumentation is still limited.
- Longer operative times can be expected because of the time spent in docking the robot. Moreover, there is a learning curve because these techniques differ from laparoscopic or thoracoscopic techniques.

Suggested Readings

Bodner J, Wykypiel H, Wetscher G, et al. First experiences with the da Vinci operating robot in thoracic surgery. Eur J Cardiothorac Surg 2004;25:844-851.

Boone J, Draaisma WA, Schipper ME, et al. Robot-assisted thoracoscopic esophagectomy for a giant upper esophageal leiomyoma. Dis Esophagus 2008;21:90-103.

D'Amico TA. Robotics in thoracic surgery: Applications and outcomes. J Thorac Cardiovasc Surg 2006;131:19-20.

Dapri G, Himpens J, Cadiere GB. Robot-assisted thoracoscopic esophagectomy with the patient in the prone position. J Laparoendosc Adv Surg Tech A 2006;16:278-285.

Elli E, Espat NJ, Berger R, et al. Robotic-assisted thoracoscopic resection of esophageal leiomyoma. Surg Endosc 2004;18:713-716.

Espat NJ, Jacobsen G, Horgan S, et al. Minimally invasive treatment of esophageal cancer: Laparoscopic staging to robotic esophagectomy. Cancer J 2005;11:10-17.

Galvani CA, Gorodner MV, Moser F, et al. Robotically assisted laparoscopic transhiatal esophagectomy. Surg Endosc 2008;22:188-195.

Giulianotti PC, Coratti A, Angelini M, et al. Robotics in general surgery: Personal experience in a large community hospital. Arch Surg 2003;138:777-784.

Kernstine KH, DeArmond DT, Shamoun DM, et al. The first series of completely robotic esophagectomies with three-field lymphadenectomy: Initial experience. Surg Endosc 2007;21:2285-2292.

Marescaux J, Rubino F. Robot-assisted remote surgery: Technological advances, potential complications, and solutions. Surg Technol Int 2004;12:23-26.

Talamini MA, Chapman S, Horgan S, et al. A prospective analysis of 211 robotic-assisted surgical procedures. Surg Endosc 2003;17:1521-1524.

van Hillegersberg R, Boone J, Draaisma WA, et al. First experience with robot-assisted thoracoscopic esophagolymphadenectomy for esophageal cancer. Surg Endosc 2006;20(9):1435-1439.

CHAPTER 29

ESOPHAGEAL RECONSTRUCTION

Adham R. Saad and Scott B. Johnson

Step 1. Surgical Anatomy

Reconstruction of the esophagus requires a detailed knowledge of the anatomy of the esophagus itself as well as the conduits used:

- ◆ Esophagus
    - ▲ The left side of the neck is preferred for reconstruction for three reasons:
        - ● The esophagus takes a slight bend toward the left in the neck.
        - ● The recurrent nerve, when aberrant, usually occurs on the right.
        - ● The recurrent nerve lies slightly farther away from the esophagus on the right side and therefore is less likely to be encircled when dissecting the esophagus from the left.
    - ▲ A cervical (as opposed to an intrathoracic) anastomosis is preferred for two reasons:
        - ● There is less reflux into the proximal esophageal segment.
        - ● Cervical anastomotic leaks are less life-threatening.
    - ▲ Reconstruction to areas proximal to or involving the cricopharyngeus (i.e., the pharynx) will undoubtedly affect the pharyngeal phase of swallowing, often necessitating the need for intense speech and swallowing therapy postoperatively.
- ◆ Stomach
    - ▲ Is the most commonly used conduit.
    - ▲ Blood supply is based on the right gastroepiploic artery.
    - ▲ The fundus of the stomach is what reaches to the neck.
- ◆ Colon
    - ▲ Is the second most commonly used conduit.
    - ▲ Is called a *left colon graft* because it is based on the ascending branch of the left colic artery, a branch of the inferior mesenteric artery.
    - ▲ Actual colon transposed is the transverse colon, along with portions of the right.

Step 2. Preoperative Considerations

1. Indications for Esophageal Reconstruction

- ◆ After resection for benign disease
  - ▲ Chronic acid reflux, multiple failed antireflux operations
  - ▲ Traumatic or iatrogenic injury
  - ▲ End-stage motility disorders (e.g., sigmoid esophagus)
  - ▲ End-stage connective tissue disorders (e.g., scleroderma)
  - ▲ Undilatable stricturing from chemical (e.g., lye ingestion), infectious, or drug-induced injury
  - ▲ Others
- ◆ After resection for malignant disease

2. Choice of Conduit

- ◆ Stomach
  - ▲ Simplest, requires only one anastomosis
  - ▲ Usually reaches to the cervical esophagus without difficulty but may have trouble reaching more proximally (i.e., pharynx)
  - ▲ Might not be usable because of extensive resection or injury to the pedicle (e.g., from G-tube placement)
  - ▲ Usually functions well early, as opposed to the colon, which may require an extensive "break-in" period
  - ▲ When placed in the substernal tunnel may have trouble reaching to the neck or demonstrate significant reflux and regurgitation
- ◆ Colon
  - ▲ More complicated surgery, requires three anastomoses (interposed colon to proximal esophagus or pharynx; colon to stomach or small bowel; and colon to colon to complete gastrointestinal continuity)
  - ▲ Good size match
  - ▲ Durable blood supply
  - ▲ Usually requires a "break-in" period but functions well long-term
  - ▲ Can reach farther than the stomach to the most proximal portions of the pharynx
  - ▲ Does well in the substernal tunnel
  - ▲ Used when the stomach is unavailable as first choice

3. Route

- Posterior mediastinal route preferred (more physiologic, less length required)
- Substernal tunnel should be used in cases of delayed reconstruction (e.g., because of extensive scarring due to previous esophagectomy)
- Location of anastomoses
  - ▲ Proximal and distal "targets" depend on underlying disease and extent of resection
  - ▲ Proximal
    - Most commonly the conduit ("neoesophagus") is anastomosed to the cervical esophagus.
    - Anastomosis to the pharynx or piriform sinus may be necessary when extensive scarring of the esophagus and cricopharyngeus is present (e.g., lye ingestion). Anastomosis to the intrathoracic esophagus may be necessary when the patient has had previous extensive neck surgery or radiation.
    - Operative surgeon should perform his or her own endoscopy preoperatively to "map out" the exact location to maximize function and remove all disease (e.g., Barrett, strictures).
  - ▲ Distal
    - When stomach is used, not an issue
    - When the colon is interposed, usually the distal colon conduit is anastomosed to the antrum of the stomach (leaving additional stomach is not necessary and may actually cause extensive stasis long term).
    - Roux-en-Y loop of the small bowel is preferred when the stomach has been resected in its entirety.

4. Useful Preoperative Studies

- Endoscopy
  - ▲ Esophagoscopy should be performed by the operative surgeon, preferably before any planned operation, but can be performed at the time of surgery if uncomplicated reconstruction is anticipated.
- Video esophagogram
  - ▲ Gives information about both function and structure
  - ▲ Conventional barium swallow gives less information concerning function.
- Mesenteric angiogram
  - ▲ Not always necessary but useful if compromised blood flow to conduit is suspected due to previous surgery or underlying disease (e.g., peripheral vascular disease, previous aneurysm repair)
- Physiologic evaluation
  - ▲ History and physical examination
  - ▲ Renal, hepatic, nutritional, and hematologic laboratory assessment
  - ▲ Echocardiogram or stress test (if cardiac disease is suspected)
  - ▲ Pulmonary function tests (if pulmonary disease suspected)
  - ▲ Consider the integrity of the pharyngeal phase of swallowing (reconstruction of the esophagus would be of questionable benefit in a patient unable to swallow because of, e.g., irreversible stroke, neuromuscular disorder)

Step 3. Operative Steps

1. Access to the Esophagus in the Neck

- The neck should be prepped from the anterior chest to the earlobe.
- The patient's head should be slightly turned to the right and slightly extended to expose the sternocleidomastoid muscle.
- An incision is made along the anterior border of the muscle and carried through the platysma.
- The strap muscles (sternothyroid and sternohyoid) are divided close to the clavicle-sternum.
- The plane between the carotid sheath (retracted laterally) and the trachea-larynx (retracted medially) is developed and the tracheoesophageal groove identified.
- Dissection should proceed posteriorly to the anterior cervical fascia; just anterior to this the muscular fibers of the tubular esophagus can be identified.
- The esophagus is then carefully dissected and encircled, making sure that the recurrent laryngeal nerve is protected.

2. Stomach as Conduit

- The abdominal incision should be carried quite superiorly with resection of the xiphoid process.
- Lap packs should be placed gently behind the spleen to move it forward.
- A self-retaining retractor should be placed to retract the abdominal incision apart as well as under the left rib cage to retract it upward and outward to expose the undersurface of the left hemidiaphragm.
- The lesser sac should be entered between the transverse colon and the greater curvature of the stomach, well away from the right gastroepiploic artery, approximately midline (not too close to the spleen and not too close to the duodenum, i.e., where it is "easy").
- The gastrocolic ligament should be divided away from the greater curvature, protecting the vascular pedicle, moving toward the left side, approaching the spleen and its short gastric arteries.
- The short gastrics should be divided as close to the spleen as possible.
- The gastrohepatic ligament should then be divided toward the right side, beginning where it was originally entered (i.e., where it was "easy").
- As the stomach is freed in this direction, both the right gastroepiploic artery and vein can be identified and followed proximally.
- A Kocher maneuver is performed to allow additional length to the gastric graft.
- As the most superior attachments to the spleen are divided, the lap packs behind the spleen are removed, thereby allowing the spleen to fall away and facilitate this portion of the dissection (Fig. 29-1).

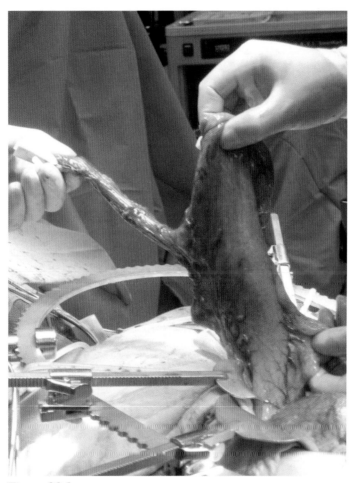

Figure 29-1

- The left crural attachments are divided and the mediastinum accessed.
- Division of the central portion of the diaphragm directly superior to the esophagus allows better access to the mediastinum if esophageal resection is performed at the same time as reconstruction.
- As the dissection proceeds from left to right, the gastrohepatic ligament, as well as the right crus, is identified.
- The gastrohepatic ligament is divided, preserving the right gastric artery.
- If there is an aberrant left hepatic branch coursing from the celiac axis, this vessel should be preserved if possible.
- The left gastric artery is ligated.
- The esophagogastric junction should be divided if not already done, usually through serial firings of a GIA stapler along the lesser curve (Fig. 29-2).
- A gastric tube is then created, and the staple line is oversewn with 3-0 braided suture (Fig. 29-3).
- A pyloric relaxing maneuver should be performed in the form of a pyloroplasty or pyloromyotomy before advancement of the graft.
- The gastric tube is brought up through the mediastinum using soft rubber drains and a plastic bowel bag to minimize friction on the graft (see Figs. 29-12 and 29-13).
- Once the graft is brought up through the cervical incision, the bowel bag is cut away.

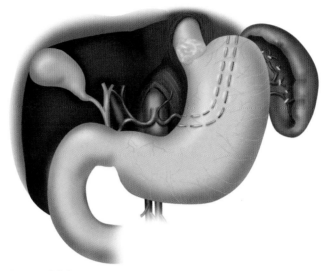

Figure 29-2

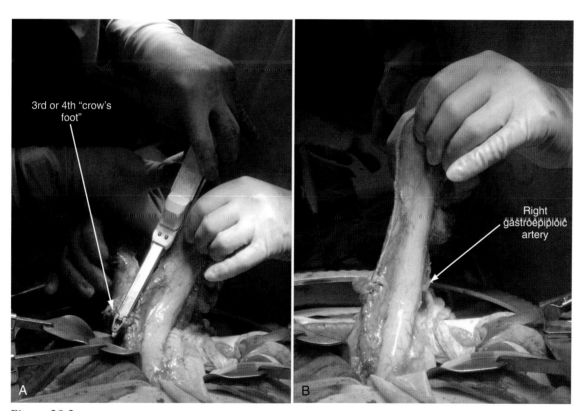

Figure 29-3

◆ A side-to-side, functional end-to-end, anastomosis is then created by laying the gastric graft alongside the proximal esophagus and inserting a 45-mm GIA stapler through a small gastrotomy created in the fundus (Figs. 29-4 and 29-5).

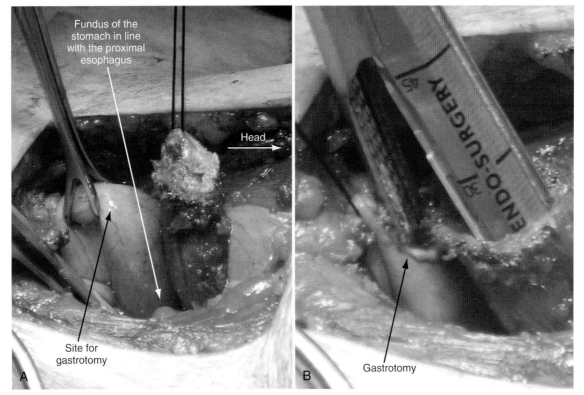

Figure 29-4

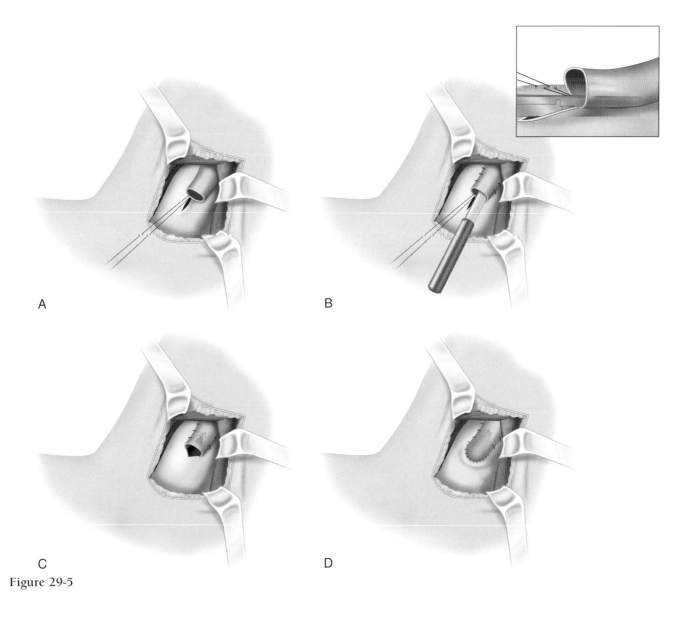

Figure 29-5

- The resultant common enterotomy is closed with interrupted 3-0 or 2-0 silk suture (Fig. 29-6).
- The gastric graft is gently pulled from below to straighten the anastomosis.
- A small, soft rubber drain is laid alongside the anastomosis and brought out through a separate stab wound.
- The gastric graft is sutured to the surrounding diaphragmatic hiatal tissue to prevent subsequent bowel herniation into the chest.

3. Colon as Conduit

- The upper abdomen is opened from umbilicus to xiphoid; extension below the diaphragm may be necessary depending on the patient's body habitus.
- The left colon is carefully mobilized from its retroperitoneal position, making sure not to injure its mesentery.
- The splenic flexure is mobilized.
- The gastrohepatic ligament is divided and the greater omentum carefully dissected off the transverse colon and resected.
- The hepatic flexure is freed, as is the right colon from its retroperitoneal attachments.
- The colon is essentially now freed on its central mesentery.
- The transverse colon is now stretched caudally as far as possible over the xiphoid based on the blood supply from the ascending branch of the left colic artery and a marking stitch placed at the apex (Fig. 29-7).
- An umbilical tape is then used to measure the distance from the apical marking stitch to the neck.
- The same length is then mapped out proximally on the colon to determine the colon interposition length needed and a second marking stitch is placed (Fig. 29-8).

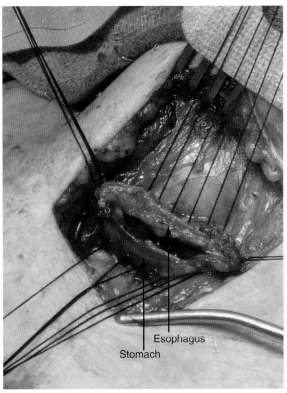

Figure 29-6

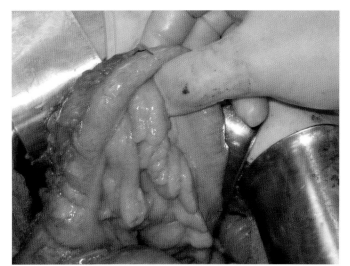

Figure 29-7

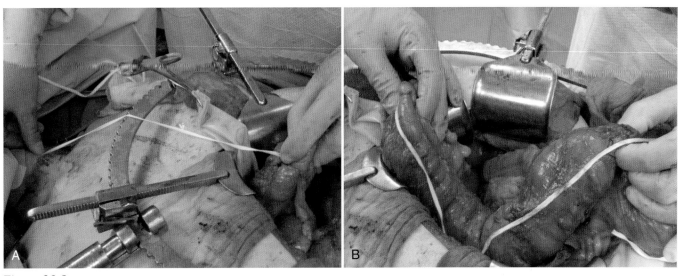

Figure 29-8

- The blood supply to the colon is now identified by carefully dissecting to the origin of the middle colic artery and vein proximal to its left and right branches (Fig. 29-9).
- The marginal artery is likewise dissected carefully at the proximal site of planned colon division.
- The middle colic artery and vein, as well as marginal artery (and any other accessory branches that would need division to allow complete transposition), are test clamped with atraumatic clamps, and blood flow to the graft is assessed before division of the colon (Fig. 29-10).
- Once blood flow to the graft is determined to be adequate based solely on the ascending branch of the left colic artery, the colon is divided proximally using a single firing of the 75-mm GIA stapler, corresponding to the second marking stitch.
- The colonic graft is placed on the anterior chest wall to ensure adequate length (Fig. 29-11).
- The proximal colon is then brought up through the mediastinum atraumatically in a similar fashion as described earlier for the gastric graft (Figs. 29-12 and 29-13).

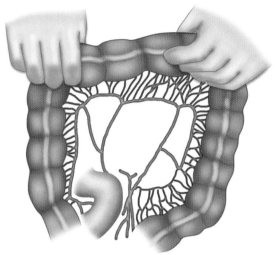

Figure 29-9

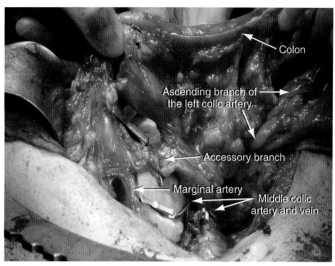

Figure 29-10

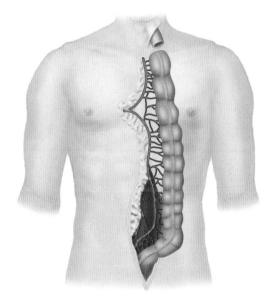

Figure 29-11

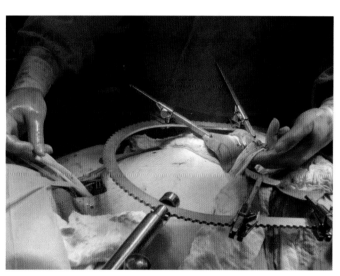

Figure 29-12

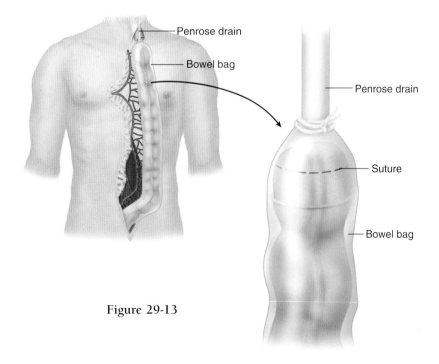

Figure 29-13

- The proximal esophagus (or pharynx, as the case may be) is anastomosed to the colon using a side-to-side, functional end-to-end, stapled anastomosis as described earlier or, alternatively, hand sewn using an end-to-end technique using interrupted 4-0 suture (necessary when attaching to the pharynx).
- A small, soft rubber drain is laid alongside the anastomosis and brought out through a separate stab wound.
- The colon is then gently pulled taught through the hiatus (or substernal tunnel as the case may be) to straighten the graft.
- At least 5 cm distal to its entrance into the abdomen, and at the planned area of distal transection of the interposition graft, the mesentery is then carefully dissected from the colon for a distance of approximately 1 cm to allow the introduction of a GIA stapler.
- The colon is then divided distally, carefully preserving the marginal artery and ascending branch of the left colic, thereby completely isolating the interposed segment.
- The distal interposition anastomosis is then created to either the gastric antrum or a Roux-en-Y segment of small bowel using a standard hand-sewn two-layered anastomosis of inner running 3-0 absorbable suture and outer layer of interrupted 3-0 silk.
- The proximal and distal colons are then anastomosed using a standard stapled, side-to-side, functional end-to-end, technique.
- The apices of the staple line(s) are reinforced with two or three interrupted 3-0 silk sutures (Fig. 29-14).
- Several interrupted 3-0 silk sutures are placed between the hiatal diaphragmatic soft tissues and the interposed colon to prevent subsequent herniation.
- Mesenteric defects are closed using running 3-0 absorbable sutures.

4. General Operative Points

- A nasogastric tube should be placed and manually confirmed to be just proximal to the pylorus before exiting the operating room.
- A feeding catheter jejunostomy should be performed for enteral feeding access on all esophageal reconstruction cases.
- When performing a colon interposition, an incidental appendectomy should be performed before transposing the colon.
- An incidental cholecystectomy should be performed if gallstones are palpated at the time of surgery.

5. Special Case of Substernal Reconstruction

- The cervical incision is extended down to the suprasternal notch.
- The suprasternal ligament is divided, and the undersurface of the manubrium is bluntly dissected with the fingertip.
- The midline of the manubrium is scored with the electrocautery inferiorly down to correspond to the first intercostal space.
- The manubrium is then scored laterally to the first intercostal space.
- The reciprocating saw is then used to divide the manubrium down and right-angled toward the first intercostal space, as previously scored (Fig. 29-15).
- Using blunt and sharp dissection, the clavicle is then carefully encircled, being careful not to injure adjacent vascular structures.

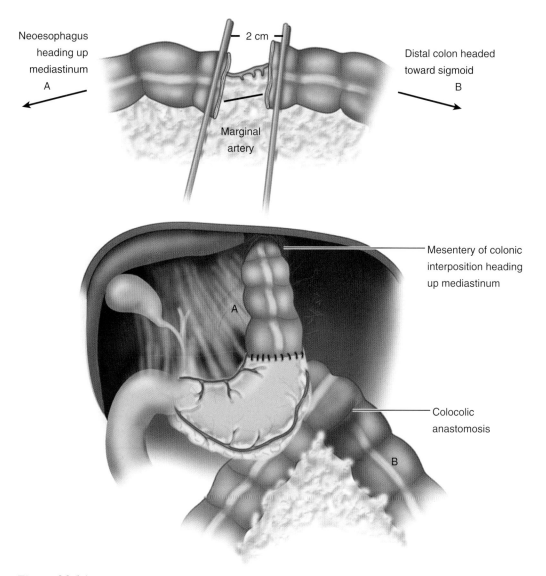

Neoesophagus
heading up
mediastinum
A

2 cm

Distal colon headed
toward sigmoid
B

Marginal
artery

Mesentery of colonic
interposition heading
up mediastinum

Colocolic
anastomosis

Figure 29-14

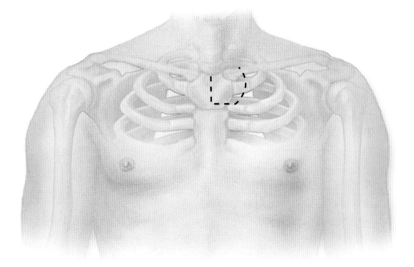

Figure 29-15

- The clavicle is then divided using the Gigli saw, making sure to preserve some of the costo-clavicular ligaments laterally.
- The first rib is likewise divided using the bone cutter close to the manubrium.
- The hemimanubrium, partial first rib, and partial clavicular head are then removed en bloc from any remaining soft tissues.
- The substernal tunnel is then created beginning inferiorly, dividing any diaphragmatic attachments that might be present by using the electrocautery.
- Using blunt dissection, the substernal tunnel is then created up to the neck.
- The neoesophagus can then be brought up this tunnel and anastomoses performed both proximally and distally as described earlier.

6. Special Case of Reconstruction to the Hypopharynx or Pharynx

- Potential proximal anastomotic sites may include either the left or right piriform sinus or the posterior pharynx.
- Additional opening to the hypopharynx may be necessary, in which case portions of the hyoid bone laterally, as well as portions of the thyroid shield laterally, may be resected to allow a wider anastomosis.
- The cricopharyngeus may be opened posteriorly and carried superiorly into the inferior constrictor muscle and the neoesophagus anastomosed to this location.
- Similarly the inferior constrictor muscle and underlying mucosa may be entered and divided just off the midline posteriorly above the cricopharyngeus.

Step 4. Postoperative Care

1. Immediate or Early

- Hydration and fluid replacement should be a primary concern the first 24 to 48 hours and diuretics specifically avoided.
- Arterial blood gases obtained to monitor the base deficit; a worsening deficit is indicative of graft ischemia.
- Visceral blood flow—constricting agents should be avoided if at all possible.
- Perioperative intravenous antibiotics should be given.
- Nasogastric tube should be kept to low wall suction and may need occasional irrigation or manipulation to remain patent.
  - ▲ If the tube becomes dislodged or accidentally pulled, it can usually be gently reinserted; however, if this is necessary, it should be done by the operative surgeon, not by the nurse.
- Slow, trophic jejunostomy tube feeds can be started on postoperative day 1, provided its intraluminal position is confirmed via contrast study.
- Deep venous thrombosis prophylaxis should be used via pneumatic compression devices on the legs and low-dose subcutaneous anticoagulation once internal bleeding is deemed not to be an issue.
- Rectal aspirin suppository is given until the patient is ambulatory to help prevent small-vessel thrombosis in the graft.
- Up in chair postoperative day 1

2. Short Term

- Intravenous fluids should be gradually tapered as enteral feeds are equally advanced via the feeding catheter jejunostomy to full goal (usually over several days).
  - ▲ Enteral feeds should be advanced only if the abdomen remains nondistended.
- Central lines should be discontinued, in addition to bladder catheters, after fluid status is no longer an issue (usually postoperative day 3).
- Begin ambulation on postoperative day 2.
- Continue nasogastric tube until the patient has return of bowel function (passage of flatus, bowel movement) *and* the abdomen is flat and soft, *and* output is minimal (usually less than 400 mL/day for an adult).
- After discontinuation of the nasogastric tube, do not begin feedings for a day.
- Once the patient has demonstrated that he or she is able to tolerate discontinuation of the nasogastric tube for 24 hours, begin clear liquid diet (if no problems with pharyngeal phase of swallowing).
  - ▲ If the patient has had reconstruction to or above the cricopharyngeus, a more conservative advancement of oral feeds is recommended, and speech pathology should be alerted to begin working with the patient before the initiation of feeds.
  - ▲ Special exercises may be given and initiated.
  - ▲ In this case, oral feeding may be delayed for several weeks as exercises are performed and therapy is continued; feeding may begin with semisolids rather than liquids.
- Once the patient has been started on a clear liquid diet and tolerates it well, a swallow study is performed consisting of thin barium.
- If no cervical leak is noted, the soft rubber drain is removed and the patient is started on a soft mechanical diet.
- Jejunostomy tube feeds are switched to nighttime only, allowing the patient to be free from all lines and tubes during the day.
- All oral medicines should be given either crushed or in liquid form.

3. On Discharge

- Avoid any foods that are hard, sharp, or crusty.
- All medicines should continue to be given either in liquid form or crushed.
- Home jejunostomy tube feeds may be given at nighttime to supplement nutrition, depending on oral intake at the time of discharge.
- Feeding jejunostomy should be continued and kept open via regular irrigation for 6 to 8 weeks, regardless of the patient's ability to eat at the time of discharge.

Step 5. Pearls and Pitfalls

- Gastric advancement
  - ▲ Mobilize the greater curve well away from the stomach.
  - ▲ Divide short gastrics close to the spleen, preserving any collaterals that may be present near the stomach.
  - ▲ Begin mobilization medially away from the spleen, between the transverse colon and the stomach, where the lesser sac can be entered easily.

▲ Be careful to preserve mesenteric blood flow to the transverse colon when mobilizing the greater curvature of the stomach away from the colon.

▲ The abdominal incision should be carried quite superiorly to remove the xiphoid process and to provide direct access to the gastroesophageal junction.

▲ Surgical clips should be avoided when ligating vessels because they can become a nidus for tearing and ripping when transposing the gastric graft into the chest.

▲ There is little reason to ligate the right gastric artery, even though the gastric graft is theoretically based on the right gastroepiploic artery.

▲ A search for an accessory left hepatic artery should be done and this artery preserved if present. It usually originates from the celiac axis or the left gastric artery directly (most common).

▲ The left gastric artery should be divided distal to the accessory left hepatic artery when present.

▲ The stomach should be handled with care and kept warm during its mobilization.

▲ Remove the lap pads as you mobilize the greater curve of the stomach near the hiatus to allow the spleen to fall back.

▲ The stomach should be pulled up into the neck atraumatically, using a bowel bag to take friction off the graft (i.e., pull up the bowel bag—not the graft—and let the graft go along for the ride).

▲ The anastomosis between the proximal esophagus and the gastric graft should be done end-to-side using a stapler.

◆ Colon interposition

▲ The splenic and hepatic flexures need to be mobilized completely, as do the right and left colons, which are usually retroperitoneal.

● The colon should be mobilized as much as possible on its mesentery to the midline.

▲ The middle colic artery and vein need to be carefully dissected near its origin, proximal to its left and right branches.

● Typically the middle colic vein easily tears near its juncture with the superior mesenteric vein, and manipulation of the colon tends to facilitate this and therefore needs to be done carefully.

▲ The proximal marking stitch is usually located somewhere along the right colon, sometimes even approaching the cecum, even though the graft is called a *left colon interposition.*

▲ A careful search for "cheater" vessels should be made because it is disappointing after dividing the colon only to find a large mesenteric vessel that is feeding the graft that was not previously identified and for that artery to inhibit the colon's transposition up to the neck.

▲ If the mesentery needs to be divided to allow more length, it should be done as proximally as possible (i.e., near the root of the mesentery) to allow as much collateralization as possible, and it should be divided through avascular planes when possible.

▲ Once temporary clamps are placed, the colon graft can be visually inspected (to see mesenteric pulsations), palpated (to confirm mesenteric pulse), or checked with a Doppler to make sure its blood supply is ensured.

● If there is any question of colon viability, it should not be divided or transposed.

▲ The colocolic anastomosis will by necessity be very close, if not immediately below, the distal interposition anastomosis by virtue of its shared mesentery.

◆ Substernal reconstruction
  ▲ It is important to take only a small piece of the clavicle, attached to the first rib close to the manubrium, to maintain ligaments laterally between the two; otherwise winging of the clavicle will occur.
  ▲ The xiphoid should be removed.
  ▲ A space posterior to the sternum and anterior to the pericardium can easily be made bluntly with the hand and fingers to allow transposition of the neoesophagus.
  ▲ When using the substernal tunnel, all else equal, it is best to leave as much proximal cervical esophagus intact as possible to allow bolus injection into the thoracic inlet.
◆ Complications
  ▲ Cervical leak
    ● Usually becomes evident between postoperative days 7 and 10
    ● Usually manifests itself clinically as enteric output from the soft cervical rubber drain
    ● May require additional opening of the cervical wound
    ● Usually closes with time so long as distal obstruction is not present
    ● Endoscopy might be helpful in determining graft viability.
    ● Prone to late stricturing
    ● Oral intake may or may not be curtailed, depending on the degree of leak.
    ● Sugar-free liquids may be helpful in flushing the wound and minimizing bacterial overgrowth.
    ● Need for reoperation is very rare in the absence of ischemic problems with the graft.
  ▲ Necrosis of neoesophagus
    ● Most feared complication
    ● Manifests by leak, sepsis, worsening base deficit
    ● Usually requires resection of the failed interposition graft with creation of an end cervical esophagostomy

Suggested Readings

DeMeester TR, Johansson K-E, Franze I, et al. Indications, surgical technique, and long-term functional results of colon interposition and bypass. Ann Surg 1988;208:460-474.
Johnson SB, DeMeester TR. Esophagectomy for benign disease: Use of the colon. Adv Surg 1994;27:317-334.
Orringer MB. Transhiatal esophagectomy without thoracotomy. In Pearson FG, Cooper JD, Deslauriers J, et al, eds. Esophageal Surgery. Toronto: Churchill Livingstone; 1995:683-701.
Orringer MB, Orringer JS. Esophagectomy without thoracotomy: A dangerous operation? J Thorac Cardiovasc Surg 1983;85:72-80.
Scott-Conner CEH. Operations to replace or bypass the esophagus. In Scott-Conner CEH, ed. Chassin's Operative Strategy in General Surgery. New York: Springer; 2002:139-150.
Thomas P, Fuentes P, Giudicelli R, Reboud E. Colon interposition for esophageal replacement: Current indications and long-term function. Ann Thorac Surg 1997;64:757-764.

CHAPTER 30

Techniques of Esophageal Preservation for High-Grade Barrett Esophagus

Aaron B. House and Joseph B. Zwischenberger

Step 1. Surgical Anatomy

- A comprehensive understanding of the anatomy of the esophagus before undertaking surgical procedures on the esophagus is critical.
- Figure 30-1 illustrates the anatomic layers of the esophagus that must be considered when performing endoscopic mucosal resection (EMR) of high-grade Barrett esophagus.

Step 2. Preoperative Considerations

- Ten percent of patients with symptomatic gastroesophageal reflux disease (GERD) will develop Barrett esophagus, typically after the sixth decade of life. More alarmingly, there is an associated 40-fold increase in risk for developing esophageal carcinoma in these patients. Although the pathophysiologic mechanism is still being investigated, it is thought to be exposure to bile and other reflux materials, not necessarily acid, that encourages the progression of dysplasia to cancer. Many patients with intestinal metaplasia of the distal esophagus are asymptomatic. Other patients have the typical symptoms of heartburn, regurgitation, acid or bitter taste in the mouth, excessive belching, and indigestion that are associated with GERD.
- The diagnosis of Barrett esophagus is made on endoscopic visualization of any segment of columnar mucosa within the esophagus that on pathology identifies intestinal metaplasia.
- Limited data and an incomplete understanding of the mechanisms leading to Barrett esophagus have made treatment of this disease controversial. Current treatment options include surveillance endoscopy, antireflux surgery, ablative therapy, EMR, and esophageal resection. EMR serves as both a diagnostic and possibly curative treatment option that also preserves

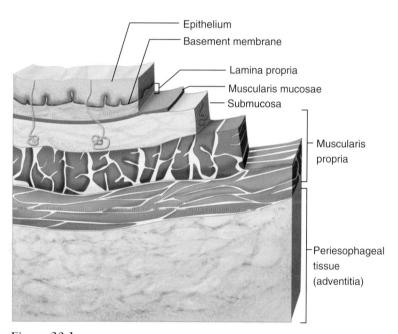

Figure 30-1

the esophagus. Further, it is a possible treatment option for patients with high-grade Barrett esophagus who are not acceptable candidates for esophagectomy.

- Several techniques have been developed for EMR; the most commonly used and technically feasible methods are the EMR cap and EMR band ligation techniques that are discussed here.
- The anesthetic approach is dictated by the co-morbidities of the patient, length of the procedure, as well as patient tolerance. The anesthesia for this procedure can range from conscious sedation to a general anesthetic.
- The patient is placed in the left lateral decubitus position and prepped in typical endoscopic fashion.
- For EMR in the esophagus, a large, soft cap (D-206-01-06, Olympus America, Center Valley, PA) is generally used for the first resection intending to acquire a large sample. The conventional hard-type transparent cap is preferably used just in case it is needed for additional resections or for resecting a small lesion. The outer diameter of the large, soft cap is 18 mm. There is an inner circular rim at the tip of the large, soft cap for the prelooping process. The scope used is the normal observation endoscope (e.g., −240 and so on).

Step 3. Operative Steps

1. Isolation of Mucosal Layers

♦ This initial step in isolating the lesion to be excised is common to all techniques of EMR. Using a standard upper endoscope, the lesion is visualized. Depending on physician preference, the margins of the lesion may then be marked using electrocautery. Submucosal injection allows elevation of the mucosa from the muscular layers to avoid perforation of the esophagus. An injection needle is passed into the endoscope to inject, most commonly, a diluted epinephrine in saline solution into the submucosa. This injection has a duration of approximately 5 minutes and may require repeating to avoid muscular damage. Alternative solutions for submucosal injection are discussed in Table 30-1.

♦ Puncturing the mucosa at an angle less than 45 degrees is the most important factor in this step to prevent transmural puncture of the esophagus. Total volume of solution injected depends on the size of the lesion, but it is necessary to inject enough to lift the whole lesion. Normally, saline injection first occurs in the normal mucosa just distal to the lesion. Accurate injection into the submucosa is confirmed with bulging and whitish swelling of the injected area.

♦ Alternatively, one may use a lift-and-cut biopsy technique in which the mucosal lesion may be lifted away from the muscular layers with endoscopic forceps without the need for saline injection and then cauterized.

TABLE 30-1. **Alternative Solutions for Submucosal Injection**

SOLUTION	CUSHION DURATION	ADVANTAGES	DISADVANTAGES
Normal saline solution (0.9%) w/epinephrine	+	Easy to inject, cheap, readily available	Quickly dissipates
Hypertonic solution of sodium chloride (3.0%)	++	Easy to inject, cheap, readily available	Tissue damage, local inflammation at injection sites
Hyaluronic acid	+++	Longest-lasting cushion	Expensive, not readily available, storage requirements, might stimulate residual tumor cell growth
Hydroxypropyl methylcellulose	+++	Long-lasting cushion, relatively inexpensive	Tissue damage, local inflammation at injection sites
Glycerol	++	Cheap, readily available	
Dextrose	++	Cheap, readily available	Tissue damage, local inflammation at injection sites
Albumin	++	Easy to inject, readily available	Expensive
Fibrinogen	+++	Easy to inject, long-lasting cushion	Expensive, not readily available
Autologous blood	+++	Clotting in syringe if injection delayed	Religious beliefs may preclude, limited human data

2. Prelooping Process

◆ Following the submucosal injection described earlier, a specially designed small-diameter endoscopic snare is passed through the scope and into the cap for what is known as the prelooping process. The snare wire is fixed along the rim of the EMR cap, and an area of normal mucosa is aspirated into the cap to create a seal. The snare wire is then opened and fixed along the rim of the cap, and the outer sheath of the snare is placed onto the rim of the cap.

3. Excision of Lesion

◆ The target mucosa, including the lesion, is then approached and fully sucked into the cap. It is then strangulated by simple closure of the prelooped snare wire. This action will create a pseudopolyp of strangulated mucosa. This pseudopolyp is then cut using electrocautery and then removed by simply removing the endoscope with the specimen still in the cap (Fig. 30-2).
◆ Alternatively, a special cap equipped with a band ligation device can be used to create the aforementioned pseudopolyp, much like a variceal ligation procedure, without the need for a prelooping step. Typically equipped with six ligation bands, this method allows the physician to perform multiple resections without removal of the endoscope. This is in contrast to the EMR cap technique, which requires removal of the scope following all resections. These steps are then repeated as needed until the lesion has been completely resected and specimens sent for pathology. Before removal of the scope assess the area of resection for active bleeding or perforation. A full sequence of procedural images can be found in Figure 30-3.

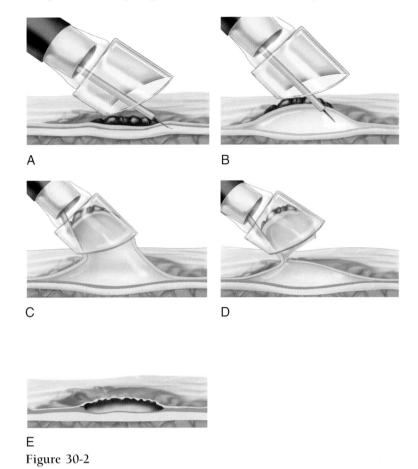

Figure 30-2

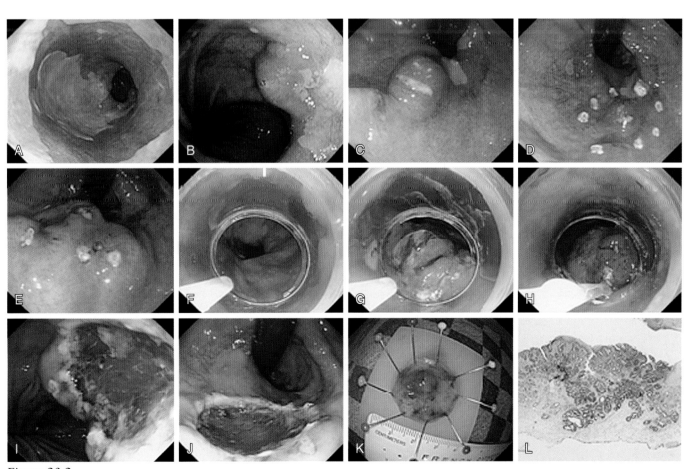

Figure 30-3
(Reproduced with permission from: www.Barrett.nl. Copyright © Amsterdam Esophageal Research Foundation.)

Step 4. Postoperative Care

- EMR is performed as an outpatient procedure, and patients may be discharged following recovery from sedation.
- Patients should be placed on acid-suppressing medications to promote appropriate healing of the procedurally induced ulcer with a normal squamous mucosa. This ulcer should heal over the next few weeks.
- The patient should be instructed to have a liquid diet the day of the procedure, which should be advanced to a soft mechanical diet the following day and regular diet thereafter.
- Patients must then be followed up with repeat upper endoscopy at 6 months to confirm complete excision of abnormal mucosa as well as for possible recurrence.

Step 5. Pearls and Pitfalls

- Although several techniques for EMR of high-grade Barrett esophagus are available, there is currently little agreement or data on which techniques are best used. Therefore current practice depends on physician preference and equipment availability.
- Complications of the procedure include perforation, bleeding, and stricture formation. These are all issues that can be corrected through endoscopic methods as well.
- The success of EMR depends on complete excision of abnormal mucosa. If this is not achieved, dysplasia may continue to progress to carcinoma. Therefore it is crucial to follow up patients with routine endoscopy. The length of this follow-up has yet to be determined.
- EMR is both diagnostic and possibly curative. If EMR is not curative, the tissue provided through EMR may provide the information needed to make further treatment decisions.
- EMR may also have a role when used in conjunction with laser ablative or photodynamic therapy to increase the chances of complete excision and eradication of abnormal mucosa.

Suggested Readings

Ahmadi A, Draganov P. Endoscopic mucosal resection in the upper gastrointestinal tract. World J Gastroenterol 2008;14(13):1984-1989.

ASGE Technology Committee, Kantsevoy SV, Adler DG, et al. Endoscopic mucosal resection and endoscopic submucosal dissection. Gastrointest Endosc 2008;68(1):11-18.

Chen L, Crawford J. The gastrointestinal tract. In Kumar V, ed. Robbins and Cotran: Pathologic Basis of Disease, 7th ed. Philadelphia: Saunders; 2005.

Inoue H. Endoscopic mucosal resection for entire gastrointestinal mucosal cancers. In Tytgat G, ed. Practice of Therapeutic Endoscopy, 2nd ed. Philadelphia: WB Saunders; 2000:117-125.

Maish M. Esophagus. In Townsend CM Jr, ed. Sabiston Textbook of Surgery: The Biological Basis of Modern Surgical Practice, 18th ed. Philadelphia: Saunders; 2007.

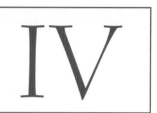

Esophageal Benign

CHAPTER 31

Laparoscopic Myotomy and Fundoplication for Achalasia

Virginia R. Litle and Thomas J. Watson

Step 1. Surgical Anatomy

- A comprehensive understanding of foregut anatomy and physiology is critical to undertaking surgical procedures on the esophagus for benign disease.
- Figure 31-1 demonstrates the key anatomic structures that must be considered in the surgical treatment of achalasia.

Step 2. Preoperative Considerations

- *Achalasia* is a motility disorder of the esophagus caused by destruction of ganglion cells in Auerbach myenteric plexus, leading to impaired relaxation of the lower esophageal sphincter (LES). Esophageal body aperistalsis is believed to be a secondary event. Progressive dysphagia to both solids and liquids is the symptomatic hallmark of achalasia.
- The barium esophagogram typically demonstrates loss of peristalsis in the smooth muscle of the distal two thirds of the esophagus as well as the classic "bird's beak" tapering at the LES. Upper endoscopy helps eliminate a pseudoachalasia diagnosis if no tumor is identified. Esophageal manometry establishes the diagnosis by showing failure of LES relaxation and esophageal body aperistalsis.
- Oral intake is restricted to clear liquids for 2 to 3 days before surgery.
- The patient is placed supine on the operating room table with arms abducted and a footboard in position.
- After general anesthetic induction with a single-lumen endotracheal tube, flexible esophagoscopy is performed to assess the adequacy of foregut preparation. If this assessment is inadequate, the surgeon may elect to reschedule the procedure. The endoscope may be left in the stomach during the myotomy and fundoplication.

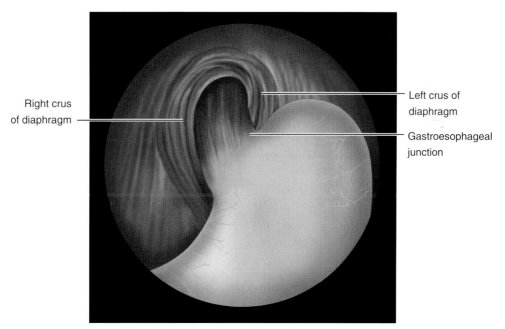

Right crus
of diaphragm

Left crus of
diaphragm

Gastroesophageal
junction

Figure 31-1

Step 3. Operative Steps

1. Incisions

- The surgeon stands on the patient's right side, the assistant on the left.
- Five abdominal ports are placed on the anterior abdominal wall, similar to our approach for a laparoscopic Nissen fundoplication: one cut-down 10-mm port in the right epigastrium and four 5-mm ports in the bilateral subcostal, left epigastric, and right flank locations (Fig. 31-2).
- A 5-mm, 30-degree laparoscope is placed through the left epigastric port.

2. Dissection

- The left lobe of the liver is lifted upward with a Diamond-Flex retractor, which is secured with a self-retaining system placed on the left side of the table. With the patient in maximal reverse Trendelenburg position, the dissection begins by dividing the gastrohepatic ligament and exposing the diaphragmatic crura bilaterally. The hiatus is circumferentially dissected, and a window is created behind the posterior vagus for subsequent passage of the fundus. The short gastric vessels are ligated using the ultrasonic shears in preparation for the partial fundoplication after the myotomy is completed.
- The anterior gastroesophageal junction (GEJ) fat pad is elevated working from left to right and from distal to proximal with preservation of the anterior vagus nerve.
- The GEJ is identified by the transition from longitudinal esophageal muscle to gastric serosa.
- The right and left crural pillars are reapproximated posteriorly using interrupted 0 nonabsorbable suture.

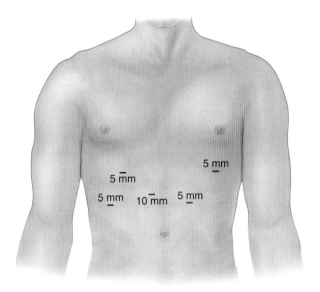

Figure 31-2

- Dilute epinephrine (1:20,000) may be injected in the submuscular plane above the GEJ using a straight cholangiogram needle (Fig. 31-3A). The esophagomyotomy is initiated using the ultrasonic shears (see Fig. 31-3B) or laparoscopic scissors and carried out as far proximally on the anterior esophagus as can be visualized (typically 6 to 8 cm above the GEJ). Endoscopic peanuts facilitate completing a 180-degree anterior myotomy (see Fig. 31-3C). The myotomy is extended 2 to 4 cm onto the gastric cardia (Fig. 31-4).
- Endoscopy is repeated to assess the completeness of myotomy and evaluate for mucosal perforation.
- A partial (Toupet) fundoplication is created by bringing the fundus posteriorly, and three interrupted 2-0 braided polyester sutures are placed: the most cephalad stitch approximating the muscle, fundus, and right crus, and the other two approximating the fundus and muscle. Similarly, three sutures are placed between the left crus, fundus, and esophageal muscle (Fig. 31-5).

3. Closing

- No nasogastric tube is placed because of risk of perforating the esophageal mucosa after the myotomy.
- The laparoscopic incisions are closed in routine manner with absorbable sutures.

Step 4. Postoperative Care

- A barium esophagogram is obtained on postoperative day 1. If no leak or obstruction occurs, a clear liquid diet is started.
- The patient is discharged home on postoperative day 1 or 2 with liquid narcotics and simethicone for pain and gas control.

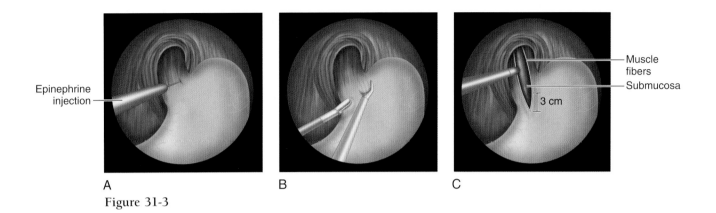

Epinephrine injection

Muscle fibers

Submucosa

3 cm

A   B   C

Figure 31-3

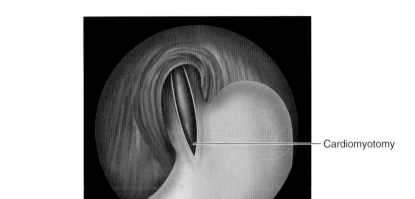

Cardiomyotomy

Figure 31-4

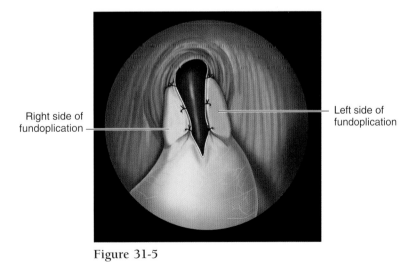

Right side of fundoplication

Left side of fundoplication

Figure 31-5

Step 5. Pearls and Pitfalls

◆ The relatively long myotomy on the gastric cardia (2-3 cm) appears to reduce postoperative dysphagia and minimize "recurrent" achalasia. Elevation of the anterior esophageal fat pad provides accurate identification of the GEJ and allows completion of at least a 2-cm-long cardiomyotomy.

◆ The surgeon should be proficient at intraoperative endoscopy or have an endoscopist available so that a perforation can be identified and immediately repaired. If a mucosal violation is detected, usually it can be repaired laparoscopically, although conversion to a laparotomy may be required. Only the minimal number of sutures (one or two) needed to reapproximate the mucosa should be placed because the injury can be easily extended during suturing. If intraoperative perforation does occur during the myotomy, an anterior partial (Dor) fundoplication should provide both an antireflux barrier and reinforcement of the repaired perforation so as to minimize the potential for postoperative leak.

◆ A Dor or Toupet partial fundoplication reduces reflux and should be a routine adjunct to laparoscopic myotomy; the choice between the two is a matter of surgeon preference. A complete 360-degree Nissen fundoplication is not advised in an aperistaltic esophagus.

◆ Perioperative mortality approaches 0%, and long-term patient satisfaction with the laparoscopic modified Heller myotomy and partial fundoplication exceeds 90%.

Suggested Readings

Donahue PE, Horgan S, Liu KJ-M, et al. Floppy Dor fundoplication after esophagocardiomyotomy for achalasia. Surgery 2002;132:716-723.

Hunter JG, Trus TL, Branum GD, et al. Laparoscopic Heller myotomy and fundoplication for achalasia. Ann Surg 1997;225:655-666.

Richards WO, Torquati A, Holzman MD, et al. Heller myotomy versus Heller myotomy with Dor fundoplication for achalasia: A prospective randomized double-blind clinical trial. Ann Surg 2004;240:405-415.

Litle VR. Laparoscopic Heller myotomy for achalasia: A review of the controversies. *Ann Thorac Surg* 2008;85:S743-746.

Luketich JD, Fernando HC, Christie NA, et al. Outcomes after minimally invasive esophagomyotomy. Ann Thor Surg 2001;72:1909-1913.

Lyass S, Thoman D, Steiner JP, et al. Current status of an antireflux procedure in laparoscopic Heller myotomy. Surg Endosc 2003;17:554-558.

Patti MG, Molena D, Fisichella PM, et al. Laparoscopic Heller myotomy and Dor fundoplication for achalasia. Arch Surg 2001;136:870-877.

Pellegrini C, Wetter LA, Patti M, et al. Thoracoscopic esophagomytomy: Initial experience with a new approach for the treatment of achalasia. Ann Surg 1992;216:291-296.

Richards WO, Torquati A, Holzman MD, et al. Heller myotomy versus Heller myotomy with Dor fundoplication for achalasia: A prospective randomized double blind clinical trial. Ann Surg 2004;240:405-415.

Shimi S, Nathanson LK, Cuschieri A. Laparoscopic cardiomyotomy for achalasia. J R Coll Surg Edinb 1991;36:152-154.

Wills VL, Hunt DR. Functional outcome after Heller myotomy and fundoplication for achalasia. J Gastrointest Surg 2001;5:408-413.

Wright AS, Williams CW, Pellegrini CA, et al. Long-term outcomes confirm the superior efficacy of extended Heller myotomy with Toupet fundoplication for achalasia. Surg Endosc 2007;21:713-718.

CHAPTER 32

TRANSTHORACIC ANTIREFLUX SURGERY PROCEDURES

John Scott Roth and Joseph B. Zwischenberger

Step 1. Surgical Anatomy

- Key anatomic structures that must be considered in antireflux surgery include the lower esophageal sphincter (LES), gastroesophageal junction (GEJ), esophageal hiatus, phrenic nerve, and vagus nerves.

Indications

- Gastroesophageal reflux disease (GERD) is a mechanical disorder associated with a defective LES mechanism, affecting as many as 2.5 million Americans.
- GERD is common in morbidly obese patients because of the high incidence of hiatal hernia and increased intra-abdominal pressure, which displaces the LES and increases the gastro-esophageal gradient.
- Typical symptoms of GERD (heartburn, regurgitation, chest pain, water brash, and occasionally dysphagia), atypical symptoms (chronic cough, hoarseness, asthma exacerbations, laryngitis, recurrent pulmonary infections, and dental lesions), and the sequelae of chronic acid reflux (esophagitis, esophageal strictures, Barrett esophagus [BE], and esophageal cancer) have been well described.
- Indications for antireflux surgery include GERD refractory to medical management, lifelong acid suppression, adverse reactions to medical therapeutic agents, and complications arising from GERD. The presence of BE may be an indication for antireflux surgery because some studies have demonstrated regression of metaplastic changes following surgery.
  - ▲ BE has been reported in up to 10% of patients with GERD, and it increases the incidence of esophageal adenocarcinoma.
  - ▲ Up to 20% of patients with BE demonstrated resolution of intestinal metaplasia, and as many as 50% to 60% show regression of low-grade dysplasia with surgical control of reflux.

Step 2. Preoperative Considerations

- A focused history and physical examination should be performed on all patients.
- Esophageal function tests should be performed. These motility studies evaluate peristalsis in the esophageal body and are useful for planning the type of fundoplication, exclusion of associated primary esophageal motor disorders, and defining the LES.
- Performance of 24-hour pH probe testing is done to quantitate the degree of acid reflux. Patients with objective evidence of reflux seen on endoscopy may not require pH probe testing.
- Esophagogastric duodenoscopy (EGD) should be performed to evaluate for mucosal changes, evaluate for the presence of a hiatal hernia, and exclude other pathologic conditions (e.g., stricture, BE, Cameron ulcers, or malignancy).
- Barium swallow provides anatomic information that may be correlated with information obtained from the other preoperative studies.
- Obese patients with reflux disease may be considered for bariatric surgery because Roux-en-Y gastric bypass performed in morbidly obese patients often achieves simultaneous goals of weight reduction and resolution of gastroesophageal reflux.
- With medical therapy, esophagitis resolves in 90% of cases; however, the underlying mechanical cause is unaltered, resulting in recurrence on withdrawal. Alkaline reflux–induced esophageal mucosal injury will not resolve with acid suppression.

Step 3. Operative Steps

Nissen Fundoplication

- Nissen fundoplication can be performed in most patients. Although esophageal dysmotility may be considered a relative contraindication to Nissen, most patients with altered motility can undergo a floppy Nissen fundoplication.
- Double-lumen intubation with right lung ventilation.
- Place patient in the right lateral decubitus position.
- A left lateral muscle-sparing thoracotomy incision is made in the seventh intercostal space.
- Exposure of the esophagus is achieved by dividing the inferior pulmonary ligament and incising the mediastinal pleura. Incision of the mediastinal pleura should continue to the level of the diaphragm. Circumferential dissection of the esophagus, encircling the esophagus with a Penrose drain, aids atraumatic retraction during dissection and avoids injury to the vagus nerves. The esophagus should be dissected down to the level of the pulmonary vein. Esophageal length is assessed following mobilization.

- The esophageal hiatus, the right and left crura, and the phrenoesophageal membrane are identified. The phrenoesophageal membrane is incised and the esophageal hiatus and crura are dissected to gain entry into the peritoneal cavity, with care being taken to preserve the left phrenic nerve.
- The stomach is retracted into the left chest, and the gastric fundus is mobilized by dividing the proximal short gastric vessels.
- The esophagogastric fat pad is excised.
- A tension-free 360-degree fundoplication is fashioned around the distal esophagus extending to the GEJ (Fig. 32-1A). The fundoplication should be 1.5 to 2.5 cm long and is created with a large esophageal Bougie (54-60 French) in place. The fundoplication is created using three interrupted sutures incorporating the esophagus and fundus (see Fig. 32-1B). The fundoplication should be adequately floppy and should easily accommodate a finger between the esophagus and the wrap while the bougie is in place.
- The stomach and Nissen gastroplasty are restored to an abdominal position.
- The hiatal defect is closed by suturing the crura posteriorly with interrupted silk sutures (see Fig. 32-1C).

Collis-Nissen Fundoplication

- The Collis-Nissen fundoplication is a modification of the Nissen fundoplication that incorporates an esophageal lengthening procedure for patients with a foreshortened esophagus generally acquired from chronic esophagitis and subsequent transmural fibrosis.
- The Collis gastroplasty can be performed either through the left chest exposure as described for the Nissen, through an upper abdominal exposure as described here, or via laparoscopic approach as described in Chapter 31. The goal is creation of a lesser curve–based gastric tube to increase esophageal length and allow for the fundoplication to be created within the abdomen.
- The abdomen is entered through a left subcostal incision, and the esophageal hiatus is exposed by detaching the triangular ligament of the left lobe of the liver. The esophagus is encircled with a Penrose drain just above the GEJ and then freed posteriorly to identify the diaphragmatic crura. Minimal dissection is performed along the anterior surface of the esophagus or within the esophageal hiatus.
- The fundus of the stomach is then mobilized by division of the uppermost short gastric vessels and the posterior attachments of the stomach to the anterior surface of the pancreas. The gastrohepatic ligament is divided with careful attention to the vagus nerves. A replaced or accessory left hepatic artery is occasionally encountered and should be preserved.
- A 48-French intraesophageal bougie is advanced through the GEJ and carefully guided along the lesser curvature of the stomach (Fig. 32-2A).
- A linear endo-GIA stapler is then applied across the gastric cardia parallel to the bougie on the left side, creating a gastric tube extending 5 cm from the GEJ inferiorly that will act as an extended neoesophagus (see Fig. 32-2B). Alternatively, a noncutting linear stapler may be used, minimizing the risk of a leak, but less length is achieved. Care should be taken to preserve the gastric fundus.
- This additional esophageal length provides an adequate segment of esophagus around which to perform a 360-degree tension-free wrap and restoration of an intra-abdominal GEJ (see Fig. 32-2C).

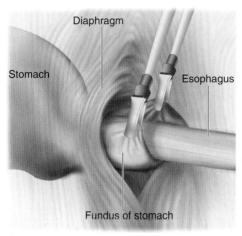

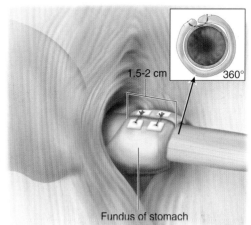

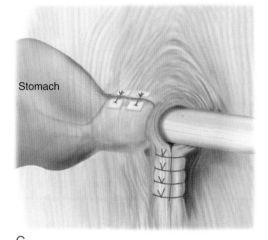

Figure 32-1

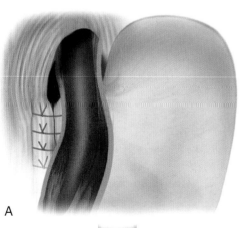

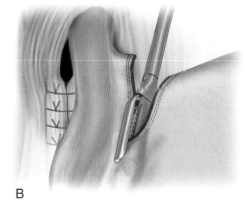

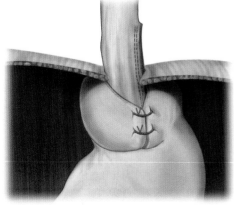

Figure 32-2

Toupet Fundoplication

- The exposure for a Toupet fundoplication is created in a manner similar to the Nissen fundoplication. The Toupet fundoplication is fashioned by creating a posterior 270-degree fundoplication, thus leaving the anterior 90 degrees of the esophagus exposed (Fig. 32-3).
- The Toupet fundoplication may be considered in patients with impaired esophageal motility. However, the incidence of dysphagia is not reduced with a Toupet fundoplication compared with a Nissen fundoplication.

Belsey Mark IV

- In contrast to the Nissen operation, the Belsey Mark IV creates a 270-degree wrap (Fig. 32-4).
- The Belsey is performed through a left posterolateral thoracotomy through the sixth interspace.
- The esophagus is mobilized from the aortic arch to the hiatus, and a two-layer suture line is created to overlap the gastric fundus around two thirds of the circumference of the lower esophagus for a distance of approximately 4 cm upward from the GEJ.
- The first row of three mattress sutures is placed between the stomach and the esophagus, and the second row incorporates the tendinous portion of the diaphragm to anchor the repair within the abdomen
- Belsey Mark IV is good option for treatment of persistent GERD after bariatric procedures because the mobilization of the GEJ via a thoracotomy incision is facilitated by avoiding the adhesions associated from prior abdominal surgery.

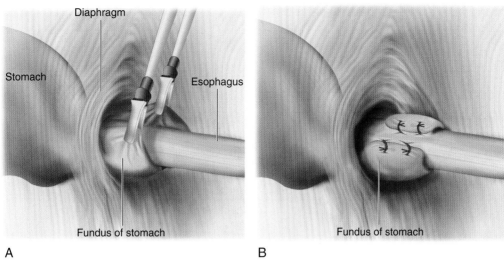

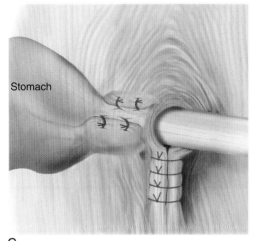

Figure 32-3

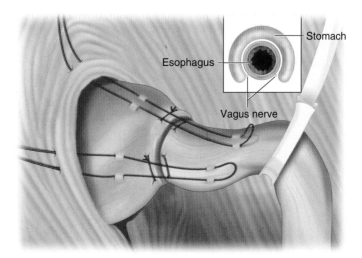

Figure 32-4

Step 4. Postoperative Care

- Transient dysphagia occurs in a small number of patients and usually resolves quickly. Long-term dysphagia occurs in less than 5% of patients.
- Precautions should be taken to avoid postoperative nausea, vomiting, and retching to avoid disruption of the fundoplication.
- Carbonated beverages, drinking straws, and chewing gum should be avoided following anti-reflux surgery to prevent gastric distention associated with swallowed gas.
- The patient is prescribed a liquid diet for 1 week and is gradually advanced to a puréed and then a soft diet. Strict adherence to a dietary regimen will minimize early dysphagia.
- Lifting restrictions may be considered to avoid disruption of the hiatal closure.
- Patients with signs and symptoms of an esophageal leak or disrupted fundoplication should undergo an esophagogram with water-soluble contrast followed by barium. Esophageal leaks require immediate reoperation. Disruption of the fundoplication or herniation of the stomach into the chest will require reoperation. When diagnosed early, immediate operation should be undertaken. Those detected in a delayed fashion should be postponed for 6 to 12 weeks postoperatively unless the patient's clinical course dictates otherwise.
- Long-term success rates occur in more than 95% of patients, with most patients avoiding the need for long-term acid suppression.
- Long-term dysphagia occurs in 5% to 7% of patients. Dietary education, including thorough chewing, eating smaller bites of food, and eating more slowly, will reduce complaints of dysphagia.
- Epidural analgesia and indwelling catheters for administration of analgesics aid in postoperative pain control.
- Postoperative medications should be administered in a liquid or crushed form whenever possible. Acid suppression is often continued for 2 to 4 weeks postoperatively to aid in the resolution of esophagitis. Long-term acid suppression is not required.

Step 5. Pearls and Pitfalls

- With proper patient selection, the outcomes of primary antireflux surgery are generally good.
- Adequate mobilization of the esophagus is required to ensure a minimum of 3 cm of intra-abdominal esophagus.
- A foreshortened esophagus will necessitate a Collis gastroplasty.
- The Nissen fundoplication should be created by using the fundus of the stomach. Creation of the fundoplication with gastric body or antrum will result in an angulated fundoplication with resultant dysphagia, reflux, or both.
- Postoperative dysphagia is minimized by creation of a floppy fundoplication. The use of a large esophageal bougie and the creation of a tension-free fundoplication will minimize postoperative swallowing complaints.
- The most common causes of failed antireflux procedures are related to technical failures, unrecognized anatomy, and inappropriate patient selection. Resection of the hernia sac and complete circumferential dissection of the esophagus and GEJ will minimize the likelihood of hernia recurrence. Failure to divide the posterior attachments between the GEJ and the diaphragm is a common reason for hiatal hernia recurrences.
- Regression of BE is strongly and inversely related to the length of the Barrett's segment and occurs in a time-dependent fashion after control of GERD.

Suggested Readings

Chen LQ, Ferraro P, Martin J, Duranceau AC. Antireflux surgery for Barrett's esophagus: Comparative results of the Nissen and Collis-Nissen operations. Dis Esophagus 2005;18:320-328.

Chen RH, Lautz D, Gilbert RJ, Bueno R. Antireflux operation for gastroesophageal reflux after Roux-en-Y gastric bypass for obesity. Ann Thorac Surg 2005;80:1938-1940.

Gurski RR, Peters JH, Hagen JA, et al. Barrett's esophagus can and does regress after antireflux surgery: A study of prevalence and predictive features. J Am Coll Surg 2003;196:706-713.

Legare JF, Henteleff HJ, Casson AG. Results of Collis gastroplasty and selective fundoplication, using a left thoracoabdominal approach for failed antireflux surgery. Eur J Cardiothor Surg 2002;21:534-540.

Krasna MJ. Surgical therapy for gastroesophageal reflux disease. In Shields TW, Locicero J, Ponn RB, Rusch VW, eds. General Thoracic Surgery, 6th ed. Philadelphia: Lippincott Williams & Wilkins; 2005:2173-2185.

Smith CD: Antireflux surgery. Surg Clin North Am 2008;88:943-958.

CHAPTER 33

LAPAROSCOPIC COLLIS GASTROPLASTY AND FUNDOPLICATION

John Scott Roth

Step 1. Surgical Anatomy

- A comprehensive understanding of the anatomy of the esophagus and stomach is essential before performing surgical fundoplication or other operations of the foregut.
- Figures 33-1 and 33-2 demonstrate the key surgical anatomy required to perform a transabdominal laparoscopic Collis gastroplasty and fundoplication successfully (see Fig. 33-1).

Step 2. Preoperative Considerations

- Gastroesophageal reflux disease (GERD) is one of the most common disorders of the gastrointestinal tract, affecting up to 40% percent of the population. Whereas most patients with GERD suffer from mild symptoms of heartburn and regurgitation, a small percentage of these patients will develop complications of reflux, including esophagitis, esophageal strictures, Barrett esophagus, hiatal hernias, and shortened esophagus. Intrinsic shortening of the esophagus is the result of the chronic inflammation associated with GERD.
- Preoperative evaluation of patients with GERD includes endoscopy, 24-hour esophageal pH monitoring, esophageal manometry, and fluoroscopic barium studies. The presence of a shortened esophagus may be suggested by a hiatal hernia greater than 5 cm in diameter, type III hiatal hernias, Barrett esophagus, a history of caustic ingestion, sarcoidosis, scleroderma, or Crohn disease.
- Indications for the surgical treatment of reflux disease include (1) patients with complications of reflux, such as esophageal stricture, Barrett esophagus, Cameron ulcers, and anemia; (2) patients with symptoms that are refractory to medical treatment; and (3) patients who are well controlled with medical therapy who wish to avoid the need to take long-term medications. The presence of a hiatal hernia alone is not generally considered an indication for repair. Hiatal hernias associated with symptoms of GERD or obstruction should undergo

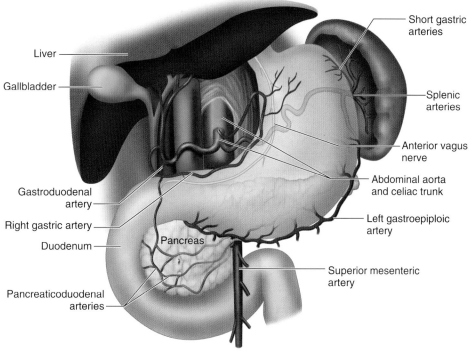

Liver

Gallbladder

Gastroduodenal
artery

Right gastric artery

Duodenum

Pancreas

Pancreaticoduodenal
arteries

Short gastric
arteries

Splenic
arteries

Anterior vagus
nerve

Abdominal aorta
and celiac trunk

Left gastroepiploic
artery

Superior mesenteric
artery

Figure 33-1

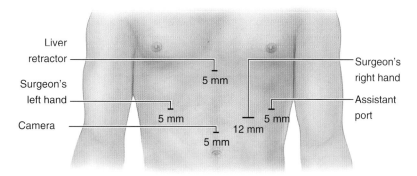

Liver
retractor

Surgeon's
left hand

Camera

5 mm

5 mm

5 mm

12 mm

5 mm

Surgeon's
right hand

Assistant
port

Figure 33-2

operative repair. However, the benefits of repairing an asymptomatic paraesophageal hernia remain an area of significant controversy.

◆ A Collis gastroplasty is a necessary adjunct to fundoplication in patients with a shortened esophagus. In most patients, the esophagus can be adequately mobilized to allow for a fundoplication without an esophageal lengthening procedure. Predicting which patients will require a Collis gastroplasty preoperatively is extremely difficult. The presence of the gastroesophageal (GE) junction at the level of the diaphragm or below on an endoscopy or other imaging study effectively excludes esophageal shortening. However, the presence of a fixed hiatal hernia does not reliably predict a shortened esophagus. In fact, most patients with large fixed hiatal hernias may undergo fundoplication without esophageal lengthening, but failure to recognize a shortened esophagus is likely to result in an early hiatal hernia recurrence.

Step 3. Operative Steps

◆ The patient is positioned on a split-leg table or in the low lithotomy position to allow the surgeon to stand between the legs. Placing the patient's arms at his or her sides allows for greater flexibility for placement of the liver retractor as well as for assistants standing at the bedside.

◆ Skin cleansing with a chlorhexidine-based preparation, as recommended by the Centers for Disease Control and Prevention, is used and extends from the nipples to the inguinal ligaments craniocaudally and should extend to the posterior axillary line on either side.

◆ Access to the peritoneal cavity is obtained by using either the Veress needle or a Hasson technique. The initial trocar should be positioned in the midline approximately 15 cm below the xyphoid process. Placement of this port at the umbilicus may limit the surgeon's ability later to dissect into the mediastinum to obtain adequate esophageal mobilization. Additional ports are placed for retraction and exposure and include 5-mm ports in the right midclavicular line, the subxyphoid position, and the left anterior axillary line. A 12-mm port is placed in the left midclavicular line, which is used for introducing the stapling device (see Fig. 33-2).

◆ A liver retractor is placed through the subxyphoid port site to retract the left lobe of the liver anteriorly and expose the esophageal hiatus.

- Gentle retraction is used to reduce the contents of the hiatal defect into the peritoneal cavity. The left lateral port site is used to maintain retraction on the stomach.
- Initial dissection is performed along the greater curvature of the stomach, approximately 1 cm lateral to the stomach, dividing the short gastric vessels. Dissection is performed along the cephalad third of the stomach and extending up to the level of the left diaphragmatic crus. Attachments between the posterior wall of the stomach and the retroperitoneum are also released.
- The hernia sac is incised along the medial border of the left crus of the diaphragm. Using blunt dissection, a plane is dissected above the hernia sac, reducing the hernia sac into the abdomen. The esophagus is identified in the mediastinum above the hernia sac. The use of an esophageal bougie may facilitate identification of the esophagus in some patients.
- The gastrohepatic ligament is incised through its avascular portion and extended up to the phrenoesophageal ligament. Care must be taken to identify an accessory left hepatic artery within the gastrohepatic ligament. The peritoneum and hernia sac over the anterior aspect of the esophagus are incised carefully to avoid injury to the underlying anterior vagus nerve. The hernia sac and preesophageal fat pad are fully reduced from the mediastinum into the abdomen.
- The esophagus is encircled with a Penrose drain to facilitate anterior retraction of the esophagus. Posterior hernia sac attachments between the esophagus and the diaphragm are carefully incised while identifying the posterior vagus nerve, which is left adherent to the esophagus to avoid injury.
- The esophagus is then circumferentially mobilized into the mediastinum to ensure a minimum of 2.5 to 3 cm of intra-abdominal esophageal length. If the GE junction does not remain below the diaphragm with an adequate tension-free intra-abdominal length, then a Collis

gastroplasty is required to prevent the postoperative migration of the stomach into the mediastinum.

◆ A stapled wedge Collis gastroplasty is performed using a reticulating endoscopic linear stapler. A 48 to 52 French bougie is placed transorally and introduced into the stomach. The fundus is marked adjacent to the bougie in the desired location of the newly created GE junction. This is typically 3 to 5 cm below the Angle of His. The reticulating stapler is introduced through the left midclavicular port and maximally angled toward the bougie. The stapler is placed along the greater curvature of the stomach with the anvil directed toward the marked location on the fundus. Two to three applications of the stapler are generally required. The stapler is then reticulated such that the anvil of the stapler is parallel to the bougie and fired in a vertical fashion to excise a wedge of fundus, thus creating a 3- to 5-cm neoesophagus (Fig. 33-3).

◆ Following completion of the Collis gastroplasty, the staple lines and stomach may be interrogated by the infusion of methylene blue and the use of intraoperative endoscopy to assess for leak. Staple-line leaks are more easily addressed at this time than after completion of the fundoplication.

◆ Closure of the hiatus is performed posterior to the esophagus, displacing the esophagus anteriorly and further increasing intra-abdominal esophageal length. Reinforcement of the crura with a biologic mesh will decrease the risk of hernia recurrence. A 4 × 6-cm piece of mesh is fashioned and sutured to the crura to reinforce the diaphragmatic closure (Fig. 33-4).

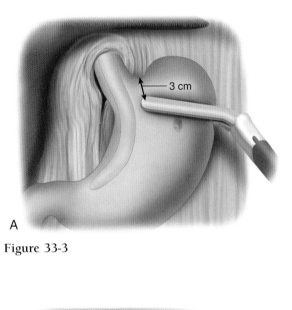
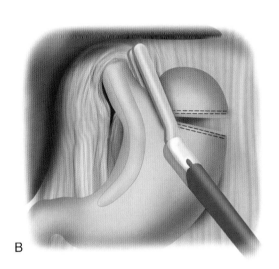

A

B

Figure 33-3

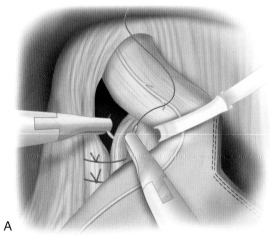
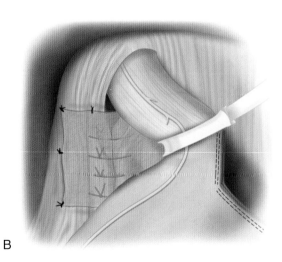

A

B

Figure 33-4

- A 360-degree fundoplication is fashioned around the neoesophagus to prevent postoperative reflux. The posterior fundus adjacent to the greater curvature of the stomach is passed posterior to the esophagus through the retroesophageal window. A "shoeshine" maneuver is performed by gently pulling the fundus on either side of the esophagus to ensure that the posteriorly wrapped fundus is contiguous with the anterior fundus to be used for creation of the wrap (Fig. 33-5).
- The bougie is advanced through the GE junction into the stomach, and the fundoplication is performed with the bougie in place. The anterior fundus is secured to the posteriorly wrapped fundus, incorporating the adjacent muscle of the esophagus in the first stitch. In patients with more significant esophageal shortening, it might not be feasible for the fundoplication to be anchored to the native esophagus, and the cephalad stitch incorporates the serosa of the neoesophagus. Generally a total of three stitches are placed to create a fundoplication that is 2.5 cm long. The fundoplication should be adequately floppy as determined by placing an instrument between the fundoplication and the esophagus while the bougie is in place. Evidence of tension on the fundoplication should prompt the surgeon to revise the procedure at this time to prevent postoperative dysphagia (Fig. 33-6).
- Completion of laparoscopic surveys is performed with removal of ports under direct visualization. Fascial closure is required only at the site of the 12-mm trocar.

Step 4. Postoperative Care

- Following recovery from anesthesia, patients are returned to a hospital room and kept "nothing by mouth" overnight. Nasogastric tubes are not required. A contrast esophagogram is performed on postoperative day 1, and a liquid diet is begun if no leak is demonstrated.
- The postoperative diet is focused on preventing ingestion of air and minimizing dysphagia. Patients are counseled to avoid foods and activities that result in the ingestion of air.
- Patients are typically discharged from the hospital on the second postoperative day on a liquid or puréed diet.

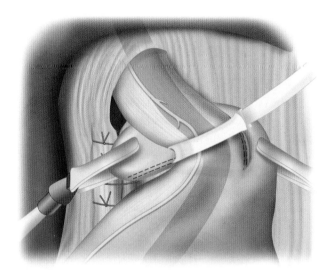

Figure 33-5

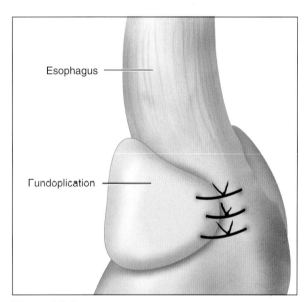

Figure 33-6

Step 5. Pearls and Pitfalls

- Trocar placement close to the costal margin dramatically facilitates conduct of the operation. Placement of the camera and working ports low on the abdomen may limit the extent of esophageal mobilization. Extended-length laparoscopic instruments are generally not required but may be helpful in selected patients.
- Assessment of intra-abdominal esophageal length can be challenging. Traction on the stomach and esophagus should be avoided to avoid overestimations of intra-abdominal esophageal length. Pneumoperitoneum displaces the diaphragm cephalad, resulting in further overestimations of esophageal length. However, closure of the crura posterior to the esophagus results in anterior displacement of the esophagus and an increase of esophageal length of 0.5 to 1 cm.
- Careful evaluation of the esophagus and stomach for evidence of injury or leak can be performed by instilling methylene blue through a nasogastric tube and by means of intraoperative endoscopy.

Suggested Readings

Chen LQ, Ferraro P, Martin J, Duranceau AC. Antireflux surgery for Barrett's esophagus: Comparative results of the Nissen and Collis-Nissen operations. Dis Esophagus 2005;18:320-328.

Collis JL. An operation for hiatus hernia with short esophagus. Thorax 1957;12:181-188.

Hoang CD, Koh PS, Maddaus MA. Short esophagus and esophageal stricture. Surg Clin North Am 2005;85:433-451.

Horvath KD, Swanstrom LL, Jobe BA. The short esophagus: Pathophysiology, incidence, presentation, and treatment in the era of laparoscopic antireflux surgery. Ann Surg 2000;232:630-640.

Houghton SG, Deschamps C, Cassivi SD, et al. Combined transabdominal gastroplasty and fundoplication for shortened esophagus: Impact on reflux-related and overall quality of life. Ann Thorac Surg 2008;85:1947-1953.

McLean TR, Haller CC, Lowry S. The need for flexibility in the operative management of type III paraesophageal hernias. Am J Surg 2006;192:e32-e36.

Pearson FG, Cooper JD, Patterson GA, et al. Gastroplasty and fundoplication for complex reflux problems. Ann Surg 1987;206:473-478.

Stylopoulos N, Gazelle GS, Rattner DW. Paraesophageal hernias: Operation or observation? Ann Surg 2002;236:492-501.

Terry ML, Vernon A, Hunter JG. Stapled-wedge Collis gastroplasty for the shortened esophagus. Am J Surg 2004;188:195-199.

Youssef YK, Shekar N, Lutfi R, et al. Long-term evaluation of patient satisfaction and reflux symptoms after laparoscopic fundoplication with Collis gastroplasty. Surg Endosc 2006;20:1702-1705.

ENDOSCOPIC TREATMENT FOR GASTROESOPHAGEAL REFLUX

Jonathan P. Pearl and Jeffrey L. Ponsky

Gastroesophageal reflux disease (GERD) affects more than 10 million Americans. Most are maintained on oral antacid medications such as histamine type 2 blockers and proton pump inhibitors (PPIs). A subset, of GERD patients are considered good candidates for antireflux procedures. At present, patients with typical symptoms, such as pyrosis and regurgitation, are commonly offered laparoscopic antireflux surgery. However, the available methods of endoscopic therapy for GERD are constantly evolving and will likely become the primary method of antireflux therapy in the future.

In April 2000, the Food and Drug Administration (FDA) approved both an endoscopic suturing device (EndoCinch; Bard, Davol Inc, Cranston, RI) and a catheter for delivering radiofrequency energy (Stretta, formerly of Curon Medical Inc, Fremont, CA) for the treatment of GERD. The initial fervor for these devices, as well as the subsequently introduced bulking agents (Enteryx; Boston Scientific Inc, Natick, MA; and Gatekeeper, Medtronic Inc, Minneapolis, MN), may have led to their clinical application before assuring efficacy and safety. As the data accumulated, the side-effect profiles of the bulking agents led to their withdrawal from the market, and the results from the suturing device were not durable. To complicate matters further, the manufacturer of the Stretta device, for which there may be reasonable data to support its use, has declared bankruptcy, and the catheters are no longer available for purchase.

Two additional endoscopic devices were recently introduced that more closely mimic laparoscopic antireflux surgery: the NDO plicator (NDO Surgical Inc, Mansfield, MA) and EsophyX (EndoGastric Solutions Inc, Redmond, WA). Both create gastric plications using full-thickness sutures. The long-term data are still being accumulated, but these devices show promise in offering an endoscopic solution to the common affliction of GERD.

Step 1. Surgical Anatomy

- The primary barrier to gastroesophageal reflux is provided by the lower esophageal sphincter (LES). This sphincter is unique in that it is a physiologic entity rather than an anatomic structure. The LES is located just above the esophagogastric junction and is identified as an area of high pressure on esophageal manometry. Additionally, an acute angulation between the esophagus and the gastric cardia, termed the *angle of His*, likely provides a barrier to reflux.

◆ Several factors contribute to the high-pressure zone of the LES. The normal anatomic location of the LES is within the abdominal cavity. The positive pressure within the abdomen and the negative pressure within the thorax are transmitted to the LES. The crura of the diaphragm may partially compress the LES, and finally, the esophageal musculature supplies tone to the distal esophagus. Normally the distal esophageal musculature is contracted. Upon swallowing, the musculature relaxes to allow passage of liquid and solid into the stomach and then returns to its normal tonic state. Patients with GERD typically have a relatively flaccid LES with inopportune transient relaxations.

◆ Most patients with GERD have a hiatal hernia. The most common hiatal hernia in GERD patients is a sliding hiatal hernia, in which the gastroesophageal junction migrates into the thorax while the fundus remains in the abdomen. The phrenoesophageal ligament, a continuation of the endoabdominal fascia, stretches to accommodate the cardia of the stomach as it migrates into the chest, thus becoming the hernia sac (Fig. 34-1). The LES is exposed to negative thoracic pressure and the angle of His is disrupted. Hence the function of the LES is compromised, and reflux of gastric contents into the distal esophagus occurs.

Step 2. Preoperative Considerations

◆ The goal of any antireflux procedure is to re-create a barrier to reflux of gastric and duodenal contents into the lower esophagus. Some of the principles of laparoscopic antireflux surgery include reduction of the hiatal hernia and its hernia sac, extensive mediastinal dissection of the esophagus to create adequate intra-abdominal length, and mobilization of the fundus with creation of a short, floppy fundoplication. Because there is no dissection or mobilization during endoscopic antireflux procedures, the indications for endoluminal procedures for GERD are limited.

◆ In general, only patients who have a small hiatal hernia (<3 cm) and an adequate resting LES pressure (>5 mm Hg) should be considered for endoscopic antireflux procedures. There should be no evidence of Barrett metaplasia, and the patient should be able to tolerate moderate sedation. Finally, the patient should be made aware of the limited available data supporting endoscopic treatment of GERD.

◆ Some might argue that the best candidates for endoscopic antireflux procedures are those who need it least—those with small hiatal hernias whose symptoms respond well to antacid medication. At present the indications are limited and will likely remain so until additional evidence is accumulated supporting widespread application of endoluminal therapies.

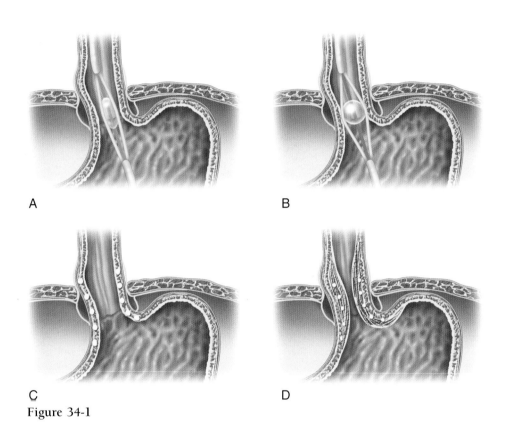

A

B

C

D

Figure 34-1

Step 3. Operative Steps

♦ The procedural details are discussed here only for Stretta, the NDO plicator, and the EsophyX endoluminal fundoplication. The mucosa-to-mucosa endoscopic suturing devices do not yield durable results, and refinements in the devices are required before they should be used clinically.

1. Stretta

♦ The Stretta catheter consists of a soft, flexible tip with a balloon-basket assembly with four radially oriented nickel titanium needle electrodes (Fig. 34-2). A generator delivers temperature-controlled radiofrequency energy to the esophagogastric junction via the electrodes. Thermocouplers on the electrodes constantly monitor temperature and impedance in the tissue. Continuous irrigation with cooled sterile water maintains temperatures below 50°C to prevent tissue injury.

♦ An upper endoscopy is performed with attention to the location of the squamocolumnar junction. A guidewire is passed into the stomach and left in place while the endoscope is removed. The Stretta catheter is advanced over the guidewire and positioned 1 cm above the Z line. The balloon is inflated to 2.5 psi, and the needles are deployed into the tissue by advancing a thumb control. The radiofrequency energy is delivered to each electrode with a target temperature of 85°C. The catheter is sequentially rotated 45 degrees, and the procedure is repeated at the same level. The same procedure is performed at 5-mm increments to the level of the Z line. Pull-back lesions are then created by advancing the catheter into the stomach. The balloon is filled with 25 mL of saline and pulled back until resistance is met at the esophagogastric junction. Energy is then delivered to this area.

♦ There are two postulated mechanisms of action of the Stretta procedure. The application of radiofrequency energy may increase the tone of the LES, and transient relaxation of the LES may be reduced. A sham-controlled study of Stretta has shown significant improvement in GERD quality-of-life measures and a substantial reduction in the percentage of patients taking antacid medication. Contrarily, Stretta does not appear to reduce the distal acid exposure.

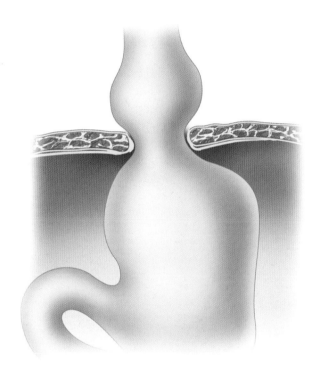

Figure 34-2

2. NDO Plicator

♦ The NDO plicator creates a full-thickness gastric plication using permanent sutures. The device is 15 mm in outer diameter and accommodates a slim (<6 mm) endoscope through an accessory channel. Initially, a diagnostic endoscopy is performed. A Savary wire is left in the stomach, and the NDO plicator is advanced over the wire into the stomach. The device is retroflexed toward the gastric cardia. The slim endoscope is used for visualization, thus requiring two endoscopists. An area 1 cm from the esophagogastric junction is chosen for plication and grasped with the plicator's retracting device. The tissue is brought into the jaws of the plicator, and a turn of a wheel deploys the sutures. The sutures comprise polypropylene with polytetrafluoroethylene bolsters. The device is then disengaged and removed, leaving behind a full-thickness serosa-to-serosa gastric plication.

♦ A sham-controlled trial showed significant improvement in GERD symptoms, a substantial reduction in PPI requirement, and improvement in distal acid exposure. The device appears to be safe, and no major complications have been noted in the published trials. Long-term data are lacking, but full-thickness endoluminal plication may serve effectively to mimic laparoscopic fundoplication.

3. EsophyX

♦ The EsophyX device is used to create an endoluminal fundoplication (ELF) using full-thickness sutures secured with T-fasteners. The device and a standard gastroscope are advanced into the stomach. The stomach is inflated, and a hinge on the device is used to position both limbs of the device in apposition. A retracting device is then advanced to grasp a portion of the fundus, which is then retracted toward the hinge on the device. The opposing limbs of the device are then approximated with the fundus intervening. A full-thickness polypropylene suture is then placed and secured with T-fasteners. Multiple sutures are placed to create a 270-degree valve 3 to 5 cm long.

♦ Short-term results from ongoing European and American studies have demonstrated both the safety and short-term efficacy of EsophyX.

Step 4. Postoperative Care

- Because these procedures are still in flux, postoperative care has not yet been standardized. In general, endoluminal treatments for GERD are outpatient procedures performed with the patient under moderate sedation. Patients receive a single dose of antibiotics before the procedure. Patients continue PPIs for 1 week and wean from the medications at that point. Acetaminophen elixir is usually adequate for pain control, although some patients require a few doses of narcotics. Most endoscopists recommend a liquid diet for 1 to 3 days after the procedure, with gradual progression to the patient's regular diet thereafter.
- Patients are typically seen in the office 2 to 4 weeks after the procedure to assess the results. Most trials have shown that 50% of patients completely stop PPI use after endoluminal GERD therapy, and another 30% are able to reduce the dose. Patients who do not respond to endoluminal therapy remain candidates for laparoscopic antireflux surgery.

Step 5. Pearls and Pitfalls

- Patient selection is critical to salutary outcomes of endoluminal therapy for GERD. The best candidates are those with small hiatal hernias, adequate LES pressures, and typical symptoms. Patient selection beyond those strict parameters may lead to diminished efficacy.
- Technical performance of endoscopic antireflux procedures requires expertise with flexible endoscopy. Before clinical application of these procedures, the endoscopist should become familiar with the devices in the laboratory.

Conclusions

◆ Endoluminal therapy for GERD will likely become the preferred therapy for patients with small hiatal hernias and competent LES. However, endoluminal therapies for GERD have yet to reach maturity. Many techniques appear promising, especially those which incorporate full-thickness endoluminal fundoplications, but lack supporting data. Before widespread application of these techniques, clinical trials with rigorous follow-up should be conducted.

◆ Endoluminal GERD treatment does not portend the demise of laparoscopic antireflux surgery. Patients with large hiatal hernias and depressed LES pressures will remain good surgical candidates. Furthermore, endoscopic treatment does not preclude a future operation if the endoscopic outcome is inadequate. Rather, endoluminal therapy for GERD will be another tool with which to treat select patients suffering from reflux.

Suggested Readings

Corley DA, Katz P, Wo JM, et al. Improvement of gastroesophageal reflux symptoms after radiofrequency energy: A randomized, sham-controlled trial. Gastroenterology 2003;125:668-676.

Pearl JP, Marks JM. Endolumenal therapies for gastroesophageal reflux disease: Are they dead? Surg Endosc 2007;21:1-4.

Pleskow D, Rothstein R, Kozarek R, et al. Endoscopic full-thickness plication for the treatment of GERD: Long-term multicenter results. Surg Endosc 2007;21:439-444.

Rothstein R, Filipi C, Caca K, et al. Endoscopic full-thickness plication for the treatment of gastroesophageal reflux disease: A randomized, sham-controlled trial. Gastroenterology 2006;131:704-712.

Torquati A, Richards WO. Endoluminal GERD treatments: Critical appraisal of current literature with evidence-based medicine instruments. Surg Endosc 2007;21:697-706.

Wolfsen HC, Richards WO. The Stretta procedure for the treatment of GERD: A registry of 558 patients. J Laparoendosc Adv Surg Tech A 2002;12:395-402.

CHAPTER 35

RESECTION OF BENIGN ESOPHAGEAL TUMORS

Priya Gaiha, James E. Lynch, and Joseph B. Zwischenberger

Step 1. Surgical Anatomy

- ◆ A comprehensive understanding of the anatomy of the esophagus is critical before undertaking surgical procedures on the esophagus (Fig. 35-1A-C).
- ◆ Indications
  - ▲ There are a variety of benign esophageal tumors. Generally arising from the muscularis propria layer with normal overlying mucosal layer, the vast majority of benign esophageal tumors are slow growing and remain undetected and asymptomatic. They are usually found incidentally during endoscopic or radiographic evaluation or at the time of operation for reflux. Large or strategically located tumors can be symptomatic, with 90% located in the middle and distal third of the esophagus. These tumors may require biopsy, regression therapy, and, in some cases, excision. About 5% of all detected benign esophageal tumors require surgery.
- ◆ Classification of tumor type helps determine the best operative approach.
  - ▲ Leiomyoma are the most common, comprising nearly two thirds of all benign esophageal tumors. Most are found in the lower one third of the esophagus and are usually intramural. Leiomyoma rarely cause symptoms when smaller than 5 cm in diameter. When symptomatic, dysphagia and vague pain are the most common complaints.
    - On barium swallow, leiomyoma characteristically appear as smooth, crescent-shaped defects covered by smooth mucosa (Fig. 35-2).
    - Esophagoscopy is performed in all cases. Characteristic endoscopic appearance is a submucosal bulge without stenosis, usually movable through the endoscope.
    - Recommended treatment is surgical excision for symptomatic leiomyoma and those larger than 5 cm. Asymptomatic leiomyoma or lesions smaller than 5 cm are followed periodically with barium swallow.
  - ▲ Intraluminal polyps are the second most commonly reported benign esophageal tumors and are more common in men than women (3 : 1). Due to the similarity of histologic findings of intraluminal polyps to fibroepithelial polyps, fibroma, fibrolipoma, and pedunculated lipomas, these are now all grouped under the name *fibrovascular polyps*. They usually occur in the upper esophagus and often are associated with the cricopharyngeous. The most common symptoms are dysphagia and regurgitation.

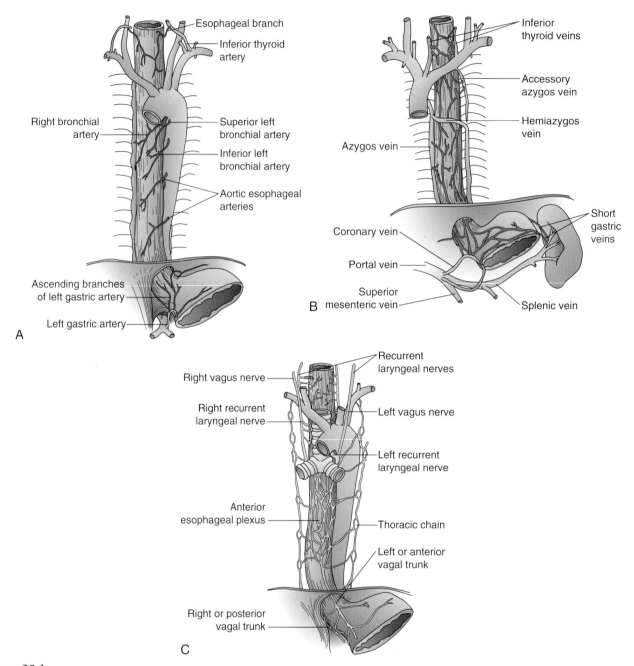

Figure 35-1
(Adapted from Hagen JA, DeMeester TR. Anatomy of the esophagus. In Shields TW, LoCicero J III, Ponn RB, eds. General Thoracic Surgery, 5th ed, vol 2. Philadelphia: Lippincott Williams & Wilkins; 2000:1599.)

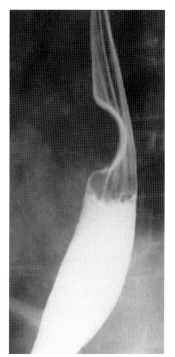

Figure 35-2
(From Zwischenberger JB,
Savage C, Bhutani MS.
Esophagus. In Townsend CM
Jr, Beauchamp RD, Evers
RM, et al, eds. Sabiston
Textbook of Surgery, 17th
ed. Philadelphia: Saunders;
2004:1116.)

BOX 35-1. Benign Esophageal Tumors

Leiomyoma
Fibrovascular polyp
Squamous cell papilloma
Granular cell tumor
Hemangioma
Congenital esophageal cyst
Bronchogenic cyst
Inflammatory fibroid polyp (eosinophilic granuloma)
Lymphangioma
Lipoma
Neurofibroma

- Barium swallow reveals the characteristic appearance of a smooth intraluminal sausage-shaped mass. Both barium swallow and esophagoscopy are recommended for diagnosis. Biopsy is not recommended because these polyps are quite vascular.
- For tumors smaller than 4 cm, observation and periodic barium swallow assessment is recommended. For tumors larger than 4 cm, not amenable to endoscopic removal, recommended treatment is surgical excision using an external approach, such as video-assisted thoracoscopic surgery (VATS) or thoracotomy.
▲ Squamous papilloma also are reported as benign esophageal tumors. They are most frequently isolated in the posterior wall of the distal third of the esophagus. They appear endoscopically as a warty, polypoid mass that is firm to the touch.
▲ Box 35-1 provides a list of reported benign esophageal tumors.

Step 2. Preoperative Considerations

- ◆ Common presenting symptoms of esophageal tumor are chest pain, dysphagia, odynophagia, regurgitation, bleeding, and respiratory compromise. Less common symptoms are thoracic pressure, anorexia, and weight loss.
- ◆ A variety of tests may be ordered to determine a diagnosis.
  - ▲ Barium swallow
  - ▲ Endoscopy
  - ▲ Computed tomography to help characterize the tumor's location and size
  - ▲ Endoscopic ultrasound (EUS)

▲ More than three of these characteristics is predictive of malignancy.
  ● Tumor diameter greater than 3 cm
  ● Nodular shape
  ● Ulceration depth greater than 5 mm
  ● Heterogeneous echo
  ● Presence of anechoic area
◆ Biopsy is not recommended if endoscopic and radiographic examinations are consistent with diagnosis of benign tumor type for the following reasons.
  ▲ Increased risk of mucosal perforation and inflammation complicates eventual surgical removal
  ▲ Possibility of massive blood if vascular mass
◆ Rationale for a surgical approach
  ▲ Presence of symptoms
  ▲ Excisional pathology excludes malignancy
  ▲ If asymptomatic, operative intervention depends on likelihood of symptom development or malignant degeneration
◆ Rationale for a nonsurgical approach
  ▲ Malignant transformation is extremely rare.
  ▲ Leiomyoma are slow growing.
  ▲ There is a benign clinical course.
◆ Contraindications to surgery
  ▲ Insufficient patient cardiopulmonary reserve
  ▲ Comorbidities that impair ability to tolerate general anesthesia
◆ Prior surgery is not a contraindication; depending on the density of adhesions, contralateral VATS approach may be needed.

Step 3. Operative Steps

1. Endoscopic Resection

◆ Ligation of tumor
  ▲ Tumor smaller than 2 cm: Resect with standard polypectomy snare.
  ▲ Tumor greater than 2 cm: Inject tumor with epinephrine (1:10,000) and then snare.
◆ If early rebleeding is suspected, then second-look endoscopy is performed 4 hours later.
◆ Reevaluate with endoscopy at 6 months and then at yearly follow-up.
◆ Complete remission
  ▲ Absence of any esophageal submucosal lesion identified by both endoscopy and EUS
  ▲ Residual thickening at lesion site consistent with scarring if biopsy negative

2. Thorascopy

◆ Confirm double lumen tube placement with bronchoscopy.
◆ Optional: Scope in proximal esophagus to verify mucosal integrity after resection
◆ Positioning
  ▲ Tumors of the middle third of the esophagus are approached through a right thoracoscopic approach.
  ▲ Tumors of the distal third of the esophagus are approached through a left thoracoscopic approach.
  ▲ If clearly favoring one or the other hemithorax, then approach from that side.
◆ Port placement
  ▲ Location of lesion will dictate port placement to achieve triangulation. For example, a lesion located at the mid-level of the esophagus would require port placement as shown in Figure 35-3.
    ● 5-mm port at eight or ninth intercostals space (ICS) post axillary line
    ● 10-mm port fourth at ICS anterior axillary line
    ● 5-mm port posterior to tip of scapula

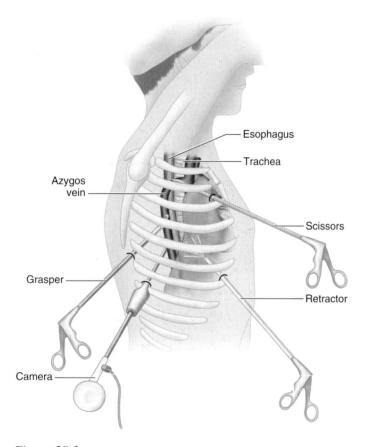

Figure 35-3

♦ Divide inferior pulmonary ligament to mobilize lung from esophagus.
♦ Use endoscopy or bougie to aid in identification of tumor location.
♦ Divide mediastinal pleura overlying esophagus.
♦ Divide azygos vein with Endo-GIA stapler for increased exposure (Fig. 35-4).
♦ Circumferentially mobilize esophagus if necessary for exposure and place a Penrose drain around for retraction.
♦ Perform myotomy over the tumor, but preserve the vagal trunks (Fig. 35-5A).
♦ Develop plane between tumor, muscularis propria, and underlying submucosa.
♦ Grasp or suture the tumor to provide retraction (see Fig. 35-5B and C).
♦ Enucleate the tumor with sharp and blunt dissection using ultrasonic shears and endoscopic peanut (see Fig. 35-5D).
♦ Close muscle layers in a transverse orientation (see Fig. 35-5E).
♦ Remove within specimen bag.
   ▲ Check integrity of submucosa with endoscope.
   ▲ Check for leak by submerging the esophagus underwater. Insufflate the lumen with air; repair primarily if leak is small. Reapproximate longitudinal muscle layer.
   ▲ Close ports sites, place chest tube.

3. Thoracotomy

♦ Posterolateral approach
   ▲ Intubate patient with double lumen tube.
   ▲ Position patient in left lateral decubitus tilted 45 degrees toward prone position.
   ▲ Use posterolateral or muscle sparing over site of tumor.
   ▲ Divide pulmonary ligament.
   ▲ Divide parietal pleura at anterior side up to azygos vein.
   ▲ Divide the azygos with Endo-GIA.
   ▲ Place Penrose drain around the esophagus to facilitate traction.
   ▲ Mobilize esophagus from thoracic inlet to diaphragmatic hiatus.
   ▲ Enucleate the tumor and close the myotomy, as described for thoracoscopic procedure earlier.

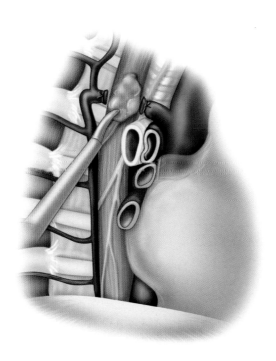

Figure 35-4

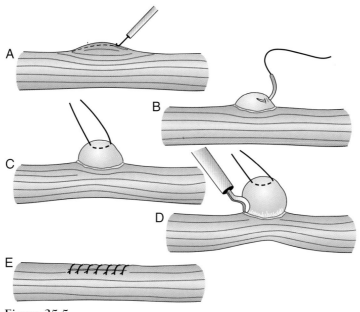

Figure 35-5
(Adapted from Lerut T. Thoracoscopic esophageal surgery. In Baue
AE, Geha AS, Hammond GL, et al, eds. Glenn's Thoracic and
Cardiovascular Surgery, 6th ed, vol 1. Norwalk, CT: Appleton &
Lange; 1996:867. With pemission of the McGraw-Hill
Companies.)

4. Esophageal Resection

- ◆ Indications
  - ▲ Large/annular leiomyoma that cannot be enucleated by VATS/open technique
  - ▲ Esophageal mucosa badly ulcerated/damaged during enucleation that cannot be easily repaired
  - ▲ Symptomatic multiple leiomyomas that cannot be enucleated
  - ▲ Diffuse leiomyomatosis
  - ▲ Leiomyosarcoma suspected and confirmed on biopsy
- ◆ See Chapters 25 and 26 for detailed descriptions of transthoracic and transhiatal procedures.

Step 4. Postoperative Care

- ◆ Remove chest tube on postoperative day 1.
- ◆ Perform barium swallow postoperatively to rule out leak (optional).
- ◆ Short-term complications: Within first 2 to 4 postoperative weeks
  - ▲ Postoperative leak due to mucosal perforation during enucleation with inadequate repair
- ◆ Late complications: Anytime after the first 4 weeks postoperative
  - ▲ New onset reflux
  - ▲ Worsening reflux
  - ▲ Development of pseudodiverticulum after enucleation (important to close myotomy)
  - ▲ Gastric tip necrosis
  - ▲ Anastamotic stricture
- ◆ Postoperative surgical complications
  - ▲ Chylothorax
  - ▲ Recurrent nerve injury
  - ▲ Wound infection

Step 5. Pearls and Pitfalls

- ◆ Surgical approach is not nearly as important as identifying location, anatomy, and structures involved.
- ◆ Division of the azygos vein is a useful adjunct to allow exposure of the mid esophagus and should be used whenever necessary.
- ◆ If a mucosal tear happens during excision, do not panic. Finish the resection, mobilize the esophagus, pass a 46 to 52 French bougie, and close esophagus primarily in layers. If primary closure is not possible, multiple options still exist, depending on location (Fig. 35-6), including pedicled pericardial fat graft (A), gastric patch (B), pleural flap (C), intercostal muscle bundle graft (D), omental onlay graft (E), and diaphragmatic pedicle graft (F).

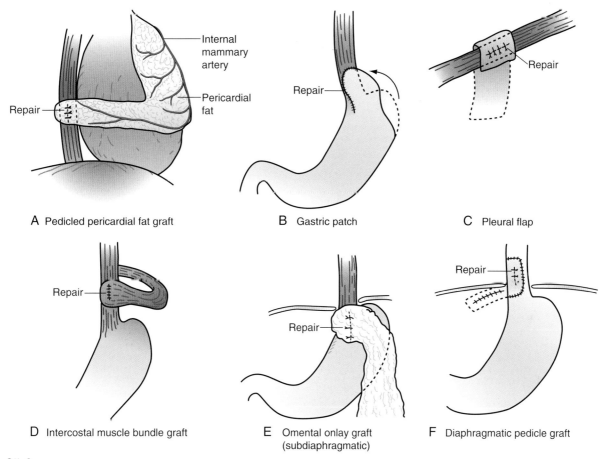

A Pedicled pericardial fat graft

Internal mammary artery

Pericardial fat

Repair

B Gastric patch

Repair

C Pleural flap

Repair

D Intercostal muscle bundle graft

Repair

E Omental onlay graft (subdiaphragmatic)

Repair

F Diaphragmatic pedicle graft

Repair

Figure 35-6
(Adapted from Brewer LA III, Carter R, Mulder GA, et al. Options in the management of perforations of the esophagus. Am J Surg 2986;152:62-69, with permission from Excerpta Medica Inc.)

Suggested Readings

Boone J, Draaisma WA, Schipper ME, et al. Robot-assisted thoracoscopic esophagectomy for a giant upper esophageal leiomyoma. Dis Esophagus 2008;21:90-93.

Giulianotti PC, Coratti A, Angelini M, et al. Robotics in general surgery: Personal experience in a large community hospital. Arch Surg 2003;138:777-784.

Honkoop P, Siersema PD, Titanus HW, et al. Benign anastomotic strictures after transhiatal esophagectomy and cervical esophagogastrostomy: Risk factors and management. J Thorac Cardiovasc Surg 1996;111:1141-1148.

Kent M, Awais O, Schuchert MJ, et al. Minimally invasive resection of benign esophageal tumors. J Thorac Cardiovasc Surg 2007;134:176-181.

Krasna MJ, Phillips SD, Gray WC, et al. Combined thorascopic/laparoscopic staging of esophageal cancer. J Thorac Cardiovasc Surg 1996;111:800-807.

Mutrie C, Donahue DM, Wain JC, et al. Esophageal leiomyoma: A 40-year experience. Ann Thorac Surg 2005;79:1122-1125.

Samphire J, Naftleux P, Luketich J. Minimally invasive techniques for resection of benign esophageal tumors. Semin Thorac Cardiovasc Surg 2003;15:35-43.

Temes R, Quinn P, Davis M, et al. Endoscopic resection of esophageal liposarcoma. J Thorac Cardiovasc Surg 1998;116:365-367.

von Rahden BH, Stein HJ, Feussner H, et al. Enucleation of submucosal tumors of the esophagus. Surg Endosc 2004;18:924-930.

Wehrmann T, Martchenko K, Nakamura M, et al. Endoscopic resection of submucosal esophageal tumors: A prospective case series. Endosc 2004;36:802-807.

CHAPTER 36

ESOPHAGEAL DIVERTICULUM EXCISION AND REPAIR

Alexandros N. Karavas and Joe B. Putnam

Zenker's Diverticulum

Step 1. Surgical Anatomy

- The upper esophageal sphincter consists of the cricopharyngeal muscle, which courses transversely along the posterior portion of the esophagus. The esophagus borders superiorly with the obliquely coursing inferior constrictor pharyngeal muscles that constitute the hypopharynx. The area between these muscles represents Killian's triangle. If abnormal relaxation and discoordination of the cricopharyngeal muscle occur during swallowing, this weak area allows the formation of a diverticulum, commonly referred to as *Zenker's*, bearing the name of the German pathologist Friedrich Albert von Zenker who first described the underlying pathophysiologic process and reported a series of patients in the 19th century.
- This is the most common diverticulum of the esophagus. It is a false pulsion diverticulum that develops as a protrusion of the mucosal layer through the Killian triangle. The pouch is usually located left posterolaterally. Access to the diverticulum is through an anterior or lateral approach, and in both cases the recurrent laryngeal nerve should be preserved as it courses along the tracheoesophageal groove and enters the larynx between the inferior cornu of the thyroid cartilage and the arch of the cricoid.
- Dysphagia is a common presentation. Halitosis from undigested food and regurgitation of undigested food particles with night cough have also been commonly reported. Because the diverticulum is above the upper esophageal sphincter, tracheobronchial aspiration is a feared complication. Barium swallow is diagnostic for its presence, and no further testing is required.

Step 2. Preoperative Considerations

- The very low morbidity and mortality of excision and myotomy of a Zenker's diverticulum justifies intervention as soon as its presence is confirmed. Potential complications (e.g., aspiration) carry a higher risk than the procedure itself.

- The pathologic substrate is dysfunction in motility and abnormal relaxation; therefore, the mainstay of the procedure is myotomy. Diverticulectomy alone is associated with a higher incidence of fistulae and should be discouraged. Depending on the size of the diverticulum, this may be left alone if it is smaller than 2 cm or resected if larger. Alternatively, the diverticulum may be fixed in an antigravity position.
- A clear liquid diet is encouraged for 2 to 3 days preceding the procedure. The patient should take nothing by mouth (NPO) after midnight before surgery.

Step 3. Operative Steps—Open Cervical Approach

- Perioperative antibiotics are administered within 1 hour from incision according to institutional policy. Ampicillin and sulbactam for up to 24 hours will provide adequate coverage. The patient is positioned supine on the operating table. General anesthesia is administered, and the airway is controlled via an endotracheal tube. A shoulder roll is placed, and the head is turned to the right side for a left lateral approach.
- An incision, about 5 cm long, is carried along the anterior border of the sternocleidomastoid (SCM) muscle, between the hyoid bone and above the clavicle. Alternatively, the head is extended in midline, and a transverse incision is performed two finger breadths below the prominence of the thyroid cartilage between the anterior borders of both SCM muscles.
- The platysma is divided sharply. Skin hooks are placed and, under gentle traction, subplatysmal flaps are developed. Self-retaining retractors are placed. The sternothyroid and sternohyoid muscles are retracted medially and the omohyoid muscle medially and superiorly (Fig. 36-1). Placement of the medial portion of the retractor should always be superficial to the thyroid gland. Avoid deep placement and injury to the recurrent laryngeal nerve. The lateral portion of the retractor is placed so that it retracts the SCM muscle laterally. The middle thyroid vein is identified just behind the deep cervical fascia over the carotid sheath and divided as lateral as possible. The thyroid gland and the trachea are manually retracted medially. The carotid sheath and the jugular vein are retracted very gently laterally.
- The retropharyngeal space and the diverticulum are exposed. If the omohyoid muscle prevents adequate exposure, it may be divided. The diverticulum is dissected off the surrounding tissue, taking care to maintain a dissection plane very close to the esophageal wall. The neck of the diverticulum is dissected in such a way that the muscle layer is visualized along its entire circumference. The content of the diverticulum is emptied intraluminally.
- A 36 to 44 French bougie is placed in the esophagus, and the myotomy is performed on the side of the diverticulum (i.e., the left posterolateral wall). It extends at least 3 cm in a caudad direction and 2 cm in a cranial direction. A fine right-angle clamp may be used to develop the plane between the mucosa and the muscle and to guide the myotomy site with the electrocautery (Fig. 36-2).
- If the diverticulum is small (i.e., <2 cm), it may be left alone. Larger diverticula are excised. Using a Babcock clamp, the diverticulum is gently lifted, and a linear stapler is fired across, ensuring that the lumen is not compromised and the recurrent laryngeal nerve is not inadvertently included in the staple line. Once the stapler is fired, the site is tested for leaks with intraluminal insufflation while warm saline is poured into the neck wound. Any leak should be repaired with fine absorbable sutures, such as 4-0 polyglactin sutures. Placement of a small drain is optional, and this is placed adjacent to the myotomy site and staple line.
- The platysma is approximated with 3-0 Vicryl interrupted sutures. Skin is approximated with a continuous subcuticular 4-0 Vicryl suture or other similar closure of choice. Steri-strips are applied over the incision, and dressing is usually applied around the drain exit site only. The patient is extubated in the operating room. Some surgeons routinely perform a laryngoscopy to ensure patency of the laryngeal nerves. This is safely accomplished with exchange of the endotracheal tube into a laryngeal mask that allows passage of a pediatric bronchoscope. As the patient becomes more awake, prompt approximation of both vocal cords is documented.

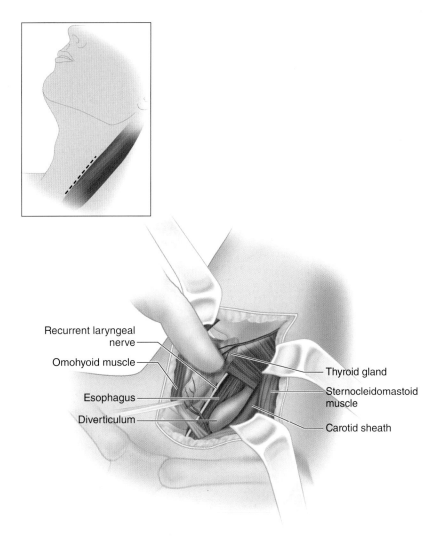

Figure 36-1

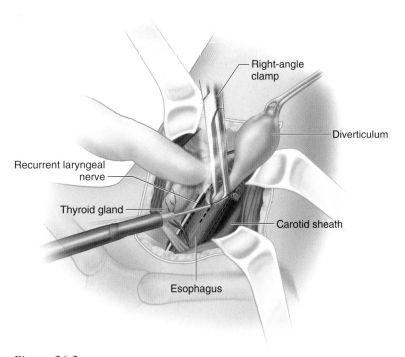

Figure 36-2

Step 3. Operative Steps—Endoscopic Approach

◆ The endoscopic approach was popularized with the advent of endoscopic staplers and coagulation devices. After general anesthesia and endotracheal intubation, the patient is placed in the supine sniffing position as for direct laryngoscopy. Adequate head extension is important to assist in smooth introduction of the stapler.

◆ A Weerda (bivalved) laryngoscope is introduced behind the endotracheal tube. The two valves are positioned in such a way that one is in the diverticulum and the other is in the esophagus, exposing the common wall ("septum") (Fig. 36-3). Visualization may be enhanced by placement of a small (5 mm or 30-degree) rigid endoscope through the laryngoscope. The esophageal lumen should be clearly seen; occasionally placement of a nasogastric tube will facilitate this and is then removed. Once adequate view is obtained, the laryngoscope is mounted to the chest with a suspension arm to allow the surgeon to work with both hands.

◆ An endoscopic GIA stapler is introduced with the smaller blade on the side of the diverticulum. Occasionally it is difficult to engage the common wall to the stapler because of inadequate fixation (see Fig. 36-3). Endoscopically placed silk sutures to the lateral walls will provide gentle traction. The stapler is then gently angulated anteriorly and fired, dividing the common wall and opening the diverticulum into the esophageal lumen. The stapler should be reapplied and fired again, if necessary, to obtain a common wall smaller than 1 cm long.

◆ Once this is accomplished, the stay sutures are removed and the laryngoscope is withdrawn. The patient is weaned off anesthesia, and the patient is extubated in the operating room.

Step 4. Postoperative Care

◆ Postoperatively, a swallow study may be obtained on the day of the surgery or on the first postoperative day. Once this confirms no leak and no risk of aspiration, liquid diet is initiated and slowly advanced as tolerated from mechanical soft to regular diet. For patients with endoscopic repair of the diverticulum, a swallow study is not usually necessary, and liquid diet is initiated on the day of surgery or the first postoperative day.

Step 5. Pearls and Pitfalls

1. Mucosal Entry

◆ Mucosal injury may be encountered during the attempt to mobilize the diverticulum at the staple line or during an attempt to fix the diverticulum in an antigravity position. This should be repaired primarily with fine absorbable sutures. The omohyoid muscle is divided as lateral as possible and brought over the repaired mucosal site and fixed to the surrounding muscle fibers using fine silk sutures. Alternatively, the mucosal defect is covered by the surrounding muscle.

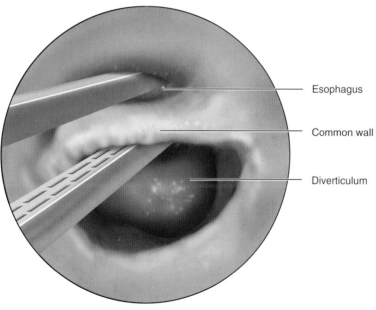

Esophagus

Common wall

Diverticulum

Figure 36-3

2. Prevertebral Fascia

- Some advocate the fixation of the diverticulum in antigravity position, which has the advantage of no suture or staple line. If this approach is elected, the diverticulum should be fixed to the superiorly lying muscle fibers, avoiding any sutures and possible contamination of the prevertebral fascia, which may result in descending mediastinitis.

3. Recurrent Laryngeal Nerve Injury

- Potential injury to the recurrent laryngeal nerves is always present, and this is prevented by avoiding any retraction in a medial direction deeper than the thyroid gland with instruments.
- Nerve injury is usually undetected until postoperatively, when voice changes are observed.
- Respiratory distress following extubation should raise suspicion of bilateral injury, which can be confirmed at reintubation. If this is suspected, endoscopy before extubation is mandatory (as described above), and the patient should remain intubated. Tracheostomy may be required to obtain control of the airway.

Epiphrenic Diverticula

Step 1. Surgical Anatomy

- Epiphrenic diverticula are the second most common diverticula of the esophagus and are considered false and pulsion in origin. The vast majority are located within 10 cm from the gastroesophageal junction. Motility disorders are the main causes of the presence of diverticula. This includes achalasia, lower esophageal sphincter (LES) spasm, or diffuse esophageal spasm. These abnormalities are addressed at the time of surgery.
- Traction diverticula are rare entities and nowadays are associated with granulomatous disease, tuberculosis, or histoplasmosis. They are true diverticula and usually located in the midesophagus. Compression symptoms, dysphagia, mucosal inflammation, or fistulization to the tracheobronchial tree are possible presentations, although many remain asymptomatic.

Step 2. Preoperative Considerations

- Many studies may be performed as part of the evaluation of the patient's symptoms before the diagnosis of esophageal diverticulum and the recommendation for surgery.

- Barium swallow study is the mainstay of evaluation and diagnosis of the esophageal diverticulum and its underlying pathology. Anteroposterior and oblique views, as well as cinematography, allow evaluation of number, size, and shape of the diverticulum and also assess the presence of esophageal dysmotility or LES dysfunction.
- Endoscopy is recommended irrespective of radiographic and manometry findings. It helps evaluate the lumen of the diverticulum and exclude the presence of cancer or ectopic tissue. Manometry and pH study are required to identify the underlying disease, whether it is esophageal motility and LES dysfunction alone, and help in the decision to perform an anti-reflux procedure.
- Because most patients are older adults, cardiopulmonary evaluation should be considered to identify patients at high risk for surgery or general anesthesia and to optimize appropriately.
- Indications for surgical excision of the diverticulum are disabling symptoms, usually dysphagia or recurrent aspiration pneumonias. Asymptomatic diverticula are preferably observed with routine annual endoscopies.
- Before the planned surgery, improvement of nutrition for patients who are debilitated and malnourished is encouraged. Any evidence of pneumonia should be treated with antimicrobials. A clear liquid diet 2 to 3 days before the procedure is encouraged. The patient is NPO beginning at midnight the night before surgery.

Step 3. Operative Steps

- Perioperative antibiotics are administered within 1 hour from incision per institutional policy. A first-generation cephalosporin for up to 24 hours will provide adequate coverage.
- The patient is positioned so as to avoid aspiration. General anesthesia is administered by the anesthesiologist, and the airway is secured using a single-lumen endotracheal tube and rapid sequence intubation, which helps prevent possible aspiration from particles that may be retained within the diverticulum. Esophagogastroscopy is performed, and the preoperative findings are confirmed, giving particular attention to localizing the diverticulum accurately in relation to the incisors and the upper esophageal sphincter. Biopsy is taken of any suspicious area at this time.
- The single-lumen tube may be exchanged at this time to a double-lumen tube to facilitate left-lung isolation. Alternatively, a bronchial blocker may be used for single-lung ventilation.
- The patient is then positioned in the right lateral decubitus position (left side up), and bony areas are appropriately padded. This involves both arms being placed away and in front of the torso. The upper arm is positioned in a padded armrest and elevated forward (anterior) so that the elbow is at the level of the shoulder and at an angle of around 90 degrees. The armrest is angulated in such a way to provide smooth distribution of pressure. The right (lower) arm is placed in 90-degree anterior (extended anteriorly) and inner rotated about 45 degrees in the shoulder. This achieves approximation of the two carpal joints. After appropriate padding, the right hand is then loosely and safely fixed using Kerlix roll or tape. The table is flexed maximally using the kidney bar while maintaining neutral head position with rolls or blankets underneath. This helps extend further the intercostal spaces. The lower extremities are padded at the knees and the ankles. A beanbag is used to maintain the position.

- A posterolateral approach is elected, and a left muscle-sparing thoracotomy is performed in the seventh intercostal space. The intercostal space is entered by separating the intercostal muscle from the lower rib. The parietal pleura is entered, collapsing the already isolated lung. This will further facilitate safe mobilization of the intercostal muscle. Care is taken to preserve the intercostal vessel and nerve bundle because this may be used as a flap to protect the site of excision. The anterior extent of intercostal muscle mobilization is the midclavicular line so as to avoid the internal mammary vessels; posteriorly it reaches the costovertebral angle. A retractor is then placed.

- The inferior pulmonary ligament is divided, and the deflated lung is retracted anteriorly and superiorly using packs. If the diaphragm obstructs the view, traction sutures may be placed in the tendinous portion and these passed through the skin via a stab incision. The mediastinal pleura is divided and the esophagus is exposed. The esophagus is mobilized bluntly and a Penrose is used to encircle the esophagus at the most proximal site of dissection and another at the most distal (Fig. 36-4). Both vagi are identified, preserved, and left together with the esophagus. The extent of the dissection is between the inferior pulmonary vein proximal and just below the LES, about 1 or 2 cm of the stomach. If there is associated hiatal hernia, this is addressed at the same time. At all times, the vagi are identified and cautiously preserved, requiring dissection and removal of the anterior fat pad at the gastroesophageal junction.

- Dissection continues toward the diverticulum, and the sac is freed from the surrounding structures. The diverticulum is usually located on the right side; gentle traction of the diverticulum with a Babcock clamp while gently rotating the esophagus with the Penrose drains will facilitate exposure and allow safe dissection. The neck of the diverticulum is dissected in such a way that the muscle layer is visualized along its entire circumference.

- Generally, a 54 French bougie for women or a 56 French bougie for men is introduced by the anesthesiologist into the esophagus under the tactile guidance by the surgeon. With mild tension to the diverticulum, a surgical stapler is fired across the diverticulum, ensuring that no compromise in the lumen of the esophagus or the vagi or any inclusion of muscle layer occurs. If the mucosa is entered, repair can be achieved primarily using absorbable sutures. The muscle layer is approximated over the staple line. If the defect is large, repair may be accomplished after the myotomy.

- A long myotomy is performed 180 degrees away from the diverticular opening in an extramucosal fashion. A fine right-angle clamp can be used to assist with proper identification of the layer between the muscle layer and the mucosa. This is then carried proximally to the level of the inferior pulmonary vein and distally 1 to 2 cm into the stomach (Fig. 36-5). The repair and myotomy sites are tested for mucosal leak by placing the end of a nasogastric tube into the esophagus above the repair site and insufflating with air while warm saline is poured into the thoracic cavity. Any leak warrants repair, which can be accomplished by primary closure with fine absorbable interrupted sutures (e.g., 4-0 polyglactin). The intercostal muscle flap is then used to cover the defect, and this is fixed on the muscle layer using 4-0 silk interrupted sutures. If gastroesophageal reflux has been documented preoperatively, a less obstructive fundoplication is recommended.

- A nasogastric tube is placed upon conclusion of the repair, and double-lung ventilation is resumed. The thoracic cavity is drained with two thoracostomy tubes placed in a superior-posterior and supradiaphragmatic position.

- A small round fluted chest tube may be placed at the area of interest, which remains longer, usually until after diet is resumed. If the right pleura has been entered during the procedure, appropriate drainage with a right-sided thoracostomy tube is performed. The retractor is removed and the ribs are loosely approximated. Layer approximation of the muscles is completed while the chest tubes are under suction. Subcutaneous and skin closure is performed per surgeon's preference.

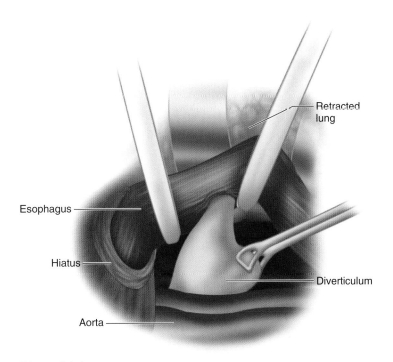

Figure 36-4

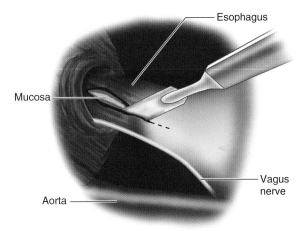

Figure 36-5

Step 4. Postoperative Care

◆ Postoperatively, the nasogastric tube remains until the second or third postoperative day. A thin barium swallow study is performed to ensure that there is no esophageal leak at the site of repair and no signs of aspiration, at which time the nasogastric tube is removed. A clear liquid diet is initiated. This is slowly advanced to mechanical soft diet, which is continued for another 10-14 days prior to advancing to regular diet. The thoracostomy tubes are removed once adequate drainage and lung expansion has been accomplished. The soft chest tube remains until after initiation of oral intake to ensure that no leak occurs and, if so, that this is being drained.

Step 5. Pearls and Pitfalls

Traction Diverticula

◆ The management of traction diverticulum is simple excision and layer closure based on the principles described in this chapter. If no preoperative esophageal motility disorder is documented, excision without myotomy is adequate if the pathogenesis is based on mediastinal inflammation and fibrosis.
◆ In the presence of a tracheobronchial fistula, closure of both esophageal and bronchial defects is performed, followed by a mandatory interposition of tissue (pleural or muscle flap) to avoid recurrence.

Mucosal Injury

◆ Mucosal injury may be encountered during dissection of the diverticulum off the surrounding tissue. If the opening is within the portion to be excluded by the stapler, this is of little significance, and simple contamination control is appropriate.
◆ If the esophageal mucosa is entered during myotomy or at the staple site, it should be repaired with simple fine absorbable sutures. The repair site should be reinforced with a flap. The intercostal muscle flap, which was mobilized during thoracotomy, is our first choice. This should be fixed with fine silk sutures to the adjacent muscle fibers under no tension. Alternatively, pericardium or pleural flaps can be used.

Vagus Injury

- Injury to one vagus is usually of little clinical importance. If both vagi are injured, there is a chance of gastric outlet obstruction, and a drainage procedure should be based on the patient's subsequent symptoms.

Postoperative Leak

- Postoperative leak is a feared complication and should be suspected early when drainage amount and/or consistency changes, or signs of sepsis are present. Adequate drainage with the tubes that are in place may occasionally be adequate for very small leaks with very small extravasation, provided they are placed at the site of leak and do not permit diffuse contamination of the mediastinum and the patient is clinically stable.
- Any clear demonstration of significant contrast leak in the thin barium study or signs of sepsis is an indication for urgent re-exploration. The basic principles at the time of re-exploration include lavage and adequate drainage of the mediastinum and the pleural cavity as well as control of contamination either by repair of the site of leak and use of a flap or by diversion and esophagostomy creation. Debridement should be performed until healthy tissue is encountered, but the latter should not be sacrificed.

Presence of Hiatal Hernia

- The presence of a large hiatal hernia should be addressed at the time of mobilization of the esophagus and dissection of the diverticulum. The hernia sac needs to be mobilized and excised, the hernia reduced, and the hiatus repaired.

Suggested Readings

Aly A, Devitt PG, Jamieson GG. Evolution of surgical treatment for pharyngeal pouch. Br J Surg 2004;91:657-664.
Cassivi SD, Deschamps C, Nichols FC 3rd, et al. Diverticula of the esophagus. Surg Clin North Am 2005;85:495-503, ix.

INDEX

Note: Page numbers followed by *f* refer to figures; page numbers followed by *t* refer to tables; page numbers followed by *b* refer to boxes.